Emergency Orthopedics
The Spine

Robert L. Galli, M.D.
Assistant Professor of Medicine and
Assistant Director
Emergency Medicine Training
UCLA School of Medicine
Attending and Director
Resident Training
Department of Emergency Medicine
Olive View—UCLA Medical Center
Sylmar, California

Daniel W. Spaite, M.D.
Assistant Professor
Section of Emergency Medicine
University of Arizona
Base Hospital Medical Director
Arizona Health Sciences Center
University Medical Center
Tucson, Arizona

Robert Rutha Simon, M.D.
Professor and Chairman
Department of Emergency Medicine
Cook County Hospital
Chicago, Illinois

With illustrations by **Susan Gilbert**

APPLETON & LANGE
Norwalk, Connecticut/San Mateo, California

0-8385-2203-3

Copyright © 1989 by Appleton & Lange
A Publishing Division of Prentice Hall

89 90 91 92 93 / 10 9 8 7 6 5 4 3 2 1

Prentice Hall International (UK) Limited, *London*
Prentice Hall of Australia Pty. Limited, *Sydney*
Prentice Hall Canada, Inc., *Toronto*
Prentice Hall Hispanoamericana, S.A., *Mexico*
Prentice Hall of India Private Limited, *New Delhi*
Prentice Hall of Japan, Inc., *Tokyo*
Simon & Schuster Asia Pte. Ltd., *Singapore*
Editora Prentice Hall do Brasil Ltda., *Rio de Janeiro*
Prentice Hall, *Englewood Cliffs, New Jersey*

Library of Congress Cataloging-in-Publication Data

Galli, Robert.
    Emergency orthopedics : the spine / Robert Galli, Daniel Spaite,
Robert Simon.
        p.   cm.
    ISBN 0-8385-2203-3
    1. Spine—Wounds and injuries—Surgery. 2. Orthopedic
emergencies.   I. Spaite, Daniel.   II. Simon, Robert R. (Robert
Rutha)   III. Title.
    [DNLM: 1. Emergency Medicine—methods.   2. Orthopedics—methods.
3. Spine. 4. Wounds and Injuries—therapy. WE 725 G168e]
RD768.G35 1989
617'.375—dc19
DNLM/DLC
for Library of Congress   88-36724
                                                        CIP

Acquisitions Editor: Stephany S. Scott
Production Editor: Karen W. Davis
Designers: M. Chandler Martylewski, Mike Kelly

PRINTED IN THE UNITED STATES OF AMERICA

To my family, especially Mom, who missed
the whole thing, but is always there.
And Frances Ann.

Robert Galli, M.D.

To Dana, my loving wife and best friend,
whose encouragement, support, and
prodding made this book a reality.

Daniel Spaite, M.D.

To Mariam, my wife, who at 1:00 AM
is there with a smile and a cup of coffee,
and to an illiterate Lebanese villager
who has been my best teacher—my Mother

Robert Simon, M.D.

Contents

Preface and Acknowledgments ix

PART I. APPROACH TO THE PATIENT WITH SPINAL INJURY **1**

1. Approach to the Patient With Spinal Injury 2

☐ Mechanisms and Pathophysiology of Spinal Trauma 2

☐ Prehospital Treatment 3

☐ Emergency Department Management 6
  Airway Management and Breathing 6
  Circulation 6
  Primary Assessment 7

Other Considerations 8
Radiographic Evaluation 9
Laboratory Tests 10

☐ Treatment 10
  Pharmacology 10

☐ References 10

☐ Bibliography 10

PART II. MEDICAL EMERGENCIES **11**

2. Cord Syndromes: Evaluation and Management **12**

☐ Introduction and Anatomic Considerations 12

☐ Complete Cord Syndrome 12

☐ Anterior Cord Syndrome 14

☐ Central Cord Syndrome 15

☐ Contusio Cervicalis Posterior 17

☐ Brown-Séquard Syndrome 17

☐ Root and Cauda Equina Syndromes 18

☐ Cord Contusion 18

☐ References 19

3. Arthridities of the Spine **20**

☐ Rheumatoid Arthritis of the Spine 20
  Incidence 20
  Pathophysiology 20
  Clinical Features 20
  Complications 21
  Diagnosis 22
  Management and Referral 23

☐ Ankylosing Spondylitis 24
  Incidence 24
  Pathophysiology 25
  Clinical Features 25
  Physical Examination 25
  Clinical Course 26
  Complications and Prognosis 26
  Diagnosis 27
  Management and Referral 28

☐ Osteoarthritis of the Spine 29
  Incidence 29
  Pathophysiology 29
  Clinical Features 29
  Complications 30
  Diagnosis 31
  Management and Referral 31

☐ References 32

4. Osteoporosis **34**

☐ Introduction 34

☐ Etiology 34

☐ Clinical Presentation 34

☐ Diagnosis 36

☐ Treatment 36

☐ References 36

5. Infections of the Spine 38

☐ Introduction 38

☐ Pyogenic Spondylitis 38
   Incidence 38
   Pathophysiology 38
   Clinical Features 38
   Complications 39
   Diagnosis 39
   Management and Referral 39

☐ Tuberculous Spondylitis 40
   Incidence 40
   Pathophysiology 40
   Clinical Features 41
   Complications 42
   Diagnosis 42
   Management and Referral 42

☐ Intervertebral Disc Infection 43

☐ References 45

PART III. THE CERVICAL SPINE 59

7. Anatomy 60

☐ Introduction 60

☐ Vertebrae 60

☐ Ligaments and Intervertebral Discs 62

☐ Stability and Mobility 64

☐ Spinal Cord and Nerve Roots 66

☐ Arteries and Veins 71

☐ Bibliography 75

8. Physical Examination 76

☐ Inspection 76

☐ Palpation 76

☐ Range of Motion 84

☐ Neurologic Examination 86
   C-1 and C-2 86
   C-3 86
   C-4 87
   C-5 87
   C-6 87
   C-7 88
   C-8 88
   T-1 89

☐ Major Peripheral Nerves 89
   Radial Nerve 90

6. Neoplasms of the Spine 46

☐ History 46

☐ Physical Examination 46

☐ Laboratory Studies 46

☐ Classification 47
   Primary Benign Tumors 47
      Osteochondroma 47
      Osteoid Osteoma 48
      Osteoblastoma 48
      Giant Cell Tumor 49
      Eosinophilic Granuloma 49
      Hemangioma 49
      Aneurysmal Bone Cysts 50
   Primary Malignant Tumors 50
      Multiple Myeloma 50
      Malignant Lymphoma 51
      Chondrosarcoma 51
      Osteosarcoma 51
      Ewing's Sarcoma 53
      Chordoma 53
   Secondary Tumors: Metastatic Disease 54

☐ Spinal Cord Compression 54

☐ References 57

   Ulnar Nerve 90
   Median Nerve 90
   Axillary Nerve 90
   Musculocutaneous Nerve 92

☐ Special Tests (Compression Test, Distraction Test, Foramenal Compression Test, Shoulder Depression Test, Vertebral Artery Test, Intermittent Claudication Test, Costoclavicular Maneuver, Hyperabduction Maneuver, Adson Maneuver, Valsalva Maneuver, Swallowing Test, Lhermitte's Sign) 93

☐ References 95

☐ Bibliography 95

9. Radiology 96

☐ Introduction 96

☐ Plain Radiography 96
   Cross-Table Lateral View 96
   Anteroposterior View 100
   Open-Mouth View 100
   Oblique View 101
   Pillar View 101
   Swimmer's View 101
   Flexion–Extension View 101
   Pitfalls 101
      Degenerative Disease 102
      Preexisting Congenital Anomaly 102

Physiologic Subluxation 102
Prominent Uncinate Process of C-3 102
Mach Effect 102
Normal Anatomic Variants 102
Artifactual Lines 103

☐ Other Imaging Modalities 102
Tomography 102
Myelography 103
Magnetic Resonance Imaging 104

☐ References 104

☐ Bibliography 104

10. Fractures, Dislocations, and Subluxations 106

☐ Classification 106

☐ Stability 107
Upper Cervical Spine 108
Lower Cervical Spine 112

☐ Neurologic Injury 114

☐ Treatment 115

☐ Flexion 116
Hyperflexion Sprain 116
Simple Wedge (Compression) Fracture 116
Clay-Shoveler Fracture 117
Bilateral Facet Dislocation 118
Flexion Teardrop Fracture 119

☐ Flexion–Rotation 120
Unilateral Facet Dislocation 120

☐ Extension–Rotation 121
Pillar Fracture 121

☐ Vertical Compression 121
Jefferson Burst Fracture 121
Burst Fracture 122

☐ Extension 122
Hyperextension Sprain 122
Avulsion Fracture of the Anterior Arch
of the Atlas 124
Extension Teardrop Fracture of the Axis 124
Fracture of the Posterior Arch of the Atlas ... 124
Laminar Fracture 125

Traumatic Spondylolisthesis of the Axis
(Hangman's Fracture) 125
Hyperextension Fracture–Dislocation 126

☐ Lateral Flexion 126
Uncinate Process Fracture 126

☐ Diverse Mechanisms 127
Atlanto-Occipital Disruption 127
Atlantoaxial Disruption, C-1 and C-2 127
Odontoid Fracture 129

☐ Pediatric Cervical Spine 130
Clinical Evaluation 130
X-ray Evaluation 130
Specific Injuries 131

☐ References 133

☐ Bibliography 134

11. Strains and Sprains 136

☐ Cervical Sprain 136

☐ Hyperextension Injury 136

☐ Hyperflexion Injury 138

☐ Cervical Disc Disorders 140

☐ References 142

12. Specific Syndromes and Disorders 144

☐ Thoracic Outlet Syndromes 144
Cervical Rib 145
Costoclavicular Syndrome 146
Scalenus Anticus Syndrome 147
Hyperabduction Syndrome 148

☐ Brachial Plexus Injuries 149

☐ "Stingers" 151

☐ Greater Occipital Nerve Syndrome
(Occipital Neuritis) 151

☐ Vertebral Artery Syndrome 152

☐ Torticollis 152

☐ References 153

☐ Bibliography 153

PART IV. THE THORACOLUMBAR SPINE 155

13. Anatomy 156

☐ Introduction 156

☐ Functional Anatomy 156

☐ Stability and Mobility 156

☐ Spinal Cord and Nerve Roots 162

☐ Vascular Supply of the Cord 163

☐ References 165

14. Physical Examination 166

☐ Introduction 166

☐ Inspection 166

☐ Range of Motion 169

☐ Palpation 174

☐ Percussion 179

☐ Auscultation 180

☐ Neurologic Examination 180
   Motor Testing 181
   Sensory Testing 182
   Reflex Testing 183
      Deep Tendon Reflexes 183
      Cutaneous Reflexes 184
      Pathologic Relfexes 184
   Special Maneuvers 184
      Tests for Sciatic Nerve and Root
        Pathology 189
      Tests for Meningeal, Dural, or Root
        Pathology 191
      Tests for Sacroiliac Joint Pathology 191
      Tests for Femoral Nerve and Root
        Pathology 196
      Tests for Innervation of the Abdominal
        Musculature 196
      Miscellaneous Tests 196
   Related Examination 198
   Determining Functional (Nonorganic) Pain . . . 198
      Special Tests 199

☐ References 201

15. Radiology **202**

☐ Introduction 202

☐ Plain Radiography 202

☐ Computed Tomography 207

☐ Tomography 210

☐ Myelography 210

☐ Pitfalls 210

☐ References 210

**16. Fractures, Dislocations, and Major
    Ligamentous Injuries** **212**

☐ Introduction and General Concepts 212

☐ Neurologic Injury 212

☐ Stability 214

☐ Classification and Mechanism of Injury 214

☐ Flexion 216
   Pure Flexion 216
      Anterior Wedge Fracture 216
   Flexion With Rotation 218
      "Slice" Fracture 218
      Fracture–Dislocation Through Disc 218
      Posterior Ligamentous Disruption
        Without Wedge Fracture 218
      Posterior Ligamentous Disruption
        With Wedge Fracture 218

☐ Distraction (Tension) 221
   "Chance" Fracture 221
   Ligamentous Disruption 221
   Ligamentous Disruption With Posterior
      and/or Middle Element Fracture 221

☐ Axial Load 225
   Pure Axial Load 225
      Burst Fracture Without Posterior Element
        Fracture 225
      Burst Fracture With Posterior Element
        Fracture 225
   Axial Load With Rotation 229
      Sagittal Slice Fracture 229

☐ Extension 230
   Extension Injury 230

☐ Shearing 230
   Type A Shear Fracture 230
   Type B Shear Fracture 230
   Type B Shear Dislocation 230

☐ Lateral Bending 233
   Pure Lateral Bending 233
      Lateral Wedge Fracture 233
   Lateral Bending With Axial Load 234
      Lateral Burst Fracture 234

☐ Minor Fractures 234

☐ Penetrating Injuries 235

☐ References 236

17. Minor Injuries **238**

☐ Introduction 238

☐ Contusions of the Thoracic and Lumbar Regions . . 238

☐ Acute Strains and Sprains of the Thoracic Region . 239

☐ Acute Strains and Sprains of the Lumbar and
   Lumbosacral Region 240

☐ References 243

18. Scoliosis and Kyphosis **244**

☐ Scoliosis 244

☐ Kyphosis 248

☐ References 250

19. Low Back Pain **252**

☐ Introduction 252

☐ Nonmusculoskeletal (Referred) Causes 252

☐ Musculoskeletal Causes 253

☐ Low Back Pain Associated With Minor Trauma . . . 253
   Myofascial Sprain 253
   Posterior Facet Syndrome 254
   Sacroiliac Sprain 255

☐ Low Back Pain With Radiation 255
   Spinal Stenosis 255
   Acute Disc Herniation 256

☐ Low Back Pain of Insidious Onset Under 50 Years
   of Age 263
   Fibrositis 263
   Infections 265

Sacroiliitis 265

Spondylolysis and Spondylolisthesis 265

☐ Low Back Pain of Insidious Onset Over 50 Years
of Age 266
Spondylosis 266
Neoplasm 268
Osteoporosis 269

☐ History and Physical Examination 269
History 269
Physical Examination 270
Standing 270
Sitting 270
Supine (Straight Leg Raising Test (Lasegue),
Fajersztan Test, Well-Leg Straight Leg
Raising Test, Hoover Test, Kern Test,
Milgram Test, Pelvic Rock Test,

Gaenslen's Sign, FABERE (Patrick)
Test 271
Neurologic Examination 272

☐ Lumbar Spine Radiography 275

☐ Treatment 275
Bedrest 275
Stretch and Spray 275
Spinal Manipulation 275
Drugs 277
Heat and Cold Applications 277

☐ References 278

☐ Bibliography 278

Index **279**

Preface

There are several texts that have been written about the spine. All of these are directed either at the orthopedic surgeon or at the medical student level. Currently, no book fully and completely covers spinal disorders from neoplasms and congenital disorders to traumatic injuries for the practicing emergency physician, family physician, or internist. Spinal disorders constitute the most common problem confronting primary care physicians in this country. As often as low back pain and cervical spine disorders occur, most primary care physicians do not feel comfortable with the current management and diagnosis of these disorders. It is ironic that something so common is so little understood.

The purpose of this text is to fill the gap by addressing spinal disease in a manner useful to the generalist with enough scope and depth to satisfy the need for a full understanding of problems related to the spine. It is divided into sections which detail anatomy, physical examination, pathology, and radiology of the spine. Medical emergencies and trauma are classified in a method which is useful to physicians who treat spinal disease nonoperatively.

As such this text will serve both as a reference and as a book which can be read from cover to cover and will provide the practitioner—emergency physician, orthopedist, neurosurgeon, family practitioner, internist, physical therapist—with sufficient knowledge to treat emergent, urgent, and chronic spinal disorders.

ACKNOWLEDGMENTS

The authors would like to thank Glenda King, Dana Sprute, Carol Schwartzman, and Kim Young for their invaluable assistance in preparing the manuscript.

We would particularly like to thank Susan Gilbert for her excellent artwork, which was often prepared from less than optimal samples under tight deadlines.

We are also indebted to Drs. Robert Scanlon, Margaret Milos, and Michael Vitullo for their expertise and participation.

For their support and patience D.S. thanks Wilbur and Pauline Spaite, and R.G. may never be able to repay his family, Bob and Jo, and Carol.

But, especially, two of us would like to thank one of us for his confidence, guidance, expertise, and faith.

PART I

Approach to the Patient With Spinal Injury

1

Approach to the Patient With Spinal Injury

It is estimated that the annual average incidence of spinal cord injury in the United States affects 11,200 people, approximately 4200 of which die before they reach the hospital, with an additional 1150 patients dying during the hospitalization.[1] Although this is a rather low incidence overall, there is a high residual morbidity for those who survive their original injury.

It is estimated that there is a total of 200,000 individuals who have survived traumatic spinal cord injury in the United States, approximately one-half quadriplegic, one-half paraplegic.[2] Half of the originally quadriplegic and 60% of the paraplegic patients remain completely paralyzed below the level of their spinal lesion. Eighty percent of the group are under the age of 40, and at the time of injury one-half are in the 15 to 35 age group.[3] Initial hospitalization costs range between $60,000 and $80,000, and estimates of lifetime costs range between 1 and 2 million dollars.[4,5] Unfortunately, it is speculated that approximately 10% of patients sustain further neurologic damage because of careless management on the part of prehospital and hospital personnel. Aggravation of the initial injury as well as complications, such as respiratory compromise, infection, and shock, can be significantly reduced by appropriate management in the phase of resuscitation.

Although there are numerous causes of spinal cord injury, by far the most common is motor vehicle accidents. Of the 55,000 people who die each year on the nation's highways, at least 40,000 die as the result of central nervous system injury, many including high cervical spine injury.[6,7] Most other causes are related to sporting injuries, including football and diving accidents, gunshot wounds, falls, and ejection from all types of moving vehicles from motorcycles to skateboards.

Regardless of etiology, most fatalities occur as the result of the initial trauma; however, it is estimated that as much as 25% of fatal complications occur within the immediate postinjury phase.[1] Despite a feeling of hopelessness often associated with spinal trauma, effective intervention on the part of emergency personnel involved in rescue, mobilization, evaluation, and resuscitation can reduce both mortality and morbidity.

☐ MECHANISMS AND PATHOPHYSIOLOGY OF SPINAL TRAUMA

Actually there is a limited number of ways in which the spinal column can be damaged, dependent on the physical forces to which it is subjected.

1. Flexion injuries: fracture vertebral bodies and cause acute disc rupture
2. Extension injuries: result in fractures of posterior bony elements and rupture of the anterior and posterior longitudinal ligaments that stabilize the vertebral bodies
3. Compression injuries: result in rupture of ligaments and burst fractures of vertebral bodies
4. Rotational injuries: rupture ligaments

Combinations of the forces at the time of injury do occur, particularly rotational forces combined with both flexion and extension injuries, resulting in fractures as well as significant ligamentous damage.

The spinal cord is injured at the moment of the accident from deformity or dislocation. Deformities seen on x-rays in the emergency department do not represent the extent of initial dislocation as bone and ligaments tend to spring back toward their normal position. Although this often reduces compression on the cord, the injury has already taken place. With persistent dislocation of the spinal column, greater damage can occur from continuous pressure on the cord and nerve roots.

The sections of the vertebral column that have the greatest mobility are also the areas of most frequent injury. The cervical spine is the most flexible portion of the vertebral column. Bounded above by the relatively heavy head and below by the more fixed thoracic spinal column, it is vulnerable to even modest energy forces. As such, the most common spinal cord injury occurs between C-5 and C-6. Relative protection to the cord is afforded at this level because the spinal canal is approximately 30% larger than the cord itself. This probably accounts for a relatively larger proportion of partial or reversible cord injuries at this level. By contrast, the thoracic spinal canal does not afford such roominess for the cord. The spinal column at this level is also less flexible and fixed by the ribs and trunk; therefore, it requires significantly more force to disrupt or dislocate the thoracic column, resulting in thoracic cord injuries that are usually complete and irreversible.

The lumbar spine includes elements of superior segments. Although heavy and relatively well fixed by the paravertebral muscles, it is still quite flexible. The canal is relatively large and the spinal cord narrows and ends opposite the L-2 vertebra. The cauda equina loosely fills the remainder of the spinal cord and tolerates compression better than the cord itself. Thus, although a T-12 to L-1 spinal cord injury at the interface of the fixed thoracic and more mobile lumbar spine is the second most common injury seen, incomplete lesions of the cord at this level and below are common.

Actual injury to the cord resulting in neurologic dysfunction rarely occurs from transection. The cord and tough meninges remain intact. Injury occurs from compression of the cord and disruption of the blood supply. Experimental studies demonstrate that trauma inflicted on the spinal cord will produce an initial increase in blood flow that later falls to 70 to 80% of the pretrauma flow.[8] It is felt that this relative cord ischemia results in neurologic cell death. Although the mechanism for these blood flow changes is unknown, present investigations show release of vasoconstrictive substances and improving mean arterial pressure. Since cell death occurs within 4 hours of the original injury, future hope of reversing permanent neurologic dysfunction will require prompt and definitive action on the part of emergency personnel.

□ PREHOSPITAL TREATMENT

Even very slight degrees of force have the potential to cause spinal injury. Therefore, any traumatized victim must be suspected of having possible spinal involvement. A high index of suspicion and caution while handling the patient can prevent future damage. As with all multiply traumatized victims, however, the basics of emergency care should not be overlooked.

Initial assessment at the scene is crucial, ensuring that airway, breathing, and circulation are adequate. Breathing should be assisted, if necessary, and major external bleeding should be controlled.

Of primary importance is an assessment of the scene of the accident to determine the extent of possible further danger either to the patient or to the rescuer. Leaking gas, fires, or falling objects have the potential to injure further all nearby. Depending on the circumstances, either the threat or the patient should be moved. If the patient must be extricated immediately, it should be done with extreme care. Although all injuries can potentially be made worse with movement, improper extrication before full assessment of patient status in the face of potential spinal injury can prove devastating. Any person with back, neck, or facial injury, impaired consciousness, unexplained neurologic deficit, tenderness, deformity, or muscle spasm in the neck, or severe neck or back pain must be suspected of having a spinal injury. If possible, the patient should not be moved until the initial assessment has been completed.

Although it is not the purpose of this text to discuss all of the details of the approach to the multiply injured patient, it is not possible to discuss the care of the spinal patient without some discussion of overall care. Likewise, whether spinal injury is suspected or obvious, primary management must focus on initial resuscitation. Thus, after immediate threat to both patient and rescuer is secured, initial assessment of the patient should be accomplished. Emergency medical technicians and paramedics should:

1. Assess airway, breathing, and circulation
2. Assess vital signs
3. Question the patient with regard to pain or numbness
4. Palpate the neck for signs of injury, record any paralysis, motor weakness, or sensory deficit
5. Assess for impaired level of consciousness
6. Check pupil size, equality, and reactivity to light
7. Examine the eyes and ears for signs of injury
8. Palpate the head, arms, legs, chest, and abdomen for injuries

Maintaining the airway in an accident victim suspected of having a cervical spine injury must be done without extending or flexing the neck as this can exacerbate neurologic damage. This is best achieved by elevating the mandible with the mandibular thrust or chin lift technique. The mouth should always be checked for debris and cleared either with suction or manually.

In a semiconscious or unconscious patient, an oropharyngeal or nasopharyngeal airway should be inserted gently, if indicated. The esophageal obturator airway can be placed in the unconscious patient who has a respiratory arrest, but is contraindicated in patients with an intact gag reflex. Endotracheal intubation at the scene is the definitive procedure for maintenance of the airway and assistance in ventilation; however, as with placement of all these devices, great caution must be taken so as not to extend or flex the neck.

Respiratory insufficiency should be expected in the patient with high cervical cord injury. Hypoventilation occurs from paralysis of the intercostal muscles. The patient will breathe with the diaphragm alone, which is innervated by the phrenic nerve originating primarily from the C-4 level. With injuries at this level, the patient will be noted to have abdominal breathing, the stomach rising and falling with each breath, but with the chest not appearing to move. A patient with a cervical cord lesion at a higher level than C-4 associated with phrenic nerve involvement will suffer complete respiratory paralysis. Assisted ventilation is imperative.

Assessment of circulation can be difficult in the neurologically impaired patient. The victim of multiple trauma can be hypotensive from hypovolemic shock. This is generally characterized by hypotension with a rapid heart rate and cool and clammy skin. Neurologic shock results from the loss of sympathetic nerve function. Vasodilatation and vascular collapse will lead to hypotension, but with a normal or slow heart rate and the skin warm and dry. In both cases, intravenous fluids by at least two large-bore intravenous lines and military anti-shock trousers (MAST suit) are indicated during early resuscitative efforts.

Extrication of a patient with a suspected spinal injury requires immobilization of the neck and normal axial alignment of the body. Soft cervical collars allow complete neck movement in all directions and can often act as a tourniquet around the neck.

Axiom: *Soft cervical collars do not prevent neck movement and have no place in cervical spine immobilization.*

If a patient is seated in a vehicle or is otherwise in a position of difficult access, rigid cervical collars can give some support. The patient should be immobilized on a half backboard for removal from the vehicle, used in a way to act as a passive splint for the spine. In all cases, the patient should be placed in the supine position on a long backboard as soon as possible by a team of at least three people. If a half backboard has been used, the patient should be placed on the long board with it still in place.

If the patient is found in the water and has sustained an injury secondary to diving, all efforts should be made to keep the person floating on the surface, supporting the head and the neck. The common error of carrying the patient to dry ground unfortunately allows the head to dangle unsupported. Extrication in the water is relatively easily accomplished by securing the floating patient to the long board while in the water.

Podolsky and associates[9] have demonstrated that appropriate immobilization can be maintained with sandbags or plastic intravenous bags placed on either side of the head and a 3-inch cloth tape placed across the forehead (Fig 1–1). For spinal immobilization that would include the head and the trunk, the latter can be immobilized with straps surrounding the patient and the board, or sheets placed under the board, torn in broad strips, and tied over the patient (Fig 1–1). In this way

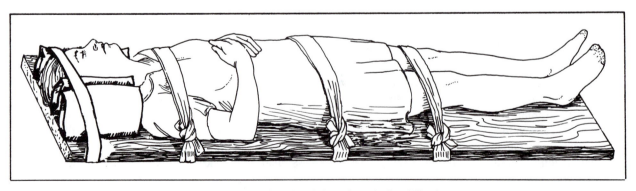

Figure 1–1. The optimal technique for spinal stabilization.

the patient is completely immobilized and will remain secured to the board, enabling rescuers to tilt the patient, even to the prone position, during extrication or to keep the airway clear while vomiting.

The motorcyclist, bicyclist, or athlete may be found at the accident site with a helmet still in place. The removal of helmets from injured patients requires two rescuers as recommended by the American College of Surgeons (Fig 1–2). In-line traction is always applied while a second rescuer is supporting the head and the neck. If the helmet cannot be removed easily, the authors recommend that it be left in place during transport. In the emergency room it can be safely removed once cervical spine radiographs demonstrate no abnormality, or bivalved along the coronal plane with a cast cutter.

Although all circumstances vary and less seriously injured patients will require less intervention, in general, the preparation for transport of the multiply injured patient with suspected spinal involvement should include:

- Spinal precautions on a long board, the head secured with sandbags and 3-inch cloth tape, and the body secured with broad straps or sheets
- Supplementary oxygen
- Assisted ventilation, as necessary, with airway esophageal obturator or endotracheal intubation as indicated
- Two large-bore intravenous lines
- MAST in place, inflated if hypotension is present
- Communications should be established with the nearest trauma facility. If the facility is a great distance away, air transport by helicopter or airplane is recommended

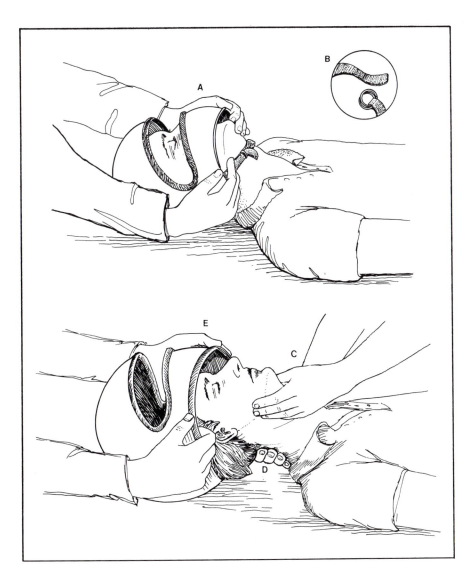

Figure 1–2. The technique for removal of a helmet from an injured patient. **A.** Apply hands to each side of helmet, fingers on victim's mandible to stablize the head. **B.** Maintain in-line traction while strap is undone or cut. **C.** A second person places the thumb on one side of the mandible and the index finger on the other side. **D.** The opposite hand is placed around the neck under the occipital region. **E.** Helmet is pulled off while traction is maintained by the second person.

☐ EMERGENCY DEPARTMENT MANAGEMENT

Initial emergency room management of the suspected spinal injury patient will vary depending on presentation. The emergency department team will approach the multiply injured patient far more aggressively than the patient with isolated neck stiffness due to a low-speed, rear-end accident, although no less carefully. Similarly, the approach to a cervical injury will require certain specific interventions not necessarily indicated with a thoracic or lumbar injury. Although the specific injury will dictate management, the overall approach to evaluation and support should be the same for all patients.

It is possible in the case of both the critically injured patient or the not so critically ill that spinal precautions might have been overlooked by prehospital personnel or that the patient may have been transported to the emergency department by friends or come in on his or her own after the accident. Any patient with one or more of the following should have spinal precautions instituted if not already in place:

- Impaired consciousness
- Obvious neurologic deficits
- Mechanism consistent with spinal injury
- Head or facial injury
- Localized deformity or swelling
- Unexplained hypotension

If brought in by prehospital personnel, an update of history and physical findings at the scene and en route to the facility should be obtained. Initial evaluation by the physician should again begin with the ABCs (airway, breathing, circulation).

Airway Management and Breathing

Respiratory complications are not uncommonly seen in cervical and high thoracic cord injuries. The incidence increases markedly when other bodily injuries are present.

As all spinal cord lesions have the potential to develop in ascending level because of increasing spinal cord edema, respiratory decompensation can occur at any time during the early stages of resuscitation. Particularly when the initial injury includes traumatic tetraplegia, close respiratory observation is imperative. With lesions at or below the C-6 segment, diaphragmatic innervation remains intact, but intercostal muscle paralysis is present. At the level of the fifth cervical segment partial diaphragmatic innervation might be involved and at levels of C-4 and above diaphragmatic function is severely impaired as the phrenic nerve is affected. Inadequate ventilation secondary to high cervical injury leads to decreased vital capacity, retention of secretions, increased PCO_2, increased dead space, anoxia, vasoconstriction, respiratory failure, and pulmonary edema. These are leading causes of death in acute traumatic tetraplegia.

As relative hypoxia can further damage an injured cord, all patients, regardless of the level of their injury, should receive supplementary oxygen. Patients with preservation of intercostal muscle and diaphragmatic function may require oxygen only by nasal cannula.

When intubation is required, it can be accomplished in a variety of ways. Nasotracheal intubation can be accomplished without manipulation of the head or neck. It may be contraindicated, however, in the setting of significant craniofacial injury. This procedure is not without risk as extensive bleeding of the nasopharyngeal mucosa can result in aspiration of blood. Patients with an intact gag reflex might vomit and aspirate gastric contents.

Orotracheal intubation is an accepted approach, but is best accomplished with the aid of an assistant. Extreme care must be taken to avoid flexion or extension of the neck. While maintaining spinal immobilization and with additional supportive in-line traction, safe orotracheal intubation can be accomplished (Fig 1–3).

If neither nasotracheal nor orotracheal intubation is successful after one or two careful attempts or contraindicated because of facial trauma or potential for further neurologic deficit due to highly suspicious mechanics or clinical presentation, a cricothyrotomy should be performed without delay. It is for this reason that hard collars that obstruct approaches to the neck are suboptimal. Spine immobilization by use of the long board, sandbags, and tape adequately support the spine without obstructing access to the neck.

As a temporizing measure, a small plastic intravenous catheter can be passed through the cricothyroid membrane and attached to high flow oxygen or high pressure jet insufflation. This is not intended for long-term use and as soon as possible should be followed by cricothyrotomy.

Tracheotomy is a relatively complicated and lengthy procedure that should not be attempted in the emergency situation.

Circulation

Associated injuries are common in spinal cord trauma. Head injuries are most frequently encountered, particularly in the patient with a cervical cord injury, followed by chest injury, notably associated with thoracic spine injuries. It is also common to have multiply traumatized areas with significant external and internal hemorrhage. Hence, cardiovascular abnormalities may have multiple etiologies. Complete traumatic cord transection can lead to spinal shock. Lesions involving the

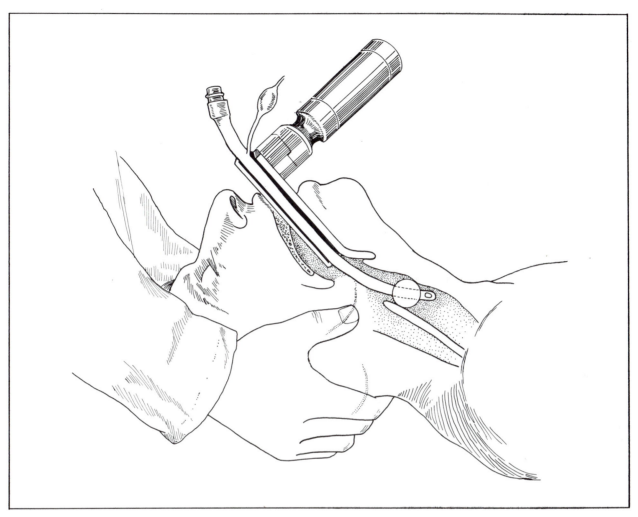

Figure 1–3. In-line traction will permit safe orotracheal intubation.

areas T-1 to L-2 with compromise to sympathetic outflow can affect blood pressure, with significant hypotension, bradycardia, and hypothermia. With a lack of sympathetic tone, response to postural changes are completely lost. It is advisable, therefore, to keep the patient as level as possible.

Hypovolemic shock secondary to significant hemorrhage, by contrast, will also manifest itself with hypotension, but generally is associated with tachycardia and cool and clammy skin. In the patient with sensory loss, significant chest or abdominal injuries might be present in the absence of pain. At least two large-bore intravenous lines and a fluid challenge of crystalloid are indicated in both scenarios of hypotension, as well as a fully inflated MAST suit. Catecholamines (once hypovolemic shock is ruled out), particularly dopamine, are frequently necessary for spinal shock, and are preferably administered under venous and pulmonary wedge pressure monitoring.

Primary Assessment

All patients who have sustained significant trauma should be completely undressed. In those who are more severely injured and immobilized, clothes should be cut away. Two temporary exceptions to complete visualization of the entire body are: (1) maintaining a MAST suit inflated in circumstances of hypotension and (2) not rolling the patient to assess the back until spinal films have been evaluated or several assistants are available to properly turn the patient.

A thorough physical examination is required in all cases with particular attention to a complete neurologic evaluation. A flow sheet with documentation of changes in the neurologic status should be maintained. Particular attention should be focused on:

- Altering level of consciousness, orientation, and cranial nerve function

- Observation of respiratory pattern noting chest wall movement versus abdominal breathing
- Vibratory sense (posterior cord) and pain and temperature (anterior cord) in extremities will demonstrate partial cord lesions (Fig 1–4)
- Motor strength of extremities
- Deep tendon, abdominal, and cremasteric reflexes
- Plantar responses
- Rectal examination to assess the presence of voluntary anal sphincter tone, anal wink, and bulbocavernosus reflex
- Sensory levels help to determine the upper level of cord involvement (Tables 1–1 and 1–2)

In many instances the level of involvement will ascend with time usually due to cord edema. When the initial involvement is a high cervical lesion, particularly C-4 to C-5, further deterioration or edema could lead to respiratory compromise or cardiopulmonary arrest.

Other Considerations

Gastrointestinal

Cervical and thoracic cord injuries will leave the patient with a sensory loss below the level of the lesion. The multiply injured victim will not complain of abdominal pain despite the possibility of significant internal hemorrhage. Most patients will develop paralytic ileus. Nasogastric suctioning is recommended. Depending on circumstances, abdominal computed tomography (CT) or peritoneal lavage might be necessary to rule out significant abdominal injury.

Genitourinary

A Foley catheter should be inserted to decompress the urinary bladder. When the catheter is required for more than 24 hours, intermittent catheterization is recommended.

Temperature Regulation

Disruption of sympathetic nerve function at T-8 or above is frequently associated with hypothermia or hyperthermia, although the former is more common. Hypothermia generally occurs due to cutaneous vasodilation and subsequent heat loss. Hyperthermia is more likely in warmer climates or in the face of infection. Since sympathetic nerve flow mediates sweating, heat loss may be disturbed. Hypothermia is best controlled with passive warming methods. Hyperthermia is usually mild. Severe cases, however, require management similar to heat stroke.

TABLE 1–1. THE SENSORY EXAMINATION

A Lesion at This Level	Causes Loss of Sensation at This Level
C-2	Occiput
C-3	Thyroid cartilage
C-4	Suprasternal notch
C-5	Below clavicle
C-6	Thumb
C-7	Index finger
C-8	Small finger
T-4	Nipple line
T-10	Umbilicus
L-1	Femoral pulse
L-2 to L-3	Medial thigh
L-4	Knee
L-5	Lateral calf
S-1	Lateral foot
S-2 to S-4	Perianal region

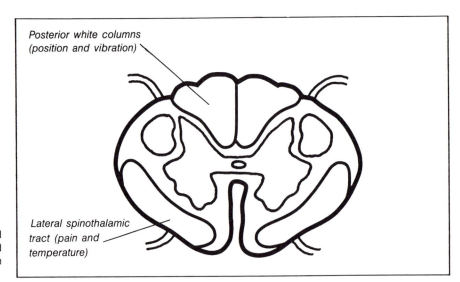

Figure 1–4. Vibration is diminished in posterior cord injury and pain and temperature sense is affected with anterior cord syndrome.

Posterior white columns (position and vibration)

Lateral spinothalamic tract (pain and temperature)

TABLE 1–2. THE MOTOR EXAMINATION

A Lesion at This Level	Causes Loss of This Function
C-4	Spontaneous breathing
C-5	Shrugging of shoulders
C-6	Flexion at elbow
C-7	Extension at elbow
C-8 to T-1	Flexion of fingers
T-1 to T-12	Intercostal and abdominal muscles[a]
L-1 to L-2	Flexion at hip
L-3	Adduction at hip
L-4	Abduction at hip
L-5	Dorsiflexion of foot
S-1 to S-2	Plantar flexion of foot
S-2 to S-4	Rectal sphincter tone

[a]Localization of lesions in this area is best accomplished with the sensory examination.

Radiographic Evaluation

Routine radiographs of the spine should be obtained as soon as possible. In the case of the cervical spine, cross-table lateral, anteroposterior, and open-mouth views will demonstrate greater than 90% of abnormalities.[10]

Indications for x-rays in patients with suspected spinal cord injury include:

- Localized pain
- Deformity
- Neurologic dysfunction
- Local crepitance or edema
- Altered mental status with inability to assess the patient

Cervical Spine

Radiographic evaluation of the cervical spine must include a cross-table lateral view that shows all seven cervical vertebrae. Fractures or dislocations of the lower cervical spine can be missed when C-6 and C-7 to T-1 are not visualized. If spinal precautionary apparatus is removed for x-rays to be taken, two assistants are required to stabilize the patient, one placed at the head to prevent movement, the second at the feet applying traction to the arms in a downward manner. The proper grasp of the head is demonstrated in Figure 1–5.

If traction is still inadequate to visualize all cervical vertebrae, a swimmer's or transaxillary view should be attempted.

Lateral views of the cervical spine will disclose approximately 75% of possible abnormalities.[10,11] Therefore, this view alone is inadequate to rule out cervical spine injury and should be followed by a complete cervical spine radiographic series.

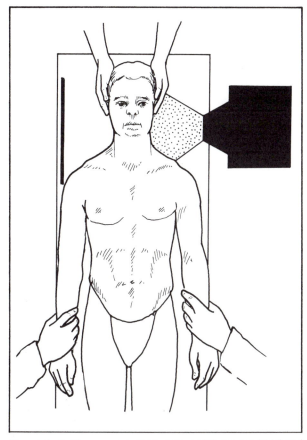

Figure 1–5. The proper technique for stabilizing the head and applying traction to the upper extremity to obtain a lateral radiograph of the cervical spine.

If any film shows an unstable fracture or if you as the emergency practitioner are uncertain of any detail, the authors recommend repeat views or CT studies.

Axiom: *If any detail of a spinal film remains uncertain, repeat the view or progress to CT evaluation.*

Refer to the specific sections of radiographic interpretation elsewhere in the text for guidelines.

If plain film radiography is inconclusive or a significant abnormality is found, a CT scan can provide valuable information. Bony alignment and spinal canal integrity can be evaluated. Fracture fragments, herniated disc material, and hematomas can be seen.

Thoracolumbar Spine

Cross-table lateral and anteroposterior views are indicated in all patients with significant spinal trauma who have mid or low back pain. These two views can be done without moving the patient off of the backboard.

Laboratory Tests

All patients with multiple trauma or neurologic deficit require the following laboratory tests:

- Serial hemoglobin, hematocrit, platelets
- Coagulation studies
- Blood type and crossmatch
- Arterial blood gases
- Blood sugar, alcohol, toxicology screen
- Urinalysis
- Electrocardiogram
- Chest x-ray (abdomen, pelvis, indicated extremity films) as required in multiple trauma

□ TREATMENT

In most instances, the particular defect involving the spinal column will require specific treatment. The authors recommend referral to the appropriate section of this text detailing the treatment of specific conditions.

Pharmacology

Emergency pharmacology of acute spinal injuries remains controversial.

Corticosteroids

Dexamethasone or corticosteroids have been used on the theory that they counteract axonal edema by stabilizing cell and vascular membranes. No substantial data, however, support their efficacy. Nevertheless, most spinal centers recommend their use early on, generally at high dose, although this too is controversial. Initial doses of 1 to 2 mg/kg of intravenous dexamethasone, repeated every 4 to 6 hours, is recommended. If clinical improvement is demonstrated, steroids are continued for approximately 1 week. If no improvement is seen early on, they should be discontinued.[12]

Diuretics

Similarly, there is no good evidence to suggest that osmotic diuretics, such as mannitol, are of any value. Nevertheless, on the theory that they reduce local edema, many spinal centers still recommend their use.

Other Drugs

Numerous other drugs are being investigated for use in the acute trauma of the spinal cord. Initial studies of some, notably naloxone and clonidine, are encouraging. Conclusive evidence that they, or other measures such as thyrotropin releasing hormone, dimethyl sulfoxide, or local spinal cord cooling, are effective is still lacking and at this time cannot be recommended.[13]

□ REFERENCES

1. Kraus JF, Franti CE, Riggins S, et al: Incidences of traumatic spinal cord lesions. J Chron Dis 28:471, 1975
2. Decker DP: Injury to the head and spine. In: Cecil Textbook of Medicine, p 2170
3. Green EA, et al: Acute spinal cord injury: Current concepts. Clin Orthop 154: 125, 1981
4. Saul TG, Ducker TB: Injuries to the spine and spinal cord. Annual Meeting, 1980, Congress of Neurological Surgeons.
5. Colohan DP: Emergency management of cervical spine injuries. Emerg Phy Series, 1977, p 3
6. Norrell H: Early management of spinal injuries. Clin Neurosurg 27:385, 1979
7. Gehweiler JA, et al: Cervical spine trauma: The common combined conditions. Radiology 130:77, 1979
8. Lohse DC, et al: Spinal cord blood flow in experimental transient traumatic paraplegic. Neurosurg 52:335, 1980
9. Podolsky S, Baraff LJ, Simon R, Hoffman JR, Larmon B, Ablon W: Efficacy of cervical spine immobilization methods. J Trauma 23:461–465, 1983
10. Swetman R: Cervical spine injuries, from Tintinalli.
11. Bladhd WH, et al: Efficacy of the post-traumatic cross-table lateral view of the cervical spine. Emerg Med 2:243, 1985
12. Sonntag V: The early management of cervical spine injuries. Arizona Med 39(10):644, 1982
13. Yashon D: Spinal injury, 2nd ed. Norwalk, Conn., Appleton-Century-Crofts, 1986, p 319

□ BIBLIOGRAPHY

Albin M: Resuscitation of the spinal cord. Crit Care Med 6(4):270, 1978

Calenoff L, et al: Multiple level spinal injuries: Incidence of early recognition. Ann J Roentgenol 130: 665, 1978

Cloward R: Acute cervical spine injury. Clinical Symposia, CIBA Series, Vol 32, No. 1, 1980

Arch. Surg., 111(6):638, 1976.

Donovan WH: Comprehensive management of spinal cord injury. Clinical Symposia, CEBA Series, Vol 34, No. 2, 1982

Hockberger RS: Spinal cord injury. Curr Therapy Emerg Med

Knopp RK: Cervical spine injury. Curr Therapy Emerg Med

Maull KI: Avoiding a pitfall in resuscitation: The painless cervical fracture. Sout Med J 70(4):477, 1977

Miller ND, et al: Significant new observations in cervical spine. Ann J Roentgenol 130: 659, 1978

Riggins RS, Kraus JF: The risk of neurologic damage with fractures of the vertebra. J Trauma 17(2):126, 1977

Scher AT: Unrecognized fractures and dislocations of the cervical spine. Paraplegia 19:25, 1981

Soderstrome CA, Brumback RJ: Early care of the patient with spine injury. Orthop Clin North Am 17(1):3, 1986

PART II
Medical Emergencies

2

Cord Syndromes: Evaluation and Management

□ INTRODUCTION AND ANATOMIC CONSIDERATIONS

Any discussion of spinal disorders must include their effect on the spinal cord, for it is this structure that gives the spine such unique importance. Although the emergency physician need not remember all of the intricate details of the cord syndromes, the knowledge of certain aspects of these entities is necessary to properly care for patients with spinal disorders.

Knowledge of the anatomy of the spinal cord is fundamental to understanding the cord syndromes. Chapters 7 and 13 cover this issue at length but a brief discussion of the cross-sectional anatomy of the cord is appropriate here. In addition, figures outlining dermatomal and motor innervation of the body are included (Fig 2–1, Tables 2–1 and 2–2).

The important cross-sectional anatomic features of the cord are shown in Figure 2–2. The function of each pathway and the level at which they cross the midline are shown in Table 2–3. It should be noted that there is evidence to support the "topographic" or laminated character of several of the tracts. That is, fibers leading to or from different parts of the body are located at different positions in the tract (Fig 2–2). Certain clinical syndromes may be explained by this phenomenon and this will be covered in the discussion of the specific syndromes.

□ COMPLETE CORD SYNDROME

There are many etiologies that result in a complete cord syndrome including congenital, infectious, neoplastic, degenerative, and vascular (see Chapters 5 and 6); however, the vast majority of acute cases presenting as emergencies are caused by trauma.

The early clinical picture is characterized by a total flaccid paralysis and loss of all sensation below the injury level. Deep tendon reflexes are absent and attempts to elicit a Babinski sign reveal no response at all. Cremasteric and bulbocavernosus reflexes are usually present. Priapism may appear and generally lasts for a day or longer before resolving. Within 1 to 3 days, spasticity, clonus, hyperactive deep tendon reflexes, and a positive Babinski sign appear. These findings, in addition to complete loss of sensory and voluntary motor function, characterize the complete cord syndrome after the first few days of the injury.

Neurologically, the specific clinical picture is determined by the exact level of the cord lesion. The sensory examination reveals deficits that correlate to the dermatomes at and below the level of the lesion (see Fig 2–1). Injuries to the C-1 to C-4 region nearly always result in immediate death due to respiratory muscle paralysis. A few patients who receive very early advanced life support may be salvaged but require continuous mechanical ventilation and generally will die within months to years of the accident even with optimum care.[1] Injuries to the C-5 to C-8 levels of the cord present with varying neurologic pictures due to the specific muscle groups that are affected (see Table 2–1). For instance, a patient with a cord injury at C-6 will present with abducted arms (unopposed deltoid action) and flexed elbows (unopposed biceps action). Similarly, complete cord syndromes in the lumbar and sacral regions of the cord produce varying neurologic deficits depending on the level of the lesion.

With regard to prognosis, complete and immediate paralysis due to cord damage that shows no recovery of

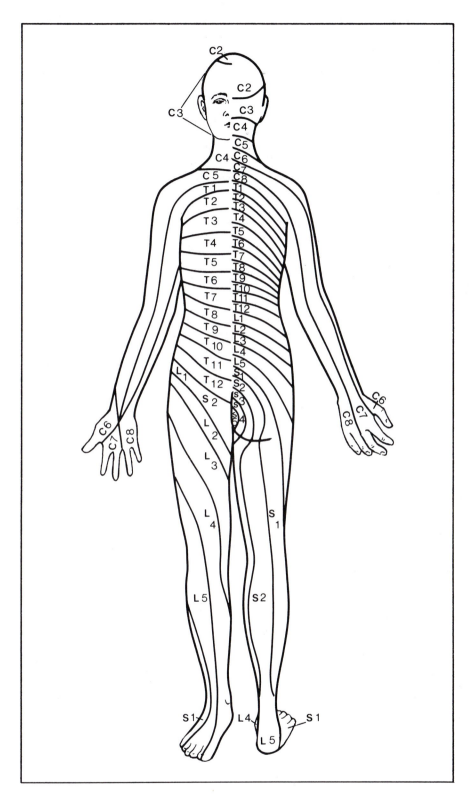

Figure 2–1. Dermatome distribution of spinal nerves.

TABLE 2–1. MOTOR INNERVATION

Body Part	Muscle Group	Action	Spinal Segment	Body Part	Muscle Group	Action	Spinal Segment
Diaphragm	Diaphragm	Respiration	C-3 to C-5	Hip (cont.)	Gluteus medius, gluteus minimus, and tensor fasciae latae	Abduction	L-4, L-5
Shoulder	Deltoid	Abduction	C-5				
	Infraspinatus	External rotation (humerus)	C-5		Gluteus maximus, and biceps femoris	Extension	L-5 to S-2
Elbow	Biceps	Flexion	C-5, C-6				
	Triceps	Extension	C-7	Knee	Quadriceps femoris	Extension	L-3, L-4
Wrist	Extensor carpi ulnaris and radialis	Extension	C-6		Semimembranosus, semitendinosus, and biceps femoris	Flexion	L-4 to S-1
	Flexor carpi radialis and palmaris longus	Flexion	C-6, C-7				
Fingers	Extensor digitorum	Extension	C-7	Ankle	Tibialis anterior and extensor digitorum longus	Dorsiflexion	L-4, L-5
	Flexor digitorum profundus and superficialis	Flexion	C-7, C-8		Gastrocnemius and soleus	Plantar flexion	S-1
	Interossei	Adduction, abduction	C-8, T-1	Foot	Peroneus longus and peroneus brevis	Eversion	L-5, S-1
Thumb	Extensor pollicis brevis and extensor pollicis longus	Extension	C-6, C-7	Toes and great toe	Extensor digitorum and hallucis longus	Extension	L-5
	Several	Flexion, adduction, abduction	C-8, T-1		Flexor digitorum, hallucis brevis, and hallucis longus	Flexion	S-1, S-2
Hip	Quadriceps femoris, sartorius, iliopsoas	Flexion	L-2 to L-4				

motor or sensory function within 24 hours is irreversible and permanent.[2,3] It should be noted, however, that the portion of the neurologic deficit due to root damage may not be readily apparent early on. This is important as impressive recovery may occur when the deficit is due to root (or cauda equina) damage even weeks after the injury.[3]

Axiom: *Complete immediate paralysis due to cord damage that lasts for 24 hours without any recovery of motor or sensory function is irreversible and permanent.*

Axiom: *Complete neurologic deficits due to root injury lasting several weeks without improvement may subsequently show impressive recovery.*

□ ANTERIOR CORD SYNDROME

The anterior cord syndrome was first described by Schneider[4] and nearly always occurs in the setting of hyperflexion injuries of the cervical spine. Rarely, hyperextension injuries may also cause the syndrome.[5] Acute disc herniation is the most common cause; how-

TABLE 2–2. REFLEXES

Reflex	Spinal Segment
Biceps	C-5, C-6
Triceps	C-7, C-8
Knee jerk	L-2 to L-4
Ankle jerk	S-1
Cremasteric	T-12
Bulbocavernosus	S-2 to S-4
Anal wink	S-2 to S-4

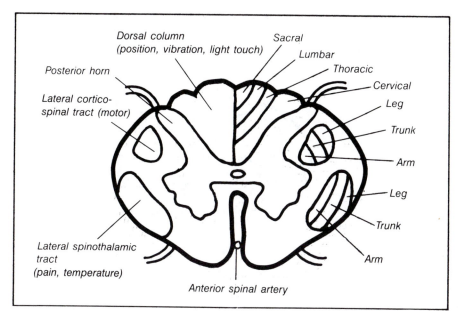

Figure 2–2. Cross-section of a normal cervical spinal cord.

ever, it is also seen with fracture-dislocations.[4,5] The damage occurs primarily in the anterior two-thirds of the cord and thus may spare much of the function of the dorsal columns (Fig 2–3).

Clinically, there is immediate, complete paralysis and loss of sensation to pain and temperature at levels below the lesion. Light touch, proprioception, and vibratory sense (dorsal columns) remain intact to a variable degree (Figs 2–2 and 2–3).[4,5] This lesion usually occurs in the cervical region but on occasion it has been noted in the thoracic cord.[6] Unlike other syndromes in which progression may be noted, the maximal neurologic deficit occurs instantaneously at the time of the injury in this syndrome.[4,5]

The prognosis for neurologic improvement in these patients is significantly greater than for those with complete cord syndrome although most patients do not attain complete recovery.[4] There is a subgroup of patients who retain some pain sensation immediately after the injury. These patients apparently have a better prognosis for recovery than those without this finding.[7] Immediate surgery has been advocated[4] and may improve neurologic outcome.[8] It should be noted that if

only a very cursory neurologic examination is carried out in these patients, their clinical picture could easily be mistaken for a complete cord syndrome. This would be very unfortunate as early surgery may alter the outcome in patients with anterior cord syndrome. In addition, the significant possibility of neurologic improvement leaves the patient, family, and physician with greater hope for recovery.

□ CENTRAL CORD SYNDROME

The central cord syndrome was first formally described by Schneider and co-workers in 1954.[9] The majority of cases are caused by hyperextension injuries of the neck, often in patients with preexisting cervical spondylosis.[2,5,9–12] In this setting the cervical cord is compressed between bony osteophytes anteriorly and areas of bulging in the ligamentum flavum posteriorly (Fig 2–4).[5,9–11] Bony damage is usually absent. Other less common mechanisms include hyperflexion (with or without fracture), facet dislocations, burst (compression) fractures, odontoid fractures, direct blows to the neck, and gunshot wounds to the neck (extremely rare).[9,11,13–16] In the vast majority of cases the lesion is in the cervical cord but apparently it occurs in the thoracic and lumbar regions on very rare occasions.[10]

Historically, it was thought that the syndrome occurred primarily in elderly persons,[2] but a more recent series has shown that the peak incidence occurs in persons in their twenties.[14] In fact, only 30% of the 99 cases in this study were patients over the age of 50. The patient's history often states that he or she has

TABLE 2–3. FUNCTION AND LEVEL OF CROSSING OF PATHWAYS

Pathway	Function	Level of Crossing
Corticospinal (pyramidal) tract	Motor	Above the cord in the medulla
Dorsal columns	Proprioception, vibration, light touch	Above the cord in the medulla
Spinothalamic tract	Pain, temperature	At the level of entry into the spinal cord

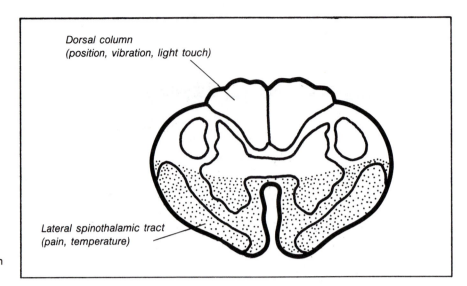

Figure 2–3. Area of cord injury in the anterior cord syndrome.

been struck on the forehead[9] or suffered a whiplash mechanism. Falls, motor vehicle accidents, pedestrians struck, diving, and sporting accidents are the most frequent causes.[14]

Clinically, the syndrome is characterized by weakness that is disproportionately greater in the upper as compared with the lower extremities with variable amounts of sensory loss and bladder dysfunction.[2,5,9,11,13–15] The weakness is generally most pronounced in the hands with the proximal arm muscles being slightly less affected. In severe forms there is immediate complete paralysis of the upper extremities, urinary retention, and sensory loss in all modalities.

Although there also may be impressive loss of lower extremity motor function, some sparing probably always occurs. This is the extreme clinical picture in a spectrum that includes essentially all gradations of severity, but always with the hallmark of relatively greater weakness in the upper extremities.

The probable explanation for this unique syndrome lies in the somatotopic character of the tracts in the spinal cord. Anteroposterior cord compression causes the greatest injury in the central region of the cord (Figs 2–4 and 2–5). Because the outer part of the cord is spared from significant injury, the fibers in the corticospinal tracts that are most peripheral sustain the least

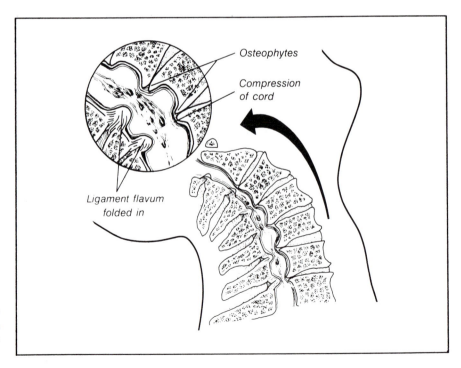

Figure 2–4. Hyperextension injury with compression of the cord due to osteophytes and bulging areas of ligamentum flavum.

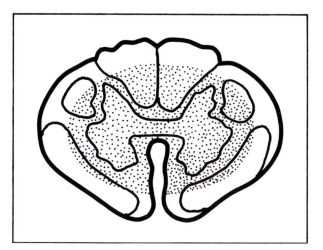

Figure 2–5. Area of cord injury in the central cord syndrome. The central cord edema and somatotopic distribution of the corticospinal tracts give rise to the greater motor weakness found in the upper extremities.

amount of damage. These are the motor fibers to the lumbosacral region of the cord, and thus lower extremity motor function is affected less than that of the upper extremity.[2]

In general, significant resolution of the neurologic deficit occurs in the days to weeks after the injury. This usually progresses in a fairly predictable pattern with the lower extremity weakness resolving first, followed by return of bladder function, and then upper extremity motor function.[5,9,11] The motor function of the fingers is the last to resolve. Recovery of sensation apparently follows no particular pattern but generally does occur.[9,11]

The prognosis for functional neurologic recovery is quite good.[2,5,11,17,18] In some patients it is indeed dramatic.[11] Knowledge of this syndrome is extremely important because the relatively good prognosis is so distinct from the hopelessness that generally surrounds most cord injured patients. Many patients who have a nearly complete quadraplegia except for minimal motor sparing of the toes may experience complete resolution of their neurologic deficits.[5] In fact, cases resulting in respiratory compromise requiring mechanical ventilation with nearly complete quadraplegia have gone on to be ambulatory with good functional recovery.[11] A truly catastrophic scenario can be conceived in which failure to diagnose this syndrome might lead to withholding life-saving interventions because of a "hopeless situation" in a patient who would have ultimately recovered.

Management of these patients is supportive. The majority of them have completely stable cervical spines. Surgery is contraindicated in most cases as improvement often occurs with conservative therapy, and laminectomy may cause some patients to worsen.[2,9]

☐ CONTUSIO CERVICALIS POSTERIOR

Contusio cervicalis posterior is a traumatic cord syndrome that was first described by Biemond[19] and is characterized by pain, tingling, and hyperesthesias of the neck, arms, hands, and to a variable extent, the trunk.[19,20] In about one-third of patients there is also mild to moderate motor involvement of one or both of the upper extremities. Pyramidial tract involvement is noted in about 10%, resulting in lower extremity findings typical of a mild upper motor neuron lesion. Hyperflexion injuries to the cervical spine are the most common cause of the syndrome, but many mechanisms have been associated with this disorder.

The syndrome is probably not caused by a distinct pathophysiologic entity but is more likely to be a mild form in the clinical spectrum of central cord syndrome.[21] Like the central cord syndrome, impressive recovery is the rule, and associated bony or ligamentous injury of the cervical spine is very uncommon.

☐ BROWN-SÉQUARD SYNDROME

Brown-Séquard syndrome is a rare cord syndrome resulting from functional or anatomic hemisection of the cord. It may be caused by penetrating spinal injuries,[22–25] blunt trauma (very rare), disc protrusion,[26,27] tumors, or epidural abscesses.

Clinically, these patients present with paralysis and loss of proprioception, vibration, and light touch on the side of the cord damage and loss of pain and temperature sensation on the contralateral side (Figs 2–2 and 2–6, Table 2–3). The likelihood of neurologic recovery is relatively small in cases caused by acute trauma. The prognosis may be significantly better, however, when the syndrome is caused by a slowly expanding lesion that is recognized relatively soon after symptoms occur.

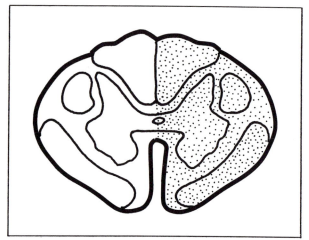

Figure 2–6. Area of cord damage in Brown-Séquard syndrome.

□ ROOT AND CAUDA EQUINA SYNDROMES

Although root and cauda equina syndromes are not cord syndromes per se, they are certainly related and clinically important and thus will be briefly discussed here.

Isolated nerve root injuries may occur at any spinal segment but are most common in the cervical region. They are less common in the lumbar region and indeed rare in the thoracic region. Unilateral or bilateral facet dislocations are the most frequent cause but various types of spinal fractures and ligamentous disruptions may lead to these injuries.[10,20]

Clinically, the motor deficit tends to be greater than the sensory component. The most common clinical syndromes involve the fifth, sixth, or seventh cervical roots unilaterally with isolated deltoid, biceps, or triceps weakness, respectively (Table 2–1).[10]

Prognosis for complete recovery is very good (about 70%) if the spinal injury is adequately reduced and anatomic restoration is accomplished.[20]

In patients with injuries to the thoracolumbar spine, neurologic injury may be due to nerve root or conus medullaris (cord) damage or a combination of both in various patterns. These mixed injuries and the specific anatomy that accounts for them are described at length in Chapter 13 and the section on neurologic injury in Chapter 16. This discussion is limited to disorders affecting solely the cauda equina.

The spinal cord terminates in most adults at the L1-2 interspace, although this varies from as high as T-12 to as low as the L3-4 interspace in a few cases.[28] Below the L1-2 interspace, the nerve roots course downward to exit at the foramen of their respective segments (see Fig 13–8). This collection of nerve roots below the termination of the cord is termed the cauda

equina. Various etiologies are responsible for the neurologic syndromes associated with the cauda equina. Neoplastic, infectious, and traumatic disorders are the most common causes.

Compression of the cauda, either acute or chronic, leads to the clinical picture of a lower motor neuron lesion. Flaccid weakness or paralysis, muscle atrophy (if chronic), fasciculations, decreased or absent deep tendon reflexes, and loss of the plantar response are noted on examination. Bladder dysfunction with incontinence is seen and sensation is impaired in a dermatomal distribution. Obviously, the clinical picture will vary based on the level of compression and whether or not some roots are spared. In the setting of trauma to the thoracolumbar region it is difficult to determine early on whether the neurologic deficit is due to cord, root, or cauda equina damage or some combination. This confusion is due to the fact that the neurologic picture indicating an upper motor neuron type lesion (cord damage) often takes 1 to 3 days to unfold. This differentiation is by no means trivial as the prognosis for root and cauda equina injuries is significantly better than for cord damage. The prognosis for recovery is similar to that for peripheral nerve injuries and thus the deficits may resolve even months after the initial injury.[2,3,28,29]

□ CORD CONTUSION

Some patients will have transient neurologic symptoms or signs after a traumatic event that begin resolving nearly immediately and rarely last longer than several hours.[20,30] In the authors' experience, the contusion can occur at nearly any level in the spine but the cervical region is by far the most common. Neither the incidence nor the pathophysiology is known, but some feel that it represents the spinal cord equivalent of a cerebral concussion.[20]

Clinically, the syndrome presents in a myriad of ways but complaints of paresthesias and mild weakness of the arms and hands are most frequent. Often the symptoms are essentially resolved by the time the patient is seen by a physician, and a "vague history" with "no objective findings" is common. The tendency may be to consider the symptoms "functional" but all of these patients should have radiographs of the appropriate spinal level as a serious "real" spinal injury may present in identical fashion. If the injury level is in the cervical region, flexion–extension films are advisable in addition to the standard views. Prognosis is excellent with essentially all patients undergoing complete recovery within hours to days of the injury.

☐ REFERENCES

1. Guttmann L: Spinal Cord Injuries: Comprehensive Management and Research. Oxford, Blackwell, 1973
2. Kahn E: On spinal-cord injuries. J Bone Joint Surg 41A:6, 1959
3. Holdsworth F: Fractures, dislocations, and fracture–dislocations of the spine. J Bone Joint Surg 52A:1534, 1970
4. Schneider RC: The syndrome of acute anterior spinal cord injury. J Neurosurg 12:95, 1955
5. Schneider RC, Crosby EC, Russo RH, et al: Traumatic spinal cord syndromes and their management. Clin Neurosurg 20:424, 1973
6. Young JS, Dexter WR: Neurological recovery distal to the zone of injury in 172 cases of closed, traumatic spinal cord injury. Paraplegia 16:39, 1978
7. Foo D, Bignami A, Rossier AB: Posttraumatic anterior spinal cord syndrome: Pathological studies of two patients. Surg Neurol 17:370, 1982
8. Brodkey JS, Miller CF, Harmony RM: The syndrome of acute central cervical cord syndrome revisited. J Bone Joint Surg 53B:3, 1971
9. Schneider RC, Cherry G, Pantek H: The syndrome of acute central cervical spinal cord injury. J Neurosurg 11:546, 1954
10. Bohlman HH, Ducker TB, Lucas JT: Spine and spinal cord injuries. In Rothman RH, Simeone FA (eds): The Spine. Philadelphia, WB Saunders, 1982
11. Mortara RW, Flanagan M: Acute central cervical spinal cord syndrome caused by missile injury: Case report and brief review of the syndrome. Neurosurgery 6:176, 1980
12. Marar BC: Hyperextension injuries of the cervical spine. J Bone Joint Surg 56A:1648, 1974
13. Schneider RC, Thompson JM, Bebin J: The syndrome of acute central cervical spinal cord injury. J Neurol Neurosurg Psychiatry 21:216, 1958
14. Shrosbree RD: Acute central cervical spinal cord syndrome: Aetiology, age incidence, and relationship to orthopaedic injury. Paraplegia 14:251, 1977
15. Hopkins A, Rudge P: Hyperpathia in central cervical cord syndrome. J Neurol Neurosurg Psychiatry 36:637, 1973
16. Marar BC: The pattern of neurological damage as an aid to the diagnosis of the mechanism in cervical spine injuries. J Bone Joint Surg 56A:1648, 1974
17. Heiden JS, Weiss MH, Rosenberg AW, et al: Management of cervical spinal cord trauma in Southern California. J Neurosurg 43:732, 1975
18. Bosch A, Stauffer ES, Nickel VL: Incomplete traumatic quadraplegia: A 10-year review. JAMA 216:473, 1971
19. Biemond A: Contusio cervicalis posterior. Ned T Geneesk 108:1333, 1964
20. Braakman R, Penning L: Injuries of the cervical spine. In Vinken PJ, Bruyn GW (eds): Handbook of Clinical Neurology. Amsterdam, North-Holland, 1976
21. Rosenberg RN (ed): The Clinical Neurosciences, Vol II. New York, Churchill Livingston, 1983
22. Cabezudo JM, Carrillo R, Areitio E, et al: Accidental stab wound of the cervical spinal cord from in front. Acta Neurochir 53:175, 1980
23. Saxon M, Snyder HA, Washington JA: Atypical Brown-Séquard syndrome following gunshot wound to the face. J Oral Maxillofac Surg 40:299, 1982
24. Gentleman D, Harrington M: Penetrating injury of the spinal cord. Injury 16:7, 1984
25. Grant JM, Yeo JD, Sears WR, et al: Arterial Brown-Séquard syndrome after a penetrating injury of the spinal cord at the cervicomedullary junction. Med J Aust 22:84, 1985
26. Schneider RC, Kahn EA: Chronic neurological sequelae of acute trauma to the spine and spinal cord. J Bone Joint Surg 38A:985, 1956
27. Verbiest H: Anterolateral operations for fractures or dislocations of the cervical spine due to injuries or previous surgical interventions. Clin Neurosurg 20:334, 1973
28. Bedbrook GM, Sedgley GI: The management of spinal injuries: Past and present. Int Rehabil Med 2:45, 1980
29. Bedbrook GM: Injuries of the thoracolumbar spine with neurological symptoms. In Vinken PJ, Bruyn GW (eds): Handbook of Clinical Neurology. Amsterdam, North-Holland, 1976
30. Benes V: Spinal Cord Injury. London, Balliere, Tindall, and Cassell Ltd., 1968

3

Arthridities of the Spine

Arthritis of the spine is encountered on a regular basis in the emergency room. Although it is often incidentally noted by history, physician examination,[1] or in radiographs as a finding unrelated to the chief complaint, there are many important clinical situations in which these disorders present to the emergency room as the primary problem or as a complicating factor directly related to the primary disease process (i.e., spinal trauma). Therefore, the emergency physician must have a complete understanding of the clinical presentation, complications, radiographic diagnosis, and management of these disorders.

□ RHEUMATOID ARTHRITIS OF THE SPINE

Incidence

The prevalence of rheumatoid arthritis in the general adult population is about 3% in women and 1% in men.[1] The spine is commonly involved in patients with rheumatoid arthritis, with the cervical spine being the most frequent target. The cervical spine is involved in about 80% of patients, with the most common site affected being the C-1 and C-2 region.[2,3] Sacroiliac joint involvement is also common (25 to 35%) but almost always asymptomatic.[4] Involvement of other portions of the spine is rare.

Pathophysiology

Rheumatoid arthritis is a systemic disorder primarily involving synovial tissue. It is this property of the disease that accounts for the nearly exclusive involvement of the upper cervical region. The joints between the atlas and the occiput, the atlas and the axis, and the atlas and the dens are lined by synovium. Thus, synovial joint effusion and synovial tissue proliferation may result in progressive destruction of the odontoid process, lateral masses of C-1, occipital condyles, and the alar and transverse ligaments. Unlike osteoarthritis, rheumatoid arthritis causes vertebral osteopenia that can further decrease stability as well as make radiographic interpretation difficult.

Clinical Features

Cervical Spine

Involvement of the cervical spine occurs primarily in four patterns, listed here in decreasing order of frequency:

1. Atlantoaxial subluxation alone
2. Atlantoaxial subluxation with subaxial subluxation
3. Subaxial subluxation alone
4. Upward migration of the dens into the foramen magnum with or without one of the above combinations.

Atlantoaxial Joint

As stated previously, C-1 and C-2 involvement in rheumatoid arthritis is very common, occurring to some degree in approximately 60% of patients.[5] The symptomatology tends to vary with the severity of the structural changes, although some patients with rheumatoid arthritis without radiologic evidence of spine involvement will have relatively severe symptoms. Of note is the fact that some rheumatoid arthritis patients can have severe destructive changes and subluxation without ever experiencing symptoms. Early on in the typical patient, mild neck pain will occur and is frequently associated with occipital headaches. The pain may also radiate to the forehead or eyes and increases with neck motion, especially rotation.

Axiom: *Severe structural changes with atlantoaxial instability may be present in rheumatoid arthritis patients without any symptoms referable to the spine.*

As C-1 and C-2 instability and destruction worsens, the pain tends to increase and the spinous process of C-2 may become more prominent by palpation. Tenderness in the suboccipital region may also be noted. The *clunk* test, described by Sharp and Purser,[6] sometimes allows the examiner to palpate the slide of the atlas on the axis. This can result, however, in complications and is less sensitive than radiographs and thus should be avoided.

Sharp and Purser[6] noted that atlantoaxial subluxation occurs in about 1 in 30 of those with minimal signs or symptoms of rheumatoid arthritis, 1 in 15 of those with definite clinical rheumatoid arthritis, and in about 20% of those with disease severity requiring hospitalization.[6] A study by Matthews[7] found atlantoaxial subluxation in 25% of 76 consecutive outpatients with the diagnosis of rheumatoid arthritis.

Atlantoaxial subluxation is due to erosion and rupture of the transverse ligament in combination with the destruction of the lateral joints of C-1 and C-2. Subluxations at C-1 and C-2 can occur in three directions. Most common is anterior subluxation of C-1 on C-2. Posterior subluxation of C-1 on C-2 can occur but is very rare. Vertical subluxation also occurs and is relatively common, although frequently missed when not symptomatic. This occurs when the apophyseal joints of the atlas are eroded allowing the skull to descend on C-1 with the odontoid protruding superiorly into the foramen magnum.

Axiom: *Vertical atlantoaxial subluxations are frequently missed when they occur in asymptomatic patients.*

Subaxial Cervical Spine
Although somewhat less common than C-1 and C-2 disease, subaxial rheumatoid involvement of the cervical spine remains a significant clinical problem. The primary anatomic target in the subaxial cervical spine remains somewhat controversial but is probably either the neurocentral[8] or the apophyseal joints[9], or both. As noted, subaxial cervical spine involvement occurs more commonly in combination with atlantoaxial subluxation than it does alone.

Patients with this problem usually have neck pain that radiates to the arms, shoulders, upper back, and chest. Radiation of the pain does not necessarily imply spinal cord or nerve root involvement. On examination, the cervical spine and paraspinous muscles are often diffusely tender.

Rheumatoid involvement of the cervical spine varies with regard to its extent. Disc space narrowing, bony erosions, and subluxations can occur at one or more levels and, in its worst form, can lead to shortening of the cervical spine by as much as 50%.

Axiom: *Rheumatoid spondylitis can cause shortening of the cervical spine by as much as 50%.*

Thoracic Spine
Involvement of this region of the spine apparently occurs secondary to rheumatoid involvement of the costovertebral articulations, which then can cause destruction of the adjacent discs. This form of the disease is of clinical significance only in rare instances. A small number of patients may have local tenderness and pain that is accentuated by inspiration.

Lumbar Spine
For practical purposes, clinically significant rheumatoid arthritis of the lumbar spine does not occur.

Sacroiliac Joints
Sacroiliac joint involvement occurs perhaps in one third of patients with clinical rheumatoid arthritis; however, symptoms occur in only a small percentage of patients. Some patients will complain of local pain that increases with motion.

Complications
Significant complications secondary to rheumatoid arthritis occur only from cervical spine disease and are primarily neurologic.

Atlantoaxial subluxation can lead to multiple neurologic symptoms. With anterior subluxation, the cord can be compressed between the posterior arch of C-1 and the odontoid process (Fig 3–1). Compression will further increase with flexion of the neck. Signs and symptoms include weakness, spasticity, hyperreflexia, a positive Babinski sign, paresthesias, incontinence, and urinary retention. In addition, if the spinothalamic tract is involved, decreased pain sensation will occur.

Vertical dislocations are caused by severe erosion of the apophyseal joints of C-1 with protrusion of the odontoid into the foramen magnum as the skull descends. Thus, in addition to compression of the upper cord, the medulla and the pons may become involved and as a result, the tracts and the nuclei of cranial nerves VII to XII as well as the medullary respiratory center may be affected. This situation obviously places the patient at risk for a catastrophic event. Fortunately, sudden death is rare.

Vascular compression is also a major contributing factor to the neurologic complications. Compression of the anterior spinal artery can cause vascular compromise to the anterior horn cells with resultant fascicula-

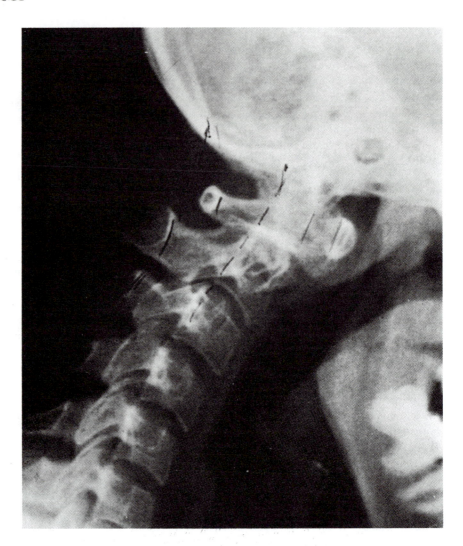

Figure 3–1. Flexion view of the cervical spine showing anterior atlantoaxial subluxation. Note the anterior displacement of the posterior aspect of the neural arch and the increased predental space. *From Sherk HH: Atlantoaxial instability and acquired basilar invagination in rheumatoid arthritis. Orthop Clin North Am 9: 1056, 1978.*

tions. Subluxation of the vertebrae can impinge on the vertebral arteries. Resultant signs and symptoms may include vertigo, nystagmus, ataxia, dysphonia, diminution or loss of vision, weakness, and loss of consciousness. Any or all of these may be precipitated or exacerbated by flexion or rotation of the neck.

Rheumatoid arthritis of the subaxial cervical spine can cause compression of the spinal cord and nerve roots either by destruction of the discs or by subluxation with the expected signs and symptoms resulting. Fortunately, neurologic complications are relatively uncommon in patients with rheumatoid spondylitis and the prognosis is quite good.[10]

Several aspects of the diagnosis and management of rheumatoid spondylitis in the emergency medicine setting are particularly important. First, the diagnosis of neurologic compromise can be very difficult in these patients. Rheumatoid patients often have contractions, weakness, and muscular atrophy. In addition, nerve entrapment syndromes are common. Signs or symptoms of incontinence, hyperreflexia, intermittent basilar artery insufficiency, and diffuse sensory loss or weakness

in the setting of rheumatoid arthritis, however, should alert the physician to the possibility of neurologic impairment. Second, due to osteopenia, as well as joint, bone, disc, and ligamentous destruction, patients with rheumatoid arthritis can have significant (or even life-threatening) spinal injuries after "trivial trauma." Thus it is incumbent upon the emergency physician to carefully evaluate any rheumatoid patient after trauma no matter how seemingly insignificant the event was.

Axiom: *Life-threatening spinal injuries can occur in rheumatoid arthritis patients during an otherwise trivial traumatic event.*

Diagnosis

In any given patient, the diagnosis of rheumatoid arthritis, based on peripheral joint involvement and laboratory data has usually been made before the onset of symptoms of rheumatoid spondylitis. This makes the diagnosis of spinal involvement relatively obvious in most cases based on the clinical picture and radiographic findings. It should be remembered that rheumatoid spondylitis can occur with minimal or no peripheral joint involvement and that significant spinal involvement may be present in patients with no signs or symptoms referable to the spine.

The diagnosis of atlantoaxial subluxation can be made with standard radiographic views in most cases. Anterior subluxations are accompanied by an enlarged predental space (the area between the odontoid process and the anterior arch of C-1) (Fig 3–1). A measurement of 3 mm is considered the upper limit of normal. When considering the diagnosis of atlantoaxial subluxation, flexion views should be obtained because it is possible to have an abnormal measurement in the flexion view despite a normal routine lateral (Fig 3–2). Lateral tomograms may also aid in the diagnosis if it is equivocal by standard views.

Involvement of the odontoid process can lead to erosion in the area adjacent to the transverse ligament leaving a fragile "peg" that provides little support to the atlantoaxial joint.

Vertical subluxation results in protrusion of the odontoid into the foramen magnum. On x-ray, the tip of the odontoid should be no more than 4.5 mm above the line extending from the most inferior aspect of the occipital curve to the posterior edge of the hard palate (McGregor's line) (Fig 3–3).

Radiographically, the subaxial cervical spine will show erosions, sclerosis, disc narrowing, and osteopenia. Subluxations may be present at multiple levels (Table 3–1).

The lumbar spine may show erosions, osteopenia, and joint space narrowing although these findings may be subtle and are often obscured by the findings of concurrent osteoarthritis.

Management and Referral

Most patients with rheumatoid spondylitis have concomitant peripheral joint involvement for which high-dose aspirin or a nonsteroidal anti-inflammatory drug is given. This often provides excellent relief of symptoms caused by spinal involvement as well. For those patients in whom these drugs prove inadequate for treat-

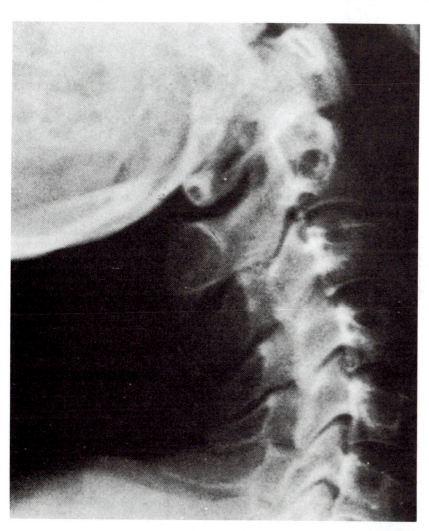

Figure 3–2. Extension view of the same patient as in Figure 3–1 showing reduction of subluxation, thus masking the problem if flexion views are not obtained. *From Sherk HH: Atlantoaxial instability and acquired basilar invagination in rheumatoid arthritis. Orthop Clin North Am 9: 1057, 1978.*

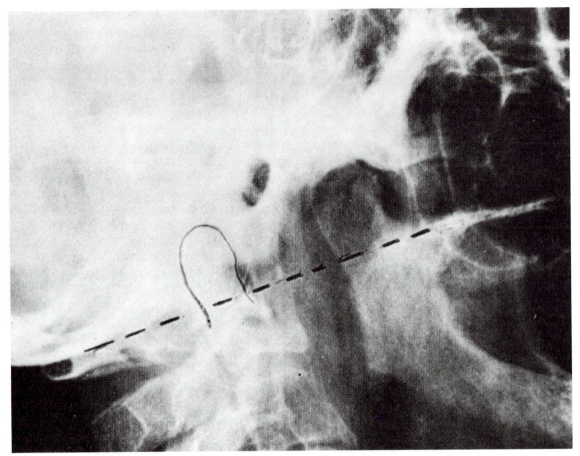

Figure 3–3. Extensive rheumatoid changes have destroyed the lateral masses of C-1 and the occipital condyles allowing vertical subluxation of the odontoid process into the foramen magnum (note McGregor's line). *From Sherk HH: Atlantoaxial instability and acquired basilar invagination in rheumatoid arthritis. Orthop Clin North Am 9: 1058, 1978.*

ing the pain, a trial of a soft or rigid collar for 2 to 6 weeks is indicated as this will sometimes provide relief. There is no evidence, however, that collars affect the progression of the disease.

Surgical stabilization of atlantoaxial subluxation is necessary in only a small percentage of patients.[11] Development of neurologic signs, severe and unremitting pain, or vertical subluxations (which are a particularly precarious situation), however, all require a consideration for open stabilization.

TABLE 3–1. RADIOGRAPHIC CHANGES OF RHEUMATOID CERVICAL SPONDYLITIS

Atlantoaxial subluxation
Anterior
Vertical
Posterior
Anterior subluxations at multiple levels
Osteopenia (osteoporosis)
Disc space narrowing
Sclerosis of vertebral end-plates
Facet joint erosions and sclerosis

For the emergency physician, there are primarily two issues regarding management: (1) as previously stated, significant fractures must be suspected with even the most trivial head or neck injury in patients with rheumatoid arthritis and (2) all patients with rheumatoid spondylitis require referral for careful follow-up.

☐ ANKYLOSING SPONDYLITIS

Incidence

The true incidence of ankylosing spondylitis in the population is unclear. Early studies estimated the prevalence of the disease to be about 1 to 3 per 1000 in the general population.[12–14] Previously, there was also thought to be a significant male preponderance for the disorder with a male to female ratio of about 4:1. These data were compiled from symptomatic patients with obvious clinical evidence of ankylosing spondylitis. Recent investigations, however, have studied groups of HLA-B27 subjects and found clinical or radiographic evidence of ankylosing spondylitis in about 20% with half of the affected persons being women.[15,16] This would suggest an overall prevalence of 1 to 2% of the general population with men and women being affected with equal frequency. It should be noted that a large portion of these patients were asymptomatic and that significant symptoms were present much more frequently in men. This fact probably accounts for the discrepancy with previous studies.

In the United States, whites have a fourfold greater prevalence of ankylosing spondylitis than blacks.[17] Of note is that whites have a greater frequency of HLA-B27 (7% vs 3%).

Pathophysiology

The cause of ankylosing spondylitis is unknown and its pathophysiology is poorly understood. The histocompatibility antigen HLA-B27 is present in approximately 80 to 95% of white patients with ankylosing spondylitis[18-20] as compared with 7% of the general population.[18-22] At present, it seems likely that a genetic predisposition in combination with some inciting factor(s) plays an important role in the pathogenesis of the disease. In any given population, the incidence of ankylosing spondylitis is closely related to the frequency of the HLA-B27 antigen in that population. This striking association is strong evidence that genetics play some key role in ankylosing spondylitis. At present, ankylosing spondylitis in not thought to be an autoimmune disease, at least in any traditional sense.

Ankylosing spondylitis causes joint fusion in contradistinction to rheumatoid arthritis, which results in joint destruction. Initially, there is an inflammatory process that occurs primarily in the joint capsule and articular cartilage. Subsequently, the ligamentous attachments to the vertebrae may also become involved. Ultimately, bony ankylosis occurs in the joints, and ligamentous ossification results in the formation of bridges between adjacent vertebral bodies (syndesmophytes).

Clinical Features

The onset of ankylosing spondylitis typically occurs between the ages of 15 and 30.[22] About 90% of cases are diagnosed before age 40 and 95% before age 50. Although cases do occur before the teenage years, they are rare.

The initial symptoms typically are isolated to the low back with most patients describing an aching pain as well as stiffness.[23] The onset of these symptoms is nearly always insidious, although on rare occasions the presentation is surprisingly acute and may compel the physician to rule out a ruptured disc. Although the pain has classically been described as unremitting, there clearly is a significant group of patients who have one or several remissions, lasting weeks to months, in the early course of the disease. Patients with ankylosing spondylitis usually experience a variation of their symptomatology throughout the course of the day with pain and stiffness typically being most severe in the morning.[23] Early in the disease course, the symptoms reflect involvement of the sacroiliac joints and lumbar region. Thus, at the time of presentation, the patient may also complain of pain that is referred either unilaterally or bilaterally to the hips, buttocks, and thighs. It should be noted that true sciatic nerve irritation accompanied by pain radiating to the calf or foot rarely, if ever, occurs.

Axiom: *True sciatica, associated with radiation of pain to the calf or the foot, is extremely rare in ankylosing spondylitis.*

Although low back pain is by far the most common presenting complaint in ankylosing spondylitis, there are a significant number of patients who initially present with other symptoms.[23] Pain and stiffness due to involvement of the cervical or thoracic spine may be the first clinical manifestation. When the disease involves the articulations between the ribs and the thoracic vertebrae, the patient may present with chest pain that is typically pleuritic in nature. A sensation of chest tightness with difficulty taking a deep breath can occur and occasionally will necessitate the exclusion of a cardiac or pulmonary etiology. Peripheral joint symptoms antedate back pain in about 20% of patients.[24] Occasionally, foot pain due to plantar fasciitis will be the initial complaint. The most common nonmusculoskeletal presentation is anterior uveitis, occurring in about 1 to 2%.

The effects of rest and exercise on the symptoms of ankylosing spondylitis are not entirely clear. It would appear that mild exercise such as that associated with simple daytime activities tends to decrease the pain and stiffness[23] with absolute rest causing an increase (so-called immobility pain). Strenuous exercise, either occupational or recreational, will definitely aggravate the symptoms. In this case, moderation or cessation of the activity will usually lessen the pain.

Physical Examination

Early on, the signs and symptoms tend to be relatively nonspecific. Evidence of an arthropathy of the spine, however, is often present even at the initial presentation. Sacroiliac joint tenderness is the most consistent finding. Despite the fact that sciatic nerve involvement does not occur, straight leg raising may produce symptoms resulting in low back and gluteal pain. A multitude of clinical tests have been described that reportedly aid in detecting inflammation of the sacroiliac joints; however, none of them are of any great diagnostic significance and thus will not be described.

As the disease progresses, several physical findings become apparent. Limited motion of the lumbar spine develops in extension, anterior flexion, and lateral bending. Loss of the normal lumbar lordosis occurs and spasm of the paralumbar musculature may be noted. To test for limitation of flexion of the lumbar spine, a mark should be made on the spinous processes of T-12 and S-1. The distance between these marks is measured with the patient standing upright and then in the position of maximum forward bending. The normal difference is 7 to 8 cm but a large variation occurs in healthy individuals. Certainly, an increase of less than 3 cm should lead the examiner to suspect lumbar pathology and, with the right history, ankylosing spondylitis.

As the disease progresses, kyphosis of the thoracic spine tends to occur as well as atrophy of the musculature of the trunk. It is thought that a "hunched over" posture partially relieves the low back pain and thus leads to the kyphotic deformity. The thoracic spinous processes and paraspinous muscles will often be tender. The costovertebral joints may be involved leading to a decrease in chest expansion. Measurement of chest expansion has been advocated and may be of some use in following the disease course;[25] however, decreased mobility of the chest wall in ankylosing spondylitis rarely, if ever, significantly compromises pulmonary function.

Involvement of the cervical spine generally occurs late in the disease course. The first signs are spinous and paraspinous tenderness as well as pain on rotation. Ultimately, decreased mobility and a flexion deformity will arise, which may eventually lead to complete ankylosis.

Peripheral joint involvement may be present at the onset of the disease or at any point in its course. The physical signs are identical to that of any peripheral arthritis with erythema, warmth, swelling, tenderness, and stiffness of the involved joints. The joints commonly involved include the hip, shoulder, knee, carpal, metacarpophalangeal, and metatarsophalangeal joints.

Clinical Course

It has become apparent from recent investigations that a very large number of patients with ankylosing spondylitis remain asymptomatic or so minimally symptomatic that they never seek medical care. This seems to be particularly true of women, who tend to have a much less aggressive course than men.

As discussed earlier, in the majority of patients initial involvement occurs at the sacroiliac joints followed by progression of the spinal arthropathy up-

ward.[22] In symptomatic patients, isolated sacroiliac joint involvement over a long period of time is very rare. Progression of the pathologic process and its concomitant spinal deformity is the norm. Despite this fact, the symptomatology of the disease tends to be intermittent, with periods during which the patient is essentially symptom-free for as long as 1 to 2 years. Surprisingly enough, a few patients do not seek medical attention until the cervical spine flexion deformity is so significant that it impairs their ability to work, drive, or carry out other daily activities. The progression from initial sacroiliac joint involvement to cervical spine deformity can take a variable period of time, but typically requires decades and only rarely takes less than 5 years.

Axiom: *The symptoms of ankylosing spondylitis are intermittent and there may be periods of disease inactivity lasting for months to years.*

Peripheral joint involvement occurs in 50 to 75% of patients at some point in their clinical course.[22] Hip or shoulder joint involvement tends to be bilateral. Although this often resolves, it may be chronic and progressive with significant disability and even complete joint fusion in some cases. Fortunately, disease of the other peripheral joints is relatively benign, lasting for weeks to months and then resolves spontaneously without residual articular damage.

Complications and Prognosis

As with rheumatoid arthritis, patients with ankylosing spondylitis are extremely vulnerable to spinal fractures, particularly in the cervical region. The combination of fusion and osteoporosis leads to a tenuous state in which minor trauma can produce catastrophic spinal injuries. The fractures are typically transverse and occur most commonly in the middle and lower portions of the cervical spine.[26] These fractures tend to be serious in that there is a relatively high incidence of dislocation and spinal cord injury. Approximately 75% of patients with cervical spine fractures will have some neurologic damage.[24] Extreme caution must be exercised in the emergency department for all patients with ankylosing spondylitis who sustain a blow to the head or spine until a fracture is ruled out.

Axiom: *As with rheumatoid arthritis, patients with ankylosing spondylitis may sustain life-threatening spinal fractures in the setting of seemingly insignificant trauma.*

Atlantoaxial subluxation also occurs in ankylosing spondylitis and may lead to cord compression, although this problem is encountered much less frequently than in rheumatoid arthritis.

Anterior uveitis occurs in up to 25% of patients with ankylosing spondylitis.[22] Generally, these episodes are short and self-limited, although visual loss can occur due to glaucoma in rare cases.[23]

Aortitis occurs in a small but significant percentage of cases.[22] The inflammatory process itself does not cause symptoms; however, aortic insufficiency often occurs years later and may result in heart failure. Conduction defects, including third degree atrioventricular block, may occur as well as pericarditis.

Pulmonary fibrosis may occur and typically involves the apical segments of both lungs. Ultimately, cavitation ensues and may predispose the patient to aspergillosis or tuberculosis.[27]

As with most diseases that result in a chronic inflammatory process, amyloidosis may develop resulting in proteinuria and renal insufficiency.

Cauda equina syndrome may develop as a complication of ankylosing spondylitis, although this association is not understood. These patients complain of incontinence as well as motor and sensory deficits in the sacral distribution.

In the past, spinal irradiation was a frequent form of therapy and resulted in a marked increase in risk for myelogenous leukemias.[28,29]

The prognosis for patients with ankylosing spondylitis to lead a relatively functional life is generally very good. Although strenuous occupations will lead to significant problems with pain and stiffness, more sedentary activities at work are generally tolerated without difficulty, particularly if the patient is compliant with a well-conceived treatment program. Except in those patients with serious systemic complications (cardiovascular, renal, pulmonary, malignancy), the life expectancy for patients with ankylosing spondylitis is normal (Table 3–2).

TABLE 3–2. COMPLICATIONS OF ANKYLOSING SPONDYLITIS

Spinal fractures/spinal cord injuries
Atlantoaxial subluxation
Hip and shoulder joint fusion
Anterior uveitis
Aortitis, pericarditis, conduction defects
Apical pulmonary fibrosis
Amyloidosis
Cauda equina syndrome
Postirradiation malignancy

TABLE 3–3. FIVE HISTORICAL CRITERIA FOR THE DIAGNOSIS OF ANKLYOSING SPONDLYITIS

Age of onset less than 40 years
Low back discomfort lasting at least 3 months
Morning stiffness
Gradual onset of symptoms
Improvement of symptoms with mild exercise

From Calin A, Fries JF: Striking prevalence of ankylosing spondylitis in "healthy" W27 positive males and females: A controlled study. N Engl J Med 293:835–839, 1975.

Diagnosis

Although the diagnosis of ankylosing spondylitis is relatively easy to make, it is often delayed for years. Calin and co-workers[15,30] found that the presence of four out of five historical criteria is 95% sensitive and 85% specific for the diagnosis of ankylosing spondylitis. The criteria are as follows: age of onset less than 40 years, gradual onset of symptoms, low back discomfort lasting at least 3 months, morning back stiffness, and improvement with mild exercise. The use of these historical criteria should be a powerful tool to aid the primary care physician in making the early diagnosis of ankylosing spondylitis and referring these patients for appropriate follow-up (Table 3–3).

Radiography is an important aspect of the diagnostic work-up. Bilateral sacroiliac joint involvement is present on x-ray in a high percentage of cases,[20] although certainly not in all.[31] Early on, the sacroiliac joints begin to lose their discrete margins. This is followed by joint space narrowing and ultimately complete fusion. The other areas of the spine show osteoporosis with "squaring" of the vertebral bodies when seen on lateral view. Marginal syndesmophytes will develop and as the disease progresses will give rise to the so-called bamboo spine (Fig 3–4). Both squaring and syndesmophytes tend to appear first in the lumbar region and progress in a cephalad direction.

X-ray findings are usually absent in the peripheral joints even when they are clinically involved. The shoulder and hip joints, however, may reveal severe changes and even fusion in longstanding disease. Atlantoaxial subluxation may occur as discussed in the section on rheumatoid arthritis.

The importance of ruling out fracture has been discussed but may be difficult to accomplish by standard radiographs due to osteopenia and fusion. At times, tomography or computed tomography (CT) may be required to insure that no acute fracture is present. The most striking laboratory finding is the 80 to 95% incidence of HLA-B27 in patients with the disease. In the individual patient, however, the presence of HLA-B27 does not make the diagnosis and its absence does not rule it out. In fact, most persons who are HLA-B27 positive do not have ankylosing spondylitis. There are

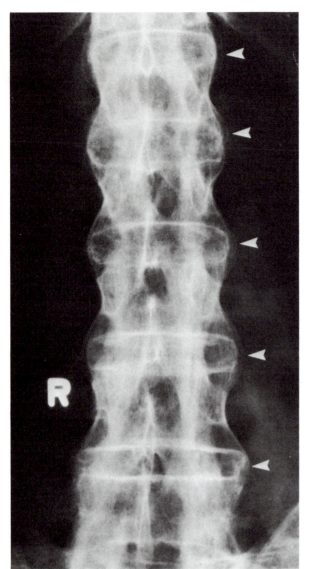 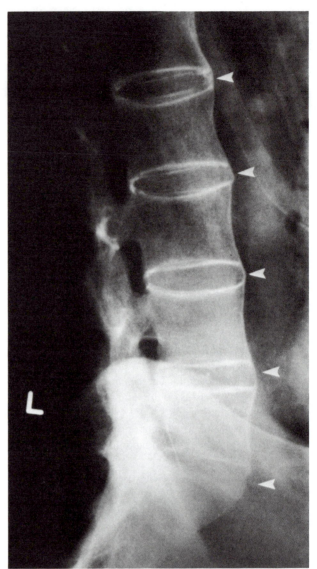

Figure 3–4. Ankylosing spondylitis. Note the joint space narrowing, squaring of the vertebral bodies, "bamboo" appearance, and fusion of the facet joints. *From Banna M: Clinical Radiology of the Spine and Spinal Cord. Rockville, Md, Aspen, 1985, p 213. Reprinted with permission of Aspen Publishers, Inc.*

multiple laboratory abnormalities that may be present. The erythrocyte sedimentation rate (ESR) is elevated in about 80% of patients. Unfortunately, there is no evidence that the ESR can be used to follow disease activity or response to treatment. A mild normocytic anemia may be present as well as minor elevations of alkaline phosphatase, serum glutamic-oxaloacetic transaminase, and creatine phosphokinase. Tests for rheumatoid factor and antinuclear antibody are negative.

It should be noted that laboratory data are of no value to the emergency physician when attempting to make the diagnosis of ankylosing spondylitis.

Management and Referral

The primary role of the emergency physician in the management of patients with ankylosing spondylitis is twofold: (1) pain relief and (2) referral to a physician who is experienced in the long-term management of these patients. With regard to pain management, as with all patients with chronic pain syndromes, the use of narcotic analgesics (particularly parenteral forms) should be avoided if at all possible. Aspirin, in adequate doses, is always the drug of choice when beginning a medication regimen for these patients because of its low cost and relatively low incidence of side effects. If proper doses are used, many patients will notice significant relief. If aspirin has been ineffective, nonsteroidal anti-inflammatory drugs such as naproxen, ibuprofen, or indomethacin should be used.[23] Steroids should be avoided because of the significant long-term complications associated with their use. Penicillamine was once thought to be a useful therapy but this has been refuted.[32]

The role of appropriate referral should not be underestimated. It is only the long-term care by experienced physicians and physical therapists that will be able to prevent or minimize the disabling effects of spinal deformity.[23] In this setting, a consistent regimen of medication, rest, exercise, and postural training can be accomplished and markedly improve the long-term functional status of the patient. Patients should be instructed to discontinue strenuous occupational or recreational activities. These should be replaced by twice or three times daily moderate exercise programs such as walking, swimming, and range of motion exercises. A firm mattress with an underlying board should be used. The use of a pillow should be discouraged as it may accelerate the formation of a cervical flexion deformity.

☐ OSTEOARTHRITIS OF THE SPINE

Incidence

Without question, osteoarthritis or degenerative joint disease is the most common disorder affecting joints. In fact, there is radiographic evidence of this disease in more than 80% of those aged 65 and over.[33] Spinal osteoarthritis is found by x-ray in about half of the population over age 50 and in nearly 75% of those over 65. Despite an extremely high incidence of the disease found by radiography, only about 5 to 10% of people over 60 have any symptoms.

Axiom: *Only about 1 in 10 patients with radiographic evidence of spinal osteoarthritis will have significant symptoms.*

Pathophysiology

At present, the etiology of osteoarthritis is unknown, although hereditary, hormonal, and metabolic factors all seem to play a role. Mechanical forces are also important and result in the lumbar and cervical spine being affected most frequently. The lumbar spine is susceptible due to the large amount of weight that it must support. The cervical spine, on the other hand, is at risk due to its great mobility. Both of these factors cause increased mechanical stress and, therefore, lead to a higher incidence of osteoarthritis in these regions.

Factors that predispose a person to osteoarthritis of the spine include trauma (resulting in sprains, fractures, or dislocations), spinal deformities (such as scoliosis), strenuous occupation, and unequal leg length. Essentially any disorder that alters the mechanics of the spine will tend to cause stress at various locations and, therefore, accelerate the degenerative process.

The pathologic process begins with the fibrocartilage of the disc being replaced by fibrous tissue over a period of years. This leads to joint space narrowing that can be noted by radiography. The result is an increase in pressure on the adjacent vertebral bodies with subsequent subchondral bone sclerosis and the formation of osteophytes at the periphery of the disc. These may occur on any part of the vertebral body, but only those that are directed toward the spinal cord or nerve roots result in any neurologic sequelae. Early on in the disease there is often a small protrusion of disc substance at the posterolateral aspect of the vertebral body on one side. This is usually directed into the intervertebral foramen and can lead to osteophyte formation that may ultimately cause nerve root compression.

Most of the movement of the spine occurs at the facet joints. Thus, these articulations are quite vulnerable to degenerative changes and subsequent osteophyte formation. The facets form the posterior aspect of the intervertebral foramen so that osteophytes directed anteriorly from the facet joint may encroach on the nerve roots. Impingement generally occurs on the posterior nerve root and its ganglion rather than on the anterior root due to their anatomic location in the neural foramen. This accounts for the high incidence of sensory symptoms relative to motor symptoms.

In the cervical and thoracic region, cord damage and myelopathy can occur. Anteriorly, the cord is compressed by the osteophytes that protrude dorsally from the margin of the disc. Posteriorly, the ligamentum flavum tends to buckle and thus encroaches on the dorsal aspect of the cord. This combination can cause cord damage directly or secondarily from compression of the anterior spinal artery although the latter mechanism is rare.

Finally, bony spurs can occur in the foramen transversarium and encroach on the vertebral artery. When the head is rotated, compression occurs on the artery contralateral to the direction of rotation and may result in complete occlusion. Osteoarthritis rarely involves the atlantoaxial joint. This is in contradistinction to rheumatoid arthritis and ankylosing spondylitis.

Clinical Features

It is important to keep in mind that the vast majority of patients with radiographic evidence of spinal osteoarthritis are asymptomatic. In fact, there is little difference in x-ray findings between symptomatic and asymptomatic patients with the disease.[34]

Cervical Spondylosis

When symptoms are present, neck pain is the primary complaint. Its onset is generally insidious although it may be relatively acute and often is first noted after a relatively minor traumatic event. The pain tends to be chronic with intermittent exacerbations that are often associated with strenuous activity or with a drop in barometric pressure (thus worsening during cold, damp weather). Stiffness is another consistent complaint and tends to be worse in the morning. In general, patients will find that aspirin and local heat give them significant relief from both the pain and the stiffness. Patients may complain of an occipital headache that tends to improve during the day. Pain in the shoulder and pectoral region may also be quite severe although it occurs infrequently. Because the lower cervical spine is affected much more frequently than the upper part, when radicular symptoms are present, they are usually in the C-6 and C-7 distribution. Nerve root impingement is almost always unilateral. Patients complain of pain and, less commonly, numbness in the thumb and the index finger (C-6) as well as the middle finger (C-7). When myelopathy occurs, the patient will complain of subtle symptoms such as mild weakness or difficulty tying shoes. If the corticospinal tract is involved, there may be lower extremity weakness and some difficulty walking. Bowel and bladder control, however, will remain intact in nearly all cases.

In a small group of patients, syncopal episodes occur. These are due to impingement on the vertebral artery, which leads to vascular compromise during rotation of the head.

Physical examination reveals tenderness of the spine and paraspinous muscles particularly low in the neck. In some instances, point tenderness will be localized at the inflamed articulation. Cervical motion tends to be limited although rotation is usually well preserved. The upper extremity may reveal sensory deficits and hyporeflexia. Weakness and muscle atrophy may also be present although at times it is difficult to determine whether the cause is compression of the cord or nerve roots. If the pyramidal tracts are involved, examination of the lower extremities will reveal clonus, hyperactive reflexes, a Babinski sign, and weakness.

Thoracic Spondylosis

Although osteoarthritis affects the thoracic spine much less commonly than the cervical or lumbar region, it does occur in a significant number of patients.

Pain is the chief complaint. Most commonly, it is located in the mid or low thoracic region and is usually, but not always, unilateral. Often the pain is located in the back, but it may radiate or be referred to the chest and the sternum if the anterior primary ramus is involved. The pain may or may not be pleuritic and, just as with other disorders of the thoracic spine, a pulmonary or cardiac etiology may need to be ruled out. Use of the arms and shoulders tends to increase the pain.

On examination, there is spinous and paraspinous tenderness that usually localizes the site of inflammation, but may be quite diffuse. Anterior chest tenderness may also be present. Sensory examination often reveals a band of hyperesthesia that may be very diffi-

cult to attribute to a single nerve root. As with cervical disease, the pyramidal tracts may be affected and thus produce the physical findings of an upper motor neuron lesion on examination of the lower extremities.

Lumbar Spondylosis

As with the other regions, pain is the cardinal symptom of osteoarthritis in the lumbar spine. Classically, the complaint is unilateral low back pain with radiation to the buttock, thigh, and calf on the affected side. The pain may be bilateral and the patient may only complain of back pain or sciatica. Stiffness is also a common symptom and tends to improve with mild activity, but is nearly always made worse by strenuous activity or heavy lifting. Both the pain and stiffness tend to be chronic with intermittent exacerbations. Numbness of the buttock and lower extremity or "electric shocks" are also frequent complaints and, in fact, on occasion are present without pain. Although the onset of all of these symptoms tends to be insidious, patients will often present after a traumatic event and attribute the onset of symptoms to that event.

On examination, there is spinous and paraspinous tenderness with spasm. This is often diffuse in the lumbar region although at times precise localization can be accomplished. The straight leg raising test is positive on the affected side if nerve root impingement is present in the lumbosacral region. While standing, the patient may slightly flex both the hip and the knee thus reducing pain. There may also be a subtle but noticeable limp while walking. There is limited motion in all directions with flexion taking place primarily at the hip. The lumbar lordosis tends to be lost due to both muscle spasm and true deformity. Nerve root compression may cause weakness, muscle atrophy, and decreased deep tendon reflexes. Both the extensor hallucis longus (dorsiflexion of the great toe) and tibialis anterior (dorsiflexion of the foot) should be tested. Recall that there may also be signs of upper motor neuron involvement due to disease in the cervical or thoracic regions. There may be decreased sensation to both pain and pin prick, but localization of affected dermatomes is not entirely reliable for determining the level of the lesion.[35]

Complications

As discussed previously, the complications of osteoarthritis of the spine are primarily neurologic. Nerve root and spinal cord compression are usually gradual with insidious onset of symptoms. On the other hand, the degenerative changes in the spine predispose these patients to acute disc herniations. Cerebrovascular accidents occur in a small number of patients due to impingement on the vertebral artery. Hyperextension injuries of the cervical spine can be catastrophic in these patients. With a bar of osteophytes protruding posteriorly from the margin of the disc and the folds of the ligamentum flavum bulging anteriorly, the spinal cord may be pinched during extension. Thus, severe cord damage can occur even without fracture or dislocation. In longstanding disease, laxity of the ligamentous attachments may allow subluxation of adjacent vertebra although significant neurologic sequelae generally do not occur. Rarely, dysphagia occurs due to a large osteophyte impinging on the esophagus.

An important complication that must be remembered in all patients with spinal disorders, and particularly with low back pain, is narcotic addiction. Every effort should be made to use other analgesics in these patients because the disorder is chronic and may require many years of therapy.

Axiom: *Hyperextension injuries may lead to severe spinal cord damage in patients with cervical spondylosis even without fracture or dislocation.*

Diagnosis

Early on in the disease, x-rays of the spine are normal. As the disease progresses, disc space narrowing occurs and subchondral bony sclerosis develops. At the margin of the discs, bony spurs (osteophytes) form and on occasion will actually fuse with osteophytes from the adjacent vertebral body (Fig 3–5). In longstanding disease, nitrogen may accumulate in the disc space and produce the so-called "vacuum sign." On x-ray, the facet joints also show loss of cartilage and narrowing with subchondral sclerosis. As joint destruction occurs, the lower facet may project into the neural foramen as seen on oblique views of the cervical or lumbar spine. Osteophytes also form around the facet. In longstanding disease, both the cervical and lumbar spine tend to be straightened. The severity of symptoms in degenerative spondylitis do not correlate with the severity of radiologic findings.

In patients with neurologic involvement of the spinal cord or nerve roots, myelography may be helpful in defining the exact site of impingement and in determining whether the lesion is amenable to surgical intervention.

In the setting of trauma, severe degenerative changes of the cervical spine may make ruling out a fracture difficult. If there is a high index of suspicion, tomography or CT should be strongly considered.

Management and Referral

Patients with radiographic evidence of disease but no symptoms require no therapy. Therapy directed at de-

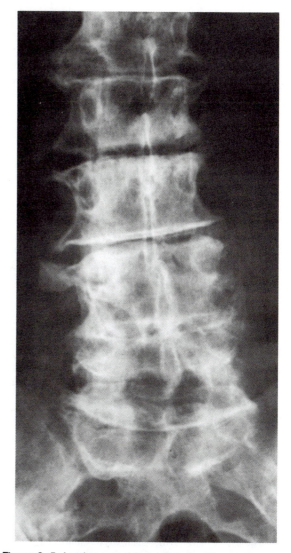

Figure 3–5. Lumbar spondylosis. Note the disc space narrowing, subchondral bony sclerosis, osteophyte formation, facet joint destruction, and secondary mild scoliosis. *From Banna M: Clinical Radiology of the Spine and Spinal Cord. Rockville, Md, Aspen, 1985, p 161. Reprinted with permission of Aspen Publishers, Inc.*

creasing pain includes bedrest, local heat, and analgesics. Aspirin is generally highly effective, but some patients will require nonsteroidal anti-inflammatory agents. At times, local injection of lidocaine and a steroid may give prompt and impressive relief from pain. This is generally only effective when a very discrete "trigger point" can be found by examination. Oral steroids should be avoided. A soft collar is sometimes useful in patients with symptoms in the neck and, on occasion, cervical traction may be of some benefit. When symptoms have stabilized, range of motion exercises for the neck and back should be taught by a physical therapist. Vigorous manipulation is contraindicated.

All patients with neurologic symptoms or signs must be referred for careful follow-up. Surgical management designed to relieve pressure on the spinal cord may be required. Patients with vertebral artery symptoms should undergo arteriography and may require anticoagulation or surgical intervention to avert the disastrous effects of complete occlusion.

□ REFERENCES

1. O'Sullivan AK, Capheart EF: The prevalence of rheumatoid arthritis. Ann Int Med 76:573, 1972
2. Bland JH, David PH, London MG: Rheumatoid arthritis of the cervical spine. Arch Intern Med 112:892, 1963
3. Bland JH: Rheumatoid arthritis of the cervical spine. J Rheumatol 1:319, 1974
4. Martel W, Duff IF: Pelvo-spondylitis in rheumatoid arthritis. Radiology 77:744, 1961
5. Conlon PW, Isdale IC, Rose BS: Rheumatoid arthritis of the cervical spine. Ann Rheum Dis 25:120, 1966
6. Sharp J, Purser DW: Spontaneous atlantoaxial dislocation in ankylosing spondylitis and rheumatoid arthritis. Ann Rheum Dis 20:47, 1961
7. Matthews JA: Atlantoaxial subluxation in rheumatoid arthritis. Ann Rheum Dis 28:260, 1969
8. Ball J: Enthesophathy of rheumatoid and ankylosing spondylitis. Ann Rheum Dis 30:213, 1971
9. Martel W: Pathogenesis of cervical discovertebral destruction in rheumatoid arthritis. Arthritis Rheum 20:1217, 1977
10. Smith PH, Benn RT, Sharp J: Natural history of rheumatoid cervical luxations. Ann Rheum Dis 21:431, 1972
11. Isdale IC, Conlon PW: Atlantoaxial subluxation: A 6-year follow-up report. Ann Rheum Dis 30:387, 1971
12. Hersh AH, Stecher RM, Solomon WM, et al: Heredity in ankylosing spondylitis. A study of 50 families. Am J Hum Gen 2:391, 1950
13. West HF: Etiology of ankylosing spondylitis. Ann Rheum Dis 8:143, 1949
14. Lawrence JS: The prevalence of arthritis. Br J Clin Pract 17:699, 1963
15. Calin A, Fries JF: Striking prevalence of ankylosing spondylitis in "healthy" W27 positive males and females. N Engl J Med 293:835, 1975
16. Cohen LM, Mittal KK, Schmid FR, et al: Increased risk for spondylitis stigmata in apparently healthy HL-AW27 men. Ann Intern Med 84:1, 1976
17. Baum J, Ziff M: The rarity of ankylosing spondylitis in the black race. Arthritis Rheum 14:12, 1971
18. Schlosstein L, Terasaki PI, Bluestone R, et al: High association of an HLA-A antigen W-27 with ankylosing spondylitis. N Engl J Med 228:704, 1973
19. Brewerton DA, Hart FD, Nicholls A, et al: Ankylosing spondylitis and HL-A27. Lancet 1:904, 1973
20. Goiethe HS, Steven MM, van der Linden, et al: Evaluation of diagnostic criteria for ankylosing spondylitis: A comparison of the Rome, New York, and modified New York criteria in patients with a positive clinical history screening test for ankylosing spondylitis. Br J Rheumatol 24:242, 1985
21. Calin A: Ankylosing spondylitis. Clin Rheum Dis 11:41, 1985
22. Deesomchok U, Tumrasvin T: Clinical study of Thai patients with ankylosing spondylitis. Clin Rheumatol 4:76, 1985
23. Calabro JJ: Sustained-release indomethacin in the management of ankylosing spondylitis. Am J Med 79:39, 1985
24. Ogryzlo MA, Rosen PS: Ankylosing (Marie-Strumpel) spondylitis. Postgrad Med 45:182, 1969
25. Gran JT, Husby G: Ankylosing spondylitis: A comparative study of patients in an epidemiologic survey, and those admitted to a department of rheumatology. J Rheumatol 11:788, 1984
26. Woodruff FV, Dewing SB: Fracture of the cervical spine in patients with ankylosing spondylitis. Radiology 80:17, 1963
27. Appelrouth D, Gottlieb N: Pulmonary manifestations of ankylosing spondylitis. J Rheumatol 2:446, 1975
28. Graham DC: Leukemia following x-ray therapy for ankylosing spondylitis. Arch Intern Med 105:51, 1960
29. Darby SC, Nakaşhima E, Kato H: A parallel analysis of cancer mortality among atomic bomb survivors and patients with ankylosing spondylitis given x-ray therapy. J Natl Cancer Inst 75:1, 1985
30. Calin A, Porta J, Schurman D, et al: Comparing HLA B27 and an appropriate history: A new look at an old perspective. In HLA and Disease—Predisposition to Disease and Clinical Implications. Baltimore, Williams & Wilkins, 1977
31. Gran JT, Husby G, Hordvik M: Spinal ankylosing spondylitis: A variant form of ankylosing spondylitis or a distinct disease entity? Ann Rheum Dis 44:368, 1985
32. Steven MM, Morrison M, Sturrock RD: Penicillamine in ankylosing spondylitis: A double blind placebo controlled trial. J Rheumatol 12:735, 1985
33. Lawrence LJ, Bremner JM, Bier F: Osteoarthrosis: Prevalence in the population and relationship between symptoms and x-ray changes. Ann Rheum Dis 25:1, 1966
34. Friedenberg Z, Miller W: Degenerative disc disease of the cervical spine. J Bone Joint Surg 45A:1171, 1963
35. Davis L, Martin J, Goldstein SL: Sensory changes with herniated nucleus pulposus. J Neurosurg 9:133, 1952

4

Osteoporosis

☐ INTRODUCTION

Osteoporosis is a clinical syndrome characterized by decreased bone mass of the axial skeleton, resulting in structural bone failure and fractures. It is a common condition estimated to affect 15 to 20 million people in the United States. Approximately 1.3 million fractures per year in persons older than 45 are attributable to osteoporosis at an estimated cost of $3.8 billion.[1]

Bone consists of an organic matrix (collagen) impregnated by minerals (calcium and phosphorus). Two predominant forms of bone, trabecular and cortical, exist in human bone in varying proportions. The vertebral bodies are largely trabecular, whereas the femur is predominantly dense cortical bone. Remodeling by osteoclasts (resorption) and osteoblasts (deposition) occurs continuously. Peak bone mass occurs by the early thirties, varying according to sex (men more than women), race (black more than white), nutrition, and overall health. Decline in bone mass occurs due to alterations in remodeling and similarly varies according to sex and race, as well as other factors. For instance, women steadily lose vertebral trabecular bone in early adulthood, overall loss being 45%,[2] fractures occurring most frequently between the ages of 55 and 75. Cortical bone mass, however, remains consistent until menopause when resorption accelerates rapidly. By contrast, men will lose only 14% of vertebral body bone mass and insignificant cortical bone mass. It is predominantly this reduction in bone mass that leads to the increased incidence of fractures in osteoporosis (Fig 4–1).

☐ ETIOLOGY

The cause of primary osteoporosis is not known. Regulation of bone mass is dependent on a number of fac-

tors. Maintenance of specific cell types, systemic hormones, local factors, diet, intestinal and renal function, and external physical forces all play a role in developing, maintaining, and renewing bone. Osteoporosis has been shown histologically and biochemically to be heterogeneous. In some, there is greater bone resorption; in others, decreased formation. It is likely, therefore, that multiple causes of the final outcome are at fault, either individually or in combination.

Two possible causes are particularly significant: estrogen and calcium deficiencies. Osteoporosis progresses rapidly after menopause and prematurely after bilateral oophrectomy. When estrogen deficiency is replaced exogenously, bone loss is prevented, both by altering skeletal remodeling and increasing calcium absorption in the gut while decreasing calcium excretion by the kidneys.[3] Calcium deficiency causes osteoporosis in experimental animals; statistical correlation between osteoporosis and low calcium intake has been shown, and calcium supplementation significantly reduces the rate of bone loss.[1–3]

Bone resorption is also increased by immobilization, alcoholism, high phosphate diets, vitamin D deficiency, corticosteroids, thyrotoxicosis, protein calorie malnutrition, multiple endocrinopathies, and tumors.[2,3]

☐ CLINICAL PRESENTATION

Patients with osteoporosis can present to the emergency department in three ways: acute pain, chronic pain, and no pain (incidental finding).

Patients with acute back pain and osteoporosis typically present with midline back pain and vertebral body fractures. Much of the pain is secondary to erector spinae muscle spasm. Trauma is usually minimal, of the kind associated with routine activities such as bend-

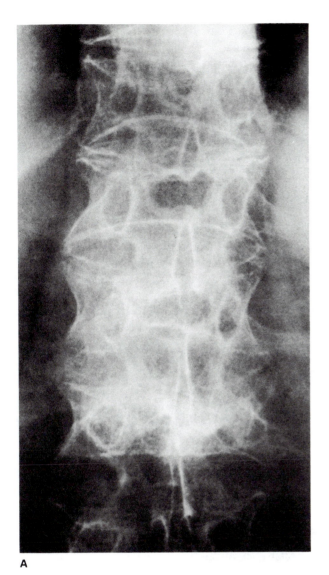 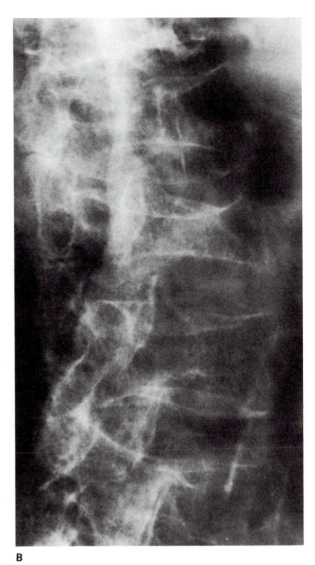

A   B

Figure 4–1. Frontal **(A)** and lateral **(B)** radiographs of the lumbar spine of an elderly patient with severe osteoporosis showing multiple codfish vertebrae. *From Banna M: Clinical Radiology of the Spine and Spinal Cord. Rockville, Md, Aspen, 1985, p 394. Reprinted with permission of Aspen Publishers, Inc.*

ing, lifting, or coughing. Vertebral body fractures range from microfractures to complete anterior wedging, sparing posterior segments and thus not involving nerve roots or spinal cord. Women are more frequently affected than men. Weight-bearing vertebrae between T-8 and L-3 are primarily involved causing loss of height. When multiple fractures occur, significant kyphosis develops, leading to a condition called *dowager's hump*.

Parfitt[4] describes four clinical types of pain: (1) Acute vertebral fracture pain is severe and usually lasts 2 to 3 months. (2) Collapse of the vertebra results in a compensatory lumbar lordosis resulting in low back pain of a more chronic nature lasting 3 to 6 months. (3) With multiple or repeated fractures, chronic back pain persists from stress on ligaments, muscles, and apophy-

seal joints. (4) As kyphosis develops, pain can actually occur from ribs resting on the iliac crests.

Keep in mind that acute vertebral collapse can be painless. The patient might present weeks to months later with chronic back pain. Significant osteoporosis might also present as an incidental finding clinically or radiographically with few or no complaints referable to the spine, i.e., constipation, bloating, urinary retention.

Femoral head and neck fractures associated with osteoporosis are second only to vertebral body fractures and have a high morbidity and mortality due to associated complications of therapy and convalescence, mortality after 1 year approaching 20%. Distal radial fractures are next in frequency and, although much better tolerated than femoral fractures, they are associated with fear of loss of independence and depression.

☐ DIAGNOSIS

Idiopathic osteoporosis is largely a diagnosis of exclusion. When decrease in bone mass is discovered in a patient, other disease states must be ruled out. A complete history and physical examination in the emergency department are mandatory and will dictate necessary serologic testing. Complete blood count, erythrocyte sedimentation rate, blood urea nitrogen, creatinine, calcium, phosphorous, alkaline phosphatase, serum protein electrophoresis, and urinalysis will elucidate other possible disease entities, but generally are inappropriate in the emergency setting.

Between 30 and 50% of bone mineral must be lost before demineralization is detected on plain radiographs. Other earlier findings on x-ray are suggestive of osteoporosis. End-plate shadows are accentuated and intervertebral discs expand causing biconcave depressions in vertebral bodies ("codfish" vertebrae). Schmorl's nodes are also concave depressions in the vertebral bodies caused by nucleus pulposus herniation. Compression fractures are common from T-8 to L-3 (rare above T-6) and may be multiple.

Numerous other diagnostic procedures (radiogrammetry, photodensitometry, photon absorptiometry, neutron activation analysis, compton scattering, and histomorphometry) have little value in the emergency setting.

☐ TREATMENT

Acute Therapy

Management of acute vertebral body compression is aimed largely at controlling pain and muscle spasm. Patients frequently require a period of bedrest, but this should be kept at a minimum as immobilization probably exacerbates bone resorption. Ice, analgesia, nonsteroidal anti-inflammatory agents, and muscle relaxants are helpful. Development of an ileus and urinary retention are relatively common and thus merit admission for 1 to 2 days. Depending on severity of symptoms, patients might require orthopedic referral. All patients should be referred to an internist for long-term therapy, including patients in whom the finding is incidental.

Long-Term Therapy

Long-term therapy is aimed at prevention of acute fractures by reducing or stopping the progress of bone loss. Treatment is still quite controversial, the discussion of which is beyond the scope of this text. Upon suspicion of the diagnosis, the emergency physician should refer the patient because long-term therapy should be tailored to the individual by an internist, an orthopedist, and often, a gynecologist. Briefly, current modalities and recommendations include[1-5]:

1. Estrogen replacement. At low doses, estrogen has been shown to reduce resorption and postmenopausal bone loss. Cyclic estrogen therapy is recommended for (white) women whose ovaries have been removed before age 50 and in postmenopausal women if they have no contraindications.
2. Calcium. 1000 to 1500 mg/day of *elemental* calcium is recommended, either by diet or supplementation. Previous history of renal stones is a relative contraindication.
3. Vitamin D. Requirements increase with age. Persons not receiving adequate sunlight (shut-ins, nursing home patients) should receive supplementation, no greater than 600 to 800 units daily.
4. Modest weight-bearing exercise.

Numerous other modalities, including sodium fluoride, calcitrol, calcitonin, anabolic steroids, and thiazides, are under investigation. Neither safety nor efficacy has been proven.

☐ REFERENCES

1. Consensus Conference: Osteoporosis. JAMA 252(6): 799, 1984
2. Lukert BP: Osteoporosis—A review and update. Arch Phys Med Rehab 63:480, 1982
3. Ullrich IH: Osteoporosis, W Va Med J 79(10):221, 1983
4. Parfitt AM: What are the causes of pain in osteoporosis? In Heaney R (ed): New York, Biomedical Information Corp., 1978, p 12
5. Lane JM, et al: Osteoporosis: Current diagnosis and treatment. Geriatrics 39(4):40, 1984

5

Infections of the Spine

□ INTRODUCTION

As with most infectious diseases, both the incidence and clinical presentation of spinal infections have been drastically altered by the advent of antimicrobial therapy. The morbidity and mortality of these diseases have declined dramatically in the past four to five decades. Unfortunately, as the prevalence of serious spinal infections has decreased, so has the clinical suspicion on the part of physicians. This has led to a significant delay in diagnosis in an increasing percentage of patients.[1-3] The pathogens responsible for spinal infections are many and include a large variety of pyogenic bacteria, *Mycobacterium tuberculosis*, *Treponema pallidum*, *Brucella*, fungi, and parasites.[1-13]

□ PYOGENIC SPONDYLITIS

Incidence

The true incidence of pyogenic osteomyelitis of the spine is not known. The disorder probably constitutes no more than 4% of all cases of osteomyelititis,[14] although it may occur more frequently than has been reported.[15] Several investigators believe that the incidence is increasing due to a greater prevalence of intravenous drug abuse and iatrogenic sepsis among hospitalized patients.[13,16,17]

Pathophysiology

In the past, these infections occurred primarily in children and had a clinical course marked by severe toxicity and rapid deterioration resulting in death in nearly 75% of those affected.[18] At present, more than 50% of the patients with this disorder are adults[2,3] and the clinical course tends to be much more indolent. Essentially every bacterial pathogen has been reported to cause spondylitis;[2] however, *Staphylococcus* is by far the most common organism.[2,13,15] The incidence of gram-negative organisms, including *Pseudomonas*, is increasing.[13] In nearly all cases, hematogenous seeding occurs[13,19] from a distant source, usually the skin, or urinary or respiratory tracts.[1-3,15] The vertebral body is the most common site of involvement.[2,15] Infection will often spread to several adjacent vertebrae and, at times, to the intervertebral discs. The thoracic and lumbar regions are most frequently affected with cervical involvement accounting for only about 10% of cases.[3,14] Generally, the infection remains low grade and localized; however, extension to other anatomic sites does occur and may lead to multiple complications.[3]

Axiom: *Pyogenic osteomyelitis of the spine occurs at all ages, but more than 50% of patients are adults.*

Clinical Features

Although the acute, toxemic form of the disease still occurs, it is quite unusual.[14] Much more common is a subacute or chronic variety with absent or minimal systemic symptoms.[14,15] Typically, patients present with an insidious onset of back pain in the region of the infected vertebra that is exacerbated by movement of the spine.[15] Some will complain of malaise or weight loss.[3,13] If the diagnosis is not made at this time, a dull, aching pain may develop and persist for months.

There are several clinical settings that are associated with an increased risk for spinal infections. These include recent or chronic urinary tract infections, prostatitis, urinary tract instrumentation, diabetes mellitus, renal failure, intravenous drug abuse, and skin infections.[2,3,13-15] In a few patients, however, no source or predisposing factors are found.[11]

Unfortunately, physical examination is often nonspecific, although in most patients there is significant tenderness on palpation of the spinous processes of the involved vertebrae. Paraspinous muscle spasm may be present as well as decreased mobility of the involved area of the spine.[2,3] Most patients have a low-grade fever, although the absence of this finding certainly does not rule out the diagnosis.[2,13,15] Recently the difficulty in making the diagnosis of cervical disease has been noted.[2,14] In patients presenting with torticollis, the diagnosis must always be entertained. If spinal tenderness and fever are present, spinal infection must be considered the diagnosis until proven otherwise. Additional signs and symtoms may occur when extension of the infection into the spinal canal or paraspinal structures takes place (see Complications). In a small number of patients, the clinical course is that of rapid deterioration due to overwhelming sepsis resulting in multisystem failure and ultimately death. Fortunately, mortality has markedly decreased in recent decades.[2,3,13,15]

Complications

Most complications occur in the setting of chronic infection that extends from the vertebral body into other structures. The infection can extend into the spinal canal resulting in an epidural abscess that may lead to nerve root or cord compression.[2,3,14,15,20] Penetration through the dura may also occur and leads to bacterial meningitis.[2] Spread of infection along myofascial planes can lead to a myriad of secondary complications. Paravertebral abscesses may occur in any area of the spine,[3,5,13,20] creating fluctuant masses that are palpable and may lead to draining sinuses. With lumbar disease, this may extend to the flank, groin, or perirectal areas and in some cases will lead to the formation of a psoas abscess.[3,21] Extension from cervical or thoracic infections may lead to retropharyngeal abscess, mediastinitis, empyema, or pericarditis. In some cases, vertebral body collapse leads to a kyphotic deformity. Rarely, in cervical spine disease, fracture–dislocation occurs without history of trauma and may lead to significant neurologic sequelae. Chronic osteomyelitis may occur and leads to long-term management problems.

Diagnosis

Laboratory findings usually are not impressive. The white blood cell count is generally normal although a mild leukocytosis may be present.[3,15] The erythrocyte sedimentation rate is often mildly elevated.[3,15] Blood cultures should always be obtained, as they may identify the infecting organism.[3,13,14] In addition, needle biopsy of the lesion should be performed and generally yields the pathogen and antibiotic sensitivities.[2,3,11,13,20,21]

Radiographic findings lag behind the clinical manifestations by 1 to 3 months and are essentially always normal at the onset of symptoms.[2,3,14,15] The first radiographic finding is generally a small focus of bone de-

struction adjacent to the intervertebral disc (Fig 5–1). As the disease progresses, disc space narrowing occurs and the bone destruction extends to the center of the vertebral body.[2,3] The body may subsequently collapse and give rise to a kyphotic deformity. Ultimately, sclerosis and new bone deposition lead to osteophyte formation and fusion of the adjacent vertebral bodies (Fig 5–2).[2,3,13,15] If large retropharyngeal or paravertebral abscesses develop, they may become evident on x-ray. A psoas abscess may present as an obscured psoas margin radiographically.

Computed tomography may be useful for evaluating paraspinous and epidural abscesses as well as for guiding needle aspiration.[20,21] Radionuclide scanning may be effective for making the diagnosis before standard radiographs are positive.[2,14,22,23]

Unfortunately, delayed or missed diagnosis has been a relatively frequent problem.[2,3,13,14] In one study, the diagnosis was made within 3 months of the onset of symptoms in only 11 of 37 patients.[3] Because early diagnosis is desirable, but laboratory and radiographic findings are nonspecific or nonexistent early in the course of the disease, a high index of suspicion in the appropriate clinical setting is mandatory.

Axiom: *When one suspects pyogenic spondylitis, a bone scan should be obtained as the clinical and radiographic presentations are nonspecific and late to evolve.*

Management and Referral

All patients with this diagnosis require hospital admission. Strict bedrest is maintained early on and cervical traction is instituted in those patients with cervical spine involvement.[3,13,15] High-dose intravenous antibiotics are administered. Because both gram-positive and gram-negative organisms are common, broad spectrum coverage should be started initially until the culture and sensitivity of the needle aspirate becomes available. Oxacillin or a first-generation cephalosporin in combination with an aminoglycoside is generally the regimen of choice. Although the optimal duration of antibiotic therapy is not known, a course of 6 to 8 weeks is supported by the literature.[2,13,15] Complications, such as spinal deformity and instability, paraspinal abscesses, or secondary visceral involvement, may require surgical intervention. With early diagnosis and appropriate antibiotic therapy, however, this should be unusual.[15] The complication of cord compression should also be rare with early diagnosis and treatment.[15]

All of these patients are subject to recurrences and long-term complications and thus must be followed by appropriate consultants.

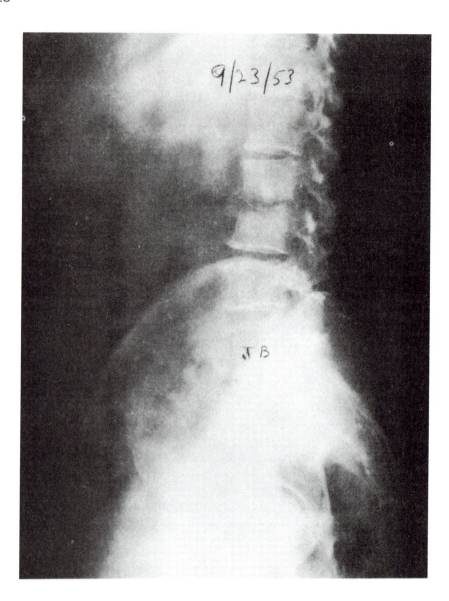

Figure 5–1. Lateral radiograph of the spine with pyogenic osteomyelitis. Destruction of the vertebral endplates is shown 3 months after the onset of symptoms. *From Ross PM, Fleming JL: Clin Orthop 118:193, 1976.*[3]

☐ TUBERCULOUS SPONDYLITIS

Incidence

As with other infections of the spine, the incidence of tuberculous spondylitis (Pott's disease) has decreased dramatically in recent decades with the advent of effective antituberculous agents. In the developed countries of the world, tuberculous infection of the spine is rare. In Third World countries, however, this disease continues to exact a massive toll of human suffering and death.

Pathophysiology

Tuberculous spondylitis is caused by *Mycobacterium tuberculosis* in the great majority of cases, although atypical mycobacterial infection does occur. The spine is the most common site of tuberculous bone involvement and generally arises from some other primary focus, usually pulmonary. The spine can become involved either by hematogenous spread or by direct extension from an adjacent focus. Spinal involvement occurs primarily in the thoracic and lumbar regions with the former being most common. Tuberculous infection of the cervical spine is extremely rare. Infection generally begins in the vertebral body and in contradistinction to pyogenic spondylitis only spreads to the disc after essentially destroying the entire body of the vertebra. Multiple levels of the spine may be affected simultaneously. As with pyogenic spondylitis, many of the significant complications are due to extension into the spinal canal or to extraspinal structures. Spinal deformity is generally much more significant with tubercu-

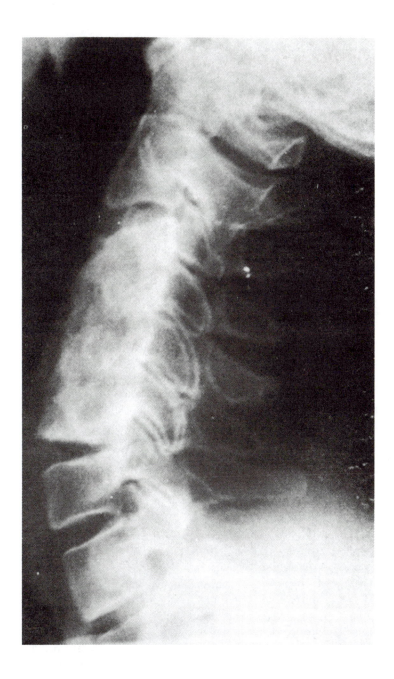

Figure 5–2. Fusion of C-3 to C-6 present 1 year after diagnosis and treatment of pyogenic vertebral osteomyelitis. The bone is stable and well aligned. *From Messer HO, Litvinoff J: Arch Neurol 33:573, 1976.*[15]

lous involvement and in some cases leads to dramatic deformities.

Tuberculous spondylitis affects all age groups, but in the United States it is primarily a disease of the elderly and the poor.

Clinical Features

When symptoms referable to spinal involvement occur, the primary focus of tuberculosis may be active or quiescent. A history of tuberculosis is generally not present. An interesting, but unexplained, association between tuberculous spondylitis and intravenous drug abuse has been reported.[13] The patient may complain of malaise, weight loss, night sweats, cough, or hemoptysis, but systemic symptoms are usually absent altogether. Typically, the initial complaint is mild back pain that may be exacerbated by movement. Unless extraspinal extension or spinal deformity have occurred, there are no other specific complaints.

Axiom: *At the onset of symptomatic tuberculous spondylitis, there is often no history or clinical evidence of active tuberculosis.*

Examination may reveal cachexia and other findings of chronic infection, although often there are no systemic signs. Tenderness of the affected level(s) of the spine is present and paraspinous muscle spasm is usually obvious. Mobility of the spine is generally decreased and attempts to document this may be described as painful. Atrophy of the trunk musculature may be present. As with pyogenic spondylitis, more impressive and specific physical findings do not occur until complications ensue.

Complications

Spinal deformity occurs frequently and may be impressive. Essentially this always occurs in the thoracic region and results in kyphosis. This angulation of the spine may become visible as a large bony prominence protruding posteriorly in the thoracic region and is known as gibbus. Marked deformities can lead to compromise of respiratory function. Destruction of the lumbar vertebral bodies may also occur, but this generally leads to compression along the axis of the spine and does not result in angulation or deformity. With significant deformity, neurologic sequelae, such as paraplegia, may occur, but this is surprisingly uncommon given the impressive angulation that may be present.[24,25] These areas, however, are relatively unstable in the setting of trauma and are prone to fracture.

As with pyogenic spondylitis, a myriad of complications may accompany the intraspinal or extraspinal extension of infection. Epidural abscesses may lead to cord compression,[2] particularly in the thoracic region where the spinal canal is narrow. The result is lower extremity weakness and spasticity with loss of sphincter control, and the examination reveals the signs of an upper motor neuron lesion. Extension of the abscess into the subarachnoid space leads to tuberculous meningitis and often results in catastrophic complications.[13,26,27] Paravertebral abscess formation is very common.[13,26,27] Spread of infection from the cervical region may lead to subcutaneous abscesses or draining fistulous tracts in the paraspinous region, supraclavicular fossa, and posterior to the sternomastoid. Retropharyngeal abscesses also occur, and collections of caseous material may lead to impingement upon the trachea or the esophagus with resultant dyspnea or difficulty swallowing. Nuchal rigidity may be present, mimicking meningeal signs, but the cerebrospinal fluid is normal. In the thoracic region, subcutaneous abscesses and cutaneous fistulae may occur. Nerve root impingement results in neuralgias that may mimic cardiac or intra-abdominal disease. As with pyogenic infections, intrathoracic extension may lead to empyema, pericarditis, and mediastinitis. Extension of lumbar disease may create abscesses and fistulae in the paralumbar region, the groin, and along the medial aspect of the thigh. Psoas abscess is not uncommon and leads to pain during extension and external rotation of the hip on the affected side. Nerve root impingement leads to referred pain in the lower extremities.

Diagnosis

Conclusive diagnosis is made only after retrieving and identifying *M. tuberculosis* from the spinal lesion. On the other hand, the entire clinical picture, including radiography, may be so compelling as to leave even the most compulsive physician without any other possibilities in the differential diagnosis. The purified protein derivative of tuberculin (PPD) is usually positive, but remains negative in a significant number of patients. A positive skin test is helpful, but by no means diagnostic. Sputum and urine specimens for acid fast stain and culture should be obtained, but are usually negative.

Chest x-ray may or may not show changes typical of tuberculosis. Paravertebral abscesses may present as apparent mediastinal widening or a retrocardiac density (Fig 5–3). In contradistinction to pyogenic spondylitis, x-ray findings of the spine are usually advanced at the time symptoms occur from tuberculous spondylitis.[15] Radiography of the spine reveals lytic lesions destroying the vertebral body while generally sparing the neural arch (Fig 5–4). Ultimately, the entire vertebral body is destroyed and the cortical margins are indistinct. Disc involvement, with disc space narrowing, generally occurs late in the course[3] and there are often multiple adjacent vertebral bodies involved, with the intervening discs remaining essentially normal. This is an important differential point with respect to tuberculosis as compared with pyogenic spondylitis. Thus, if the radiographic picture shows significant vertebral body destruction with minimal or no disc involvement, tuberculosis is much more likely to be the etiology than a pyogenic organism.[3] Another important radiographic difference is that new bone and osteophyte formation occur very late in tuberculous spondylitis relative to the pyogenic form.[3,13,28] In the lumbar region, the margins of the psoas muscle may be obscured by a psoas abscess. A lateral view of the neck may reveal a retropharyngeal abscess. If present, an abnormal thoracic kyphosis can be easily identified by x-ray.

Management and Referral

In the large majority of patients, antimicrobial therapy alone leads to excellent results and cure. The standard regimen is isoniazid and rifampin, although ethambutol and streptomycin are also frequently used. Therapy for a period of 18 to 24 months is highly effective.[2] Most cases can be managed on an outpatient basis and do not even require bedrest.[2] There are still some who advocate 1 to 2 months of bedrest even in uncomplicated cases. If there is significant deformity, large extra spinal abscesses, or evidence of cord compression, surgical intervention is necessary. In these cases, there is

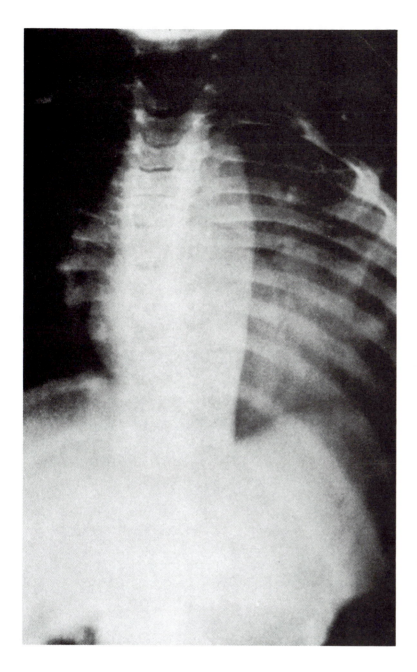

Figure 5–3. Large paravertebral abscess (left) in a child with tuberculous spondylitis at T-7 and T-8. *From La Rocca H: Spinal sepsis. In Rothman RM, Simeone FA (eds): The Spine. Philadelphia, WB Saunders, 1982, p 769.*

generally a long convalescence and body casting is often required.

☐ INTERVERTEBRAL DISC INFECTION

This uncommon disorder may occur at any age. In adults, the vast majority of cases occur after surgical disc excision, although lumbar puncture is also a rare cause. The patient generally presents 2 to 4 weeks after the procedure with severe back pain localized to the infected site. Motion significantly exacerbates the pain.

Systemic signs and symptoms are generally absent. Examination of the painful area reveals exquisite tenderness, but no other objective evidence of infection. Laboratory data are not helpful, and in fact, even when appropriate material is obtained for culture, the offending organism is difficult to culture out.[29] Radiographic changes are generally absent although bone destruction may occur weeks to months after the onset of symptoms. The diagnosis is, therefore, a clinical one. When the culture is positive, *Staphylococcus* is the most common organism retrieved, but a large number of gram-positive and gram-negative organisms has been found. Treatment includes antibiotics and bedrest until a marked clinical improvement has been noted and radio-

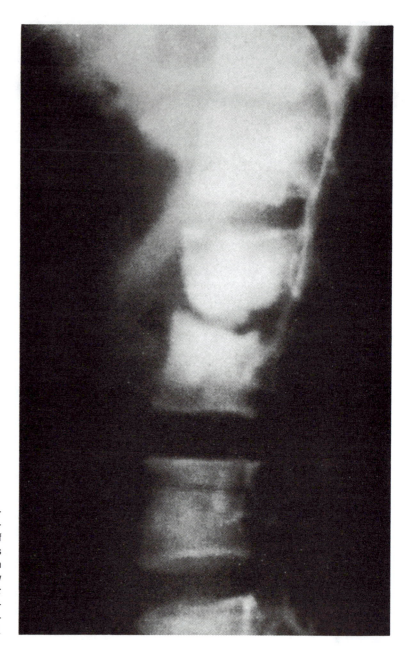

Figure 5–4. Lateral radiograph of L-1 and L-2 involvement with tuberculous spondylitis. Note destruction of the end-plates. The bony density is due to sequestration and impaction of necrotic bone rather than new bone formation. *From La Rocca H: Spinal sepsis. In Rothman RM, Simeone FA (eds): The Spine. Philadelphia, WB Saunders, 1982, p 770.*

graphic evidence of healing is present. Prognosis for cure is very good and significant complications are uncommon.

Axiom: *Severe pain at the site of a recent spinal procedure should be treated as a disc space infection until proven otherwise.*

An interesting syndrome of disc inflammation occurs in children. The average age of these patients is six and it rarely occurs after age ten.[2,30] The clinical presentation is characterized by back pain, refusal to crawl or walk, malaise, irritability, and low-grade fever, although the signs and symptoms may vary widely. Examination reveals tenderness over the involved area and straight leg raising is often positive with lumbar disease.[30] The presentation is essentially identical to that of children with spinal osteomyelitis[2,30] and, in fact, may simply reflect the least serious clinical entity in a "continuous spectrum of disease."[2] At the time of presentation, radiographs are often normal but will ultimately show disc space narrowing and end-plate irregularity.[2,30] The radionuclide scan is positive before radiographic changes can be detected.[30] Laboratory examination generally reveals a normal white blood cell count and an elevated sedimentation rate.

Optimum management for all patients is not entirely clear. Some of these cases probably represent a noninfectious inflammatory disorder. Early in the disease process, however, it is probably best to assume that all of these patients have an infectious etiology. Blood cultures and needle biopsy should be performed. Interestingly, only 20 to 35% of biopsies result in a positive culture.[2,30-32] When cultures are positive, *Staphylococcus aureus* is the offending organism in the majority of cases.[31,32] In patients with significant fever, systemic symptoms, positive blood, or biopsy cultures, antibiotic therapy should be instituted for 6 weeks.[2,30] All patients should be treated with bedrest whether they require antibiotics or not. Increasing activity can be allowed as the symptoms subside. In the vast majority of patients, the disease course is uneventful and complete recovery occurs.[2,33]

□ REFERENCES

1. Stone DB, Bonfiglio M: Pyogenic vertebral osteomyelitis. Arch Intern Med 112:491–500, 1963
2. Waldvogel FA, Vasey H: Osteomyelitis: The past decade. N Engl J Med 303:360–370, 1980
3. Ross PM, Fleming JL: Vertebral body osteomyelitis: Spectrum and natural history. Clin Orthop 118:190–198, 1976
4. Matsushita T, Suzuki K: Spastic paraparesis due to cryptococcal osteomyelitis. A case report. Clin Orthop 196:279–284, 1985
5. Chambers ST, Wilson AP, Seal DV, et al: Paratyphoid fever presenting with grand mal fits and cerebellar signs. J Infect 10:48–50, 1985
6. Smith MA, Trowers NR, Klein RS: Cervical osteomyelitis caused by *Pseudomonas cepacia* in an intravenous drug abuser. J Clin Microbiol 21:445–446, 1985
7. Petty BG, Burrow CR, Robinson RA, et al: *Hemophilus aphrophilus* meningitis followed by vertebral osteomyelitis and suppurative psoas abscess. Am J Med 78:159–162, 1985
8. Hayes WS, Berg RA, Dorfman HD, et al: Case report. Diagnosis: *Candida discitis* and verterbral osteomyelitis at L1-L2 from hematogenous spread. Skeletal Radiol 12:284–287, 1984
9. McKee DF, Barr WM, Bryan CS, et al: Primary aspergillosis of the spine mimicking Pott's paraplegia. J Bone Joint Surg 66:1481–1483, 1984
10. Anderson J, Kron IL: Treatment of aspergillus infection of the proximal aortic prosthetic graft with associated vertebral osteomyelitis. J Vasc Surg 1:579–581, 1984
11. Holzgang J, Wehrli R, von Graevenitz A, et al: Adult vertebral osteomyelitis caused by *Haemophilus influenzae*. Eur J Clin Microbiol 3:261–262, 1984
12. Masters DL, Lentino JR: Cervical osteomyelitis related to nocardia asteroides. J Infect Dis 149:824–825, 1984
13. Musher DM, Thorsteinsson SB, Minuth JN, et al: Vertebral osteomyelitis: Still a diagnostic pitfall. Arch Intern Med 136:105–110, 1976
14. Slagel SA, Skiendzielewski JJ, McMurry FG: Osteomyelitis of the cervical spine: Reversible quadraplegia resulting from Philadelphia collar placement. Ann Emerg Med 14:912–915, 1985
15. Messer HD, Litvinoff J: Pyogenic cervical osteomyelitis: Chondro-osteomyelitis of the cervical spine frequently associated with parenteral drug use. Arch Neurol 33:571–576, 1976
16. Holzman RS, Bishko F: Osteomyelitis in heroin addicts. Ann Intern Med 75:693–696, 1971
17. Griffiths HE, Jones DM: Pyogenic infection of the spine: A review of twenty-eight cases. J Bone Joint Surg 53:383–391, 1971
18. Hatch ES: Acute osteomyelitis of the spine. New Orleans Med Surg J 83:801, 1931
19. Wiley AM, Trueta J: The vascular anatomy of the spine and its relationship to pyogenic vertebral osteomyelitis. J Bone Joint Surg 41B:796–809, 1959
20. Burke DR, Brant-Zawadzki M: CT of pyogenic spine infection. Neuroradiology 27:131–137, 1985
21. McGahan JP, Dublin AB: Evaluation of spinal infections by plain radiographs, computed tomography, intrathecal metrizamide, and CT-guided biopsy. Diag Imag Clin Med 54:11–20, 1985
22. Strauss M, Kaufman RA, Baum S: Osteomyelitis of the head and neck: Sequential radionuclide scanning in diagnosis and therapy. Laryngoscope 95:81–84, 1985
23. Koren A, Garty I, Katzuni E: Bone infarction in children with sickle cell disease: Early diagnosis and differentiation from osteomyelitis. Eur J Pediatr 142:93–97, 1984
24. Yau ACMC, Hsu LCS, O'Brien JP, et al: Tuberculous kyphosis. J Bone Joint Surg 56A:1419, 1974
25. Hodgson AR, Skinsnes OK, Leong CY: The pathogenesis of Pott's paraplegia. J Bone Joint Surg 49A:1145–1147, 1967
26. Riska EB: Spinal tuberculosis treated by antituberculous chemotherapy and radical operation. Clin Orthop 119:148–158, 1976
27. Friedman B: Chemotherapy of tuberculosis of the spine. J Bone Joint Surg 48A:451–474, 1966
28. Waldvogel FA, Medoff G, Swartz MN: Osteomyelitis: A review of clinical features, therapeutic considerations and unusual aspects. N Engl J Med 282:316–322, 1970
29. Thibodeau AA: Closed space infection following removal of lumbar intervertebral disc. J Bone Joint Surg 50A:400, 1968
30. King HA: Back pain in children. Pediatr Clin North Am 31:1083–1095, 1984
31. Spiegel PG, Kengla KW, Isaacson AS: Intervertebral disc-space inflammation in children. J Bone Joint Surg 54:284–296, 1972
32. Boston HC, Bianco AJ, Rhodes KH: Disc space infections in children. Orthop Clin North Am 6:953–964, 1975
33. Smith RF, Taylor TKF: Inflammatory lesions of intervertebral discs in children. J Bone Joint Surg 49:1508–1520, 1967

6

Neoplasms of the Spine

Although spinal tumors are relatively uncommon diagnoses in emergency rooms, back pain as a primary complaint most certainly is not. Yet in their early stages, spinal neoplasms frequently present with pain and thus can mimic a variety of more common back ailments.

As early diagnosis is often the key to preserving function (particularly neurologic) and life, spinal tumors present a particular challenge to the emergency physician. Unfortunately, unlike in other areas of this text, where pathognomonic signs and symptoms provide the diagnosis, clinical evidence of spinal tumors might be quite subtle. Indeed, if there is any axiom in this chapter, it is that you might never diagnose an *early* spinal neoplasm unless you *think* of it.

☐ HISTORY

The most common symptom of spinal neoplasm (either primary or metastatic) is pain.[1] Subtle characteristics might help distinguish this from other spinal pathology.[2] The pain is more often constant. It is not necessarily worse with activity, nor relieved with rest, heat, or massage, and is often worse with rest or at night. Significant pain after minor trauma might suggest underlying neoplastic disease. Radicular symptoms might indicate a somewhat more progressive lesion. Suggestive of space occupying lesions with neurologic compromise are paresthesias, weakness, paralysis of upper or lower extremities, and disturbances of urinary, bowel, and sexual function.

Most often benign primary tumors present in children and young adults, being relatively rare over the age of 30; however, malignant tumors are far more prevalent in adults, both primary and particularly metastatic.[1]

A prior history of cancer, significant exposures (chemicals, drugs, ionizing radiation), diseases with tendency toward malignant transformation, or positive family history might suggest underlying malignancy as would systemic symptoms such as night sweats, fever, malaise, weight loss, and anorexia.

☐ PHYSICAL EXAMINATION

Careful clinical examination will not only localize the level of the lesion, but might well differentiate possible tumors from nonneoplastic diseases. Not uncommonly, the examiner may note limitation of motion, scoliosis, postural abnormalities, and muscle atrophy or fasciculations. One should palpate for maximal point tenderness or a mass at single or multiple areas if widely metastatic disease is present. Little or no muscle spasm might imply tumor. A thorough neurologic examination for sensory or motor deficits, deep tendon reflex abnormalities, clonus, or pathologic reflexes might demonstrate the level of the lesion as well as the severity of possible cord compromise.

Numerous authors have observed the relative absence of positive straight leg raising in patients with significant spinal metastatic involvement, felt by some to reflect probably a combination of large canals, compensatory flattening of the cord, and lack of inflammation.[3,4] Particularly if metastatic disease is suspected, a complete physical examination could provide a primary site. A palpable breast mass, thyroid nodule, abdominal or rectal mass, enlarged prostate, or heme positive stool might prove diagnostic and focus future work-up and treatment.

☐ LABORATORY STUDIES

In today's world of spiraling medical costs, it is particularly incumbent on the emergency physician to think before ordering a whole battery of often nondiagnostic laboratory tests. Ultimately, the definitive neoplastic diagnosis is histologic, involving procedures beyond the scope of the emergency center work-up. The emergency physician is challenged to limit the emergency evaluation to those tests that will, in general, lead to a diagnosis and, specifically, alter his or her management. Certainly the patient's presentation will determine the evaluation; an ambulatory adolescent with new onset low back pain will require a much different and less extensive emergency laboratory evaluation than a somnolent elderly man with new bladder and bowel incontinence.

With the above concerns in mind, a number of laboratory tests under certain circumstances could be considered. A complete blood count, including differential erythrocyte sedimentation rate, calcium, alkaline phosphatase, and urinalysis might prove helpful in a patient suspected of having a spinal tumor and lead to referral for further evaluation. The full extent of the primary or metastatic work-up is beyond the scope of this text and, we emphasize, generally not a part of emergency evaluation.

Routine roentgenographic studies at the initial emergency evaluation, however, should include anteroposterior, lateral, and oblique views of the spine whenever suggested by the history and physical examination. When significant neurologic defects are noted myelography and computed tomography (CT) scanning are necessary to determine the exact location and extent of spinal cord involvement (refer to Spinal Cord Compression, this chapter). When malignancy (either primary or metastatic) is suspected, technitium bone scanning provides a good skeletal survey, except in myeloma, where standard pelvic and skull x-rays provide the most information.

Definitive diagnosis of spinal neoplasms of any origin is, however, based on histology and, thus, requires biopsy.

□ CLASSIFICATION

Tumors of the spinal column can be broadly divided into two groups: (1) primary, those derived from tissues of the spinal column itself and (2) metastatic, those invading tumors of distant origin. Although primary tumors of the spine are uncommon, they are of a wide morphologic variety. It is easiest to classify them according to tissue of origin: bone, cartilage, fibrous tissue, nerve, bone marrow, and blood vessels. Table 6–1 shows a comprehensive list of possible tumors of the spinal column. A number of these are rare enough to be

TABLE 6–1. POSSIBLE TUMORS OF THE SPINAL COLUMN

Tumors originating from bone systems
Cartilage
  Osteochondroma
  Chondroma
  Chondroblastoma
  Chondrosarcoma
  Chondromyxoid fibroma
Bone
  Osteoma
  Osteoid osteoma
  Osteoblastoma
  Osteogenic sarcoma
  Parosteal ossifying fibroma
Resorptive
  Bone cyst
  Diffuse osteitis fibrosa cystica
  Fibrous dysplasia
  Giant-cell tumor

Tumors originating elsewhere
Marrow
  Ewing's endothelial myeloma
  Multiple myeloma
  Chloroma or leukemia of bones
  Reticuloendotheliosis
  Eosinophilic granuloma
  Histiocytic lymphoma (reticulum cell sarcoma)
Metastatic
  Carcinoma of thyroid, breast, prostate, and kidneys
  Lymphomas, neuroblastoma, sarcoma
Invasive
  Chordoma
  Angioma, angiosarcoma
  Fibroma and fibrosarcoma of fascia or nerve sheath
  Myosarcoma
  Synovioma

only case reports. This chapter focuses on some of the more common benign and malignant lesions.

Primary Benign Tumors

Osteochondroma

Exostoses. Spongy bone capped by cartilage (Fig 6–1).

Clinical Features. Occur in the young, during growth phase, with slight male predominance. Rarely symptomatic unless large. Neurologic symptoms by compression are rare.[5]

Radiographs. Diagnostic. Sessile or pedunculated outpouching of trabecula bone; cartilage cap is not visible, therefore, appears smaller on x-ray.

Treatment. None indicated unless symptomatic, then excised. Approximately 10% incidence of sarcomatous transformation.

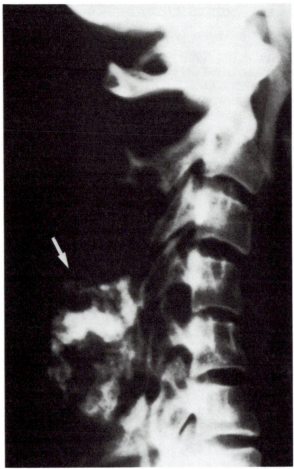

Figure 6–1. Osteochondroma. *From Banna M: Clinical Radiology of the Spine and Spinal Cord. Rockville, Md, Aspen, 1985, p 341. Reprinted with permission of Aspen Publishers, Inc.*

Osteoid Osteoma

Slowly growing, small nidus of dense compact bone (Fig 6–2).

Clinical Features. Usually in childhood and young adults with male predominance. Can be extremely painful, worse at night, relieved with aspirin. May develop scoliosis and radicular symptoms. Affects the facets and posterior elements.[6]

Radiographs. Lytic lesion less than 1 cm in diameter surrounding a small nidus, which might not be visible, requiring tomography. If scoliosis is present, the nidus is generally located at the apex of the concave side of the curve. Pain might precede any radiologic changes, and the lesion may then only be confirmed by technitium bone scanning.[7]

Treatment. Surgical resection if symptomatic. Usually remain small. No malignant transformation.

Osteoblastoma

A rare, dense lesion of bone, but commonly affects the spine (Fig 6–3).

Clinical Features. Seen in children and teenagers. Although often referred to as a giant osteoid osteoma, this painful lesion is not necessarily worse at night, nor is it relieved with aspirin. As it can be quite large and affects the posterior elements of the spine, it can be palpable on examination and produce neurologic symptoms by compression.

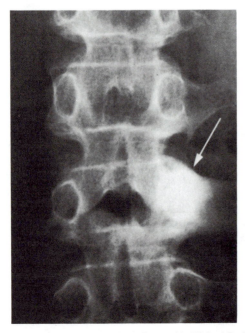
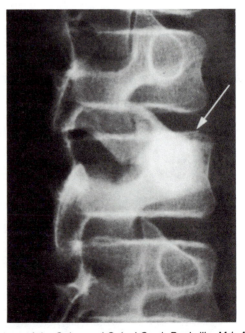

Figure 6–2. Osteoid osteoma. *From Banna M: Clinical Radiology of the Spine and Spinal Cord. Rockville, Md, Aspen, 1985, p 337. Reprinted with permission of Aspen Publishers, Inc.*

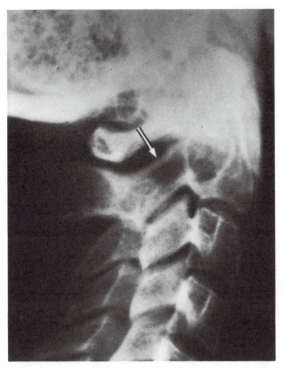

Figure 6–3. Osteoblastoma. *From Banna M: Clinical Radiology of the Spine and Spinal Cord. Rockville, Md, Aspen, 1985, p 338. Reprinted with permission of Aspen Publishers, Inc.*

Radiographs. Lytic lesion surrounded by sclerotic bone with thin rim of new bone.

Treatment. Although it is considered a benign lesion, osteoblastoma can be locally aggressive. Occasional malignant transformation (excision recommended, radiation therapy if inaccessible).[8]

Giant Cell Tumor

Osteolytic tumor (osteoclastoma) comprised of multinucleate giant cells, uncommon in the spine (Fig 6–4).

Clinical Features. Occur in young adults, with female predominance. Presents with pain and tenderness, affecting vertebral body and may lead to collapse with neurologic symptoms.[9]

Radiographs. Totally destructive to bone, with spherical, cystic appearance and little reactive bone. Multiple small lesions may give soap bubble effect.

Treatment. Histologically controversial. Although many lesions are clearly benign, up to one-half act biologically malignant with high tendency of local recurrence and occasional metastases. Surgical excision with close follow-up is recommended. Radiation therapy reserved for surgically inaccessible lesions due to significant rate of postirradiation malignant transformation.

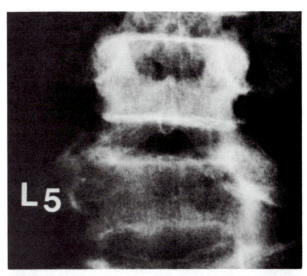

Figure 6–4. Giant cell tumor. *From Banna M: Clinical Radiology of the Spine and Spinal Cord. Rockville, Md, Aspen, 1985, p 362. Reprinted with permission of Aspen Publishers, Inc.*

Eosinophilic Granuloma

Benign variant of Hand-Schüller-Christian disease. Histiocytosis. Abnormal proliferation of histiocytes displacing bones (Fig 6–5).

Clinical Features. Most commonly seen between ages of 5 and 10, but also in young adults and elderly. Presents with pain and local tenderness, unrelieved with aspirin.

Involves the vertebral body and is the most common cause of vertebra plana, flattening of the vertebral bodies, in immature spines. Significant decrease in height results, which resolves with therapy. Involves little neurologic effects.

Radiographs. Lesion is ovoid, well demarcated, translucent. Loss of bone tissue, vertebral collapse.

Treatment. Low dose irradiation or, where feasible, local excision.

Hemangioma

Frequently silent tumors of fully developed blood vessels in as many as 12% of spines (Fig 6–6).[1]

Clinical Freatures. Can occur at any age. Rarely symptomatic (pain). When involving mid-thoracic vertebral bodies, can produce neurologic symptoms.

Radiographs. Coarse, dense, vertical striations of the vertebral body.

Treatment. May regress spontaneously. Surgery can be

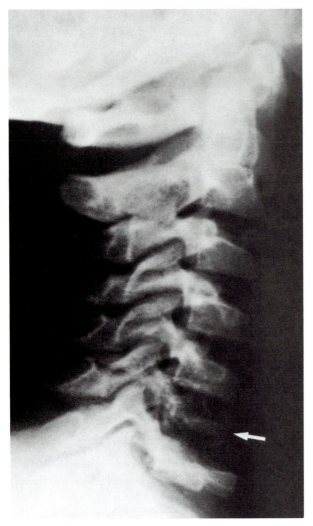

Figure 6–5. Eosinophilic granuloma. *From Banna M: Clinical Radiology of the Spine and Spinal Cord. Rockville, Md, Aspen, 1985, p 346. Reprinted with permission of Aspen Publishers, Inc.*

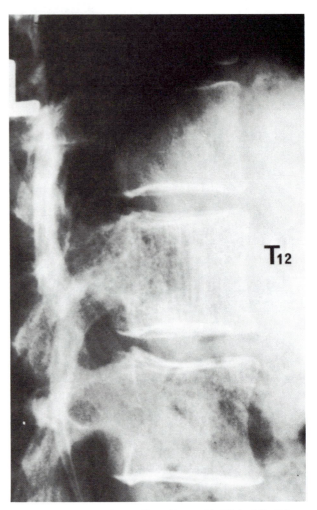

Figure 6–6. Hemangioma. *From Banna M: Clinical Radiology of the Spine and Spinal Cord. Rockville, Md, Aspen, 1985, p 344. Reprinted with permission of Aspen Publishers, Inc.*

complicated by uncontrollable bleeding. External bracing, rarely irradiation is indicated.

Aneurysmal Bone Cysts

A mass of vascular spaces, usually venous, enclosed in new bone growing outward (Fig 6–7).

Clinical Features. Usually occur in children and young adults, without sexual predominance. Common to the spine, involving the vertebral body and posterior elements. Symptoms are related to pressure from the expanding mass, including pain, ofter radicular.[10] Can involve multiple vertebrae.

Radiographs. "Blow-out" appearance caused by well-circumscribed central area of loss of bone surrounded by new reactive bone.

Treatment. Due to risk of collapse, curettage and bone grafting favored, radiation therapy if surgically inaccessible.

Primary Malignant Tumors

Multiple Myeloma

The malignant proliferation of plasma cells characterized by excessive amounts of immunoglobulins, Bence Jones proteins, and multicentric bone replacement by tumor growth (Fig 6–8).

Clinical Features. Onset usually occurs after age 50 with male predominance. Presenting complaint is of pain, described as deep and persistent, never completely relieved with rest, most often secondary to pathologic fractures (microfractures to pathologic long bone fracture). Compression fractures of the thoracic and lumbar spine are common, causing radicular pain and

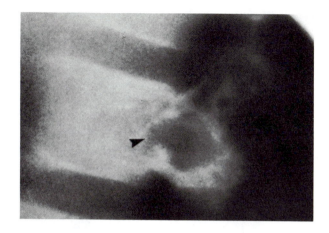

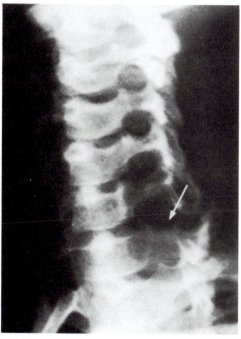

Figure 6–7. Aneurysmal bone cysts. *From Banna M: Clinical Radiology of the Spine and Spinal Cord. Rockville, Md, Aspen, 1985, p 349. Reprinted with permission of Aspen Publishers, Inc.*

restricted spinal movement. Generalized osteoporosis is felt secondary to osteoclastic activating factor from tumor cells (Fig 6–8). Anemia is always present with an increased erythrocyte sedimentation rate (from coating of red blood cells with immunoglobulins), hypercalcemia, low normal alkaline phosphatase, increased serum globulins with reversal of albumin to globulin ratio, and abnormal serum (with characteristic m-spike) and urine (with light chain, Bence Jones proteins) protein electrophoresis.

Radiographs. Multiple osteolytic areas, vertebral collapse, severe osteoporosis to point of complete dissolution of vertebrae ("disappearing vertebrae").

Treatment. Myeloma is treated with chemotherapy and supportive measures. The tumor is radiosensitive, treatment of which temporarily relieves pain. Surgical treatment of the spine is reserved for severe instability. Lightweight external bracing is beneficial.

Malignant Lymphoma
Reticulum cell sarcoma. Primary lymphoma of the bone with anaplastic reticulum cells, lymphocytes, lymphoblasts, and intercellular stroma with strands of reticulum (Fig 6–9).[11]

Clinical Features. Presents in young adults, more commonly men, with pain due to vertebral body collapse. Solitary lesion by definition (Fig 6–9).

Radiographs. Solitary, mottled, patchy areas of radiolucency, often with vertebral collapse.

Treatment. Radiation therapy is the treatment of choice in the spine, although chemotherapy may improve outcome.

Chondrosarcoma
Relatively slow growing cartilaginous tumor with variable malignant characteristics.

Clinical Features. Generally occur in older population with male predominance. The patient presents with a long history of pain, involving the vertebral bodies of the lumbrosacral area.[1] As it tends to grow locally, neurologic deficits due to compression result in bowel, bladder, and sexual dysfunction. Clinical course varies widely.

Radiographs. Bony destruction and a mass with evidence of calcification.

Treatment. Surgical excision.[12] In poorly accessible areas (i.e., sacrum), multiple (debulking) procedures may be required. Local recurrence is common, often with a more aggressive tumor.

Osteosarcoma
Highly malignant primary bone tumor characterized by neoplastic osteoid tissue, often with fibrosarcomatous and chondrosarcomatous components (Fig 6–10).

Clinical Features. After myeloma, osteogenic sarcoma is the most common primary malignancy of bone, yet rarely with the spine as origin.[1] Presents in the second decade of life with severe pain. In the spine, it affects the vertebral bodies and pedicles. Growth is rapid with early metastasis principally to lungs, liver, and other bones.

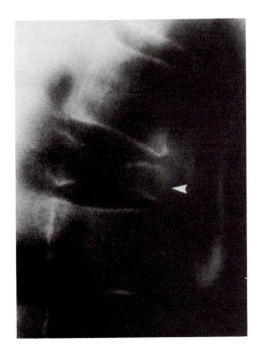

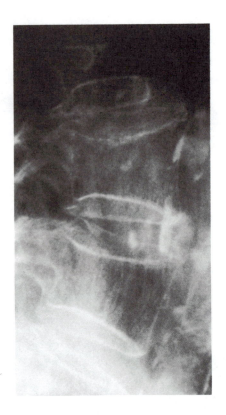

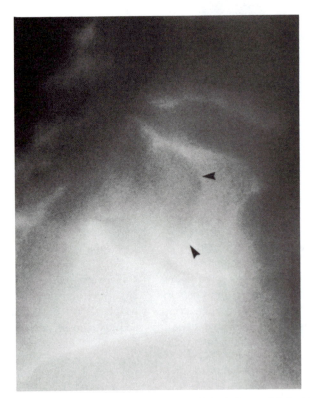

Figure 6–8. Multiple myeloma. *From Banna M: Clinical Radiology of the Spine and Spinal Cord. Rockville, Md, Aspen, 1985, p 350. Reprinted with permission of Aspen Publishers, Inc.*

Radiographs. Lytic and blastic destruction of the vertebral body or posterior elements. Reactive periosteal new bone perpendicular to the surface of the cortex ("sunburst") is more common in long bones, but not pathognomonic.

Treatment. Osteosarcoma is a systemic illness requiring combined therapies depending on presentation, most centered around combination chemotherapy.

Ewing's Sarcoma

Highly malignant tumor of uncertain origin (Fig 6–11).

Clinical Features. Most commonly occurs in childhood to young adults. Presents with pain, low-grade fever, leukocytosis, and increased erythrocyte sedimentation rate. Although not frequently originating in spine, it metastasizes to vertebral bodies, rapidly progressing to produce neurologic symptoms by compression, including paraplegia. By the time of presentation, metastases to other bones, lungs, liver, lymph nodes, and brain have already occurred (Fig 6–12).[13]

Radiographs and Treatment. Ewing's sarcoma is radiosensitive, but this is only palliative. Combination chemotherapy has recently been very effective. Surgery of the spine is indicated for decompression and stability.

Chordoma

Rare malignant tumor derived from remnants of the notochord (Fig 6–12).

Clinical Features. Most often occurs over age 30, but can occur at any age. Distribution is approximately 50% in the sacrococcygeal area, 33% in the base of the brain, and 15% vertebral, most in the cervical area. The vertebral body is always involved by a slowly growing mass. Although rectal and anal pain can occur, most symptoms are due to the mass effect: constipation, urinary incontinence with sacral tumors, cranial nerve abnormalities from increased intracranial pressure, and neurologic symptoms from nerve root compression in vertebral lesions. A mass is often palpable on rectal examination.

Radiographs. When discovered, most sacral chordomas are quite large. Five-year survival rate is approximately 10%. Although relatively radioresistant, high voltage irradiation is palliative.

Treatment. Surgical extirpation provides the best chance of survival; with recurrence, repeated debulking procedures improve quality of life. Complete resection of vertebral lesions is rarely possible due to instability, but decompression temporarily relieves some neurologic symptoms.

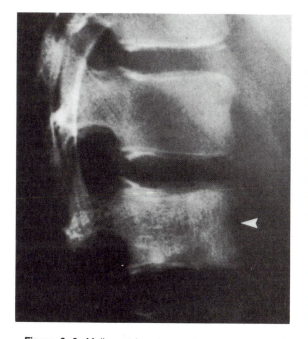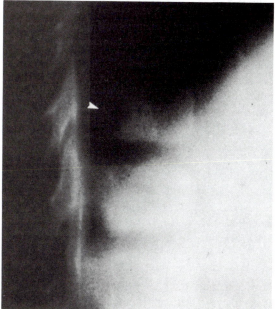

Figure 6–9. Malignant lymphoma. *From Banna M: Clinical Radiology of the Spine and Spinal Cord. Rockville, Md, Aspen, 1985, p 352. Reprinted with permission of Aspen Publishers, Inc.*

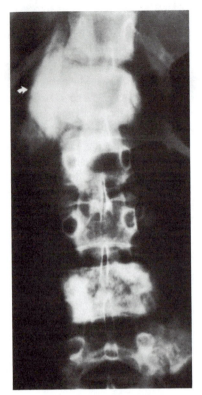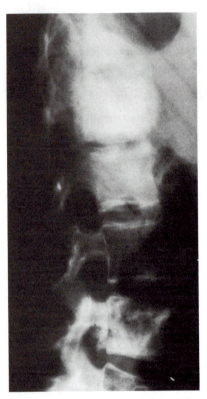

Figure 6–10. Osteosarcoma. *From Banna M: Clinical Radiology of the Spine and Spinal Cord. Rockville, Md, Aspen, 1985, p 357. Reprinted with permission of Aspen Publishers, Inc.*

Secondary Tumors: Metastatic Disease

Metastatic tumors are the most common neoplasm of bone with the greatest propensity for involvement being the spine. Principle primary organs include the breast, kidney, lung, prostate, and thyroid. Transmission is by the blood with metastases taking hold in the marrow.

Clinical Features. Primarily occur in adults, although tumors affecting all age groups can metastasize. Bone involvement can be relatively silent until tumor growth begins to destroy cortex when pain occurs, although pathologic fractures may be the first presentation, particularly in the emergency room setting. In the spine, a relatively small mass can be symptomatic.[14] The typical complaint is pain of variable quality, not fully relieved with rest. If the posterior elements are involved, a mass may be palpated. In the cervical spine, torticollis might be seen. Thoracic involvement causes radicular pain. There is often painful restriction of motion if lumbar vertebrae are affected. Despite significant low back pain, however, the straight leg test is often negative. Hypercalcemia is relatively common, both from osteolysis and production of humoral substances by the tumor. Anemia occurs with significant marrow replacement.

Radiographs. Destructive, typically lytic, but blastic lesions are seen in prostate and occasionally breast metastases. Pain can occur before the lesions are evident on x-ray, but early lesions are seen on technitium scan. Pathologic compression fractures of the vertebral bodies are common, although the disc spaces are often intact, being somewhat more resistant to tumor involvement. Pedicles may be totally absent (Fig 6–13).

Treatment. As metastatic disease is a systemic illness, treatment is specific to the primary tumor and individual case. Radiation and chemotherapy, alone or in combination, often relieve pain and decrease the size of vertebral lesions, but without increasing stability, which might require lightweight braces. Surgical intervention for decompression or stability may be required, but is controversial and highly individual.

☐ SPINAL CORD COMPRESSION

Spinal cord compression by metastatic tumor is a true oncologic emergency. Depending on its location, even a small lesion can cause severe disability. A favorable outcome is dependent on rapid diagnosis and treatment. Estimates of the frequency of cord compression in can-

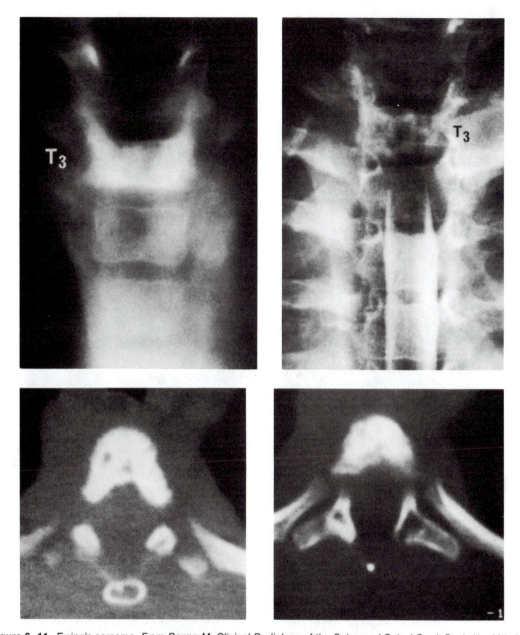

Figure 6–11. Ewing's sarcoma. *From Banna M: Clinical Radiology of the Spine and Spinal Cord. Rockville, Md, Aspen, 1985, p 358. Reprinted with permission of Aspen Publishers, Inc.*

cer patients run between 5 and 10%, most commonly from breast, lung, prostate, kidney, lymphoma, or myeloma.[15] Spread to the epidural space is by direct extension from involved vertebrae or regional lymph nodes or hematagenous spread through radicular arteries or venous plexus. Neurologic effects result from compression by involved vertebrae and tumor mass either directly to the cord or its vascular supply. The most common error of management is not considering the diagnosis, as immediate action can potentially reverse neurologic impairment.

Clinical Features. Regardless of the primary lesion, the clinical presentation is remarkably constant. Pain at the level of the lesion is usually the first complaint, with tenderness on palpation, both due to bony involvement. Radicular symptoms secondary to nerve root compression can be unilateral. Numbness, weakness, and unsteadiness are frequent vague complaints. Neurologic findings correspond to actual cord compression, and frequently occur in sequence. Corticospinal tracts are affected first with motor loss, and notable weakness below the level of the lesion.[16]

Pressure from the expanding mass on the anterior spinothalamic tracts leads to loss of light touch and pain. When the lateral tracts are compressed, tempera-

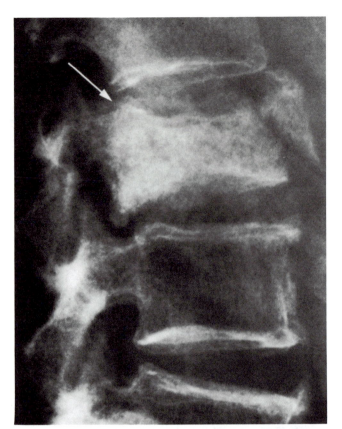

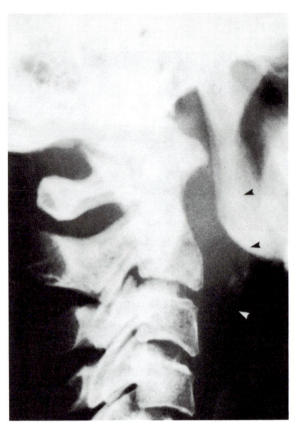

Figure 6–12. Chordoma. *From Banna M: Clinical Radiology of the Spine and Spinal Cord. Rockville, Md, Aspen, 1985, p 355. Reprinted with permission of Aspen Publishers, Inc.*

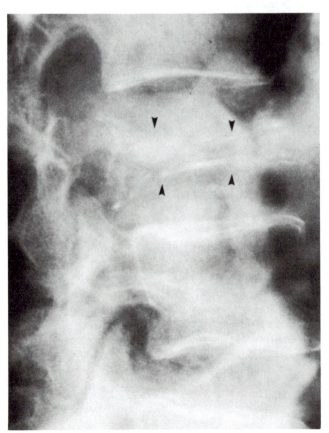

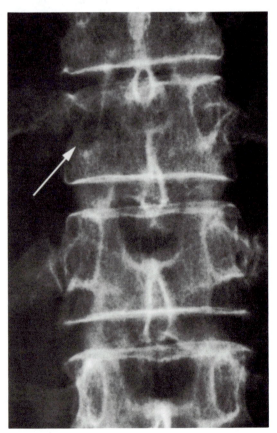

Figure 6–13. Metastatic tumor. *From Banna M: Clinical Radiology of the Spine and Spinal Cord. Rockville, Md, Aspen, 1985, p 333. Reprinted with permission of Aspen Publishers, Inc.*

ture sensation is lost. As posterior compression is a late event, proprioception and deep pressure sensation are rarely affected. Autonomic dysfunction occurs late, frequently with urinary hesitancy and constipation before actual sphincter control is lost.

Radiographs. With a suspicion of spinal cord compression from the history and physical examination, plain x-rays of the entire spine are indicated. They are often positive for osteolytic lesions involving vertebral bodies, vertebral collapse, or loss of pedicles. Osteoblastic lesions are likely with prostatic metastasis and occasionally breast tumors.

Myelography is the diagnostic study of choice to determine both the level and the extent of compression.

Cerebrospinal fluid is collected at the same time for cytology and chemical evaluation.

Treatment. Treatment of spinal cord compression requires a multidisciplinary approach. In patients with compression secondary to known radiosensitive tumors, radiotherapy has been proven to be equally effective as surgery and radiotherapy. Surgical decompression is indicated in compression of unknown cause, relapse after or progression during radiotherapy, and for lesions known to be relatively radioresistant.[17] The benefit of intravenous high-dose steroids to reverse potential compressive effects of edema is controversial, but generally recommended.

□ REFERENCES

1. Friedlaender GE, Southwick WO: Tumors of the spine. In Rothman RH, Simeone FA (eds): The Spine, 2nd ed. Philadelphia, WB Saunders, 1982, p 1022
2. McNab I: Backache. Baltimore, Williams & Wilkins, 1977, p 105
3. Macgee DJ: Cervical, thoracic, lumbar spine. Orthopedic Physical Assessment. Philadelphia, WB Saunders, 1987
4. Francis KP, Hutter VP: Neoplasms of the spine in the aged. Clin Orthop 26:54, 1963
5. Inglis AE, et al: Osteochondroma of the cervical spine: A case report. Clin Orthop 126:127, 1977
6. Fielding JW, et al: Osteoid osteoa of the cervical spine. Clin Orthop 128:163, 1977
7. Goldstein GS, et al: Cervical osteoid osteoa: A cause of chronic upper back pain. Clin Orthop 129:177, 1977
8. Schajowicz F, Lemos D: Malignant osteoblastoma. J Bone Joint Surg 58B:202, 1976
9. Larsson SE, et al: Giant cell tumors of the spine and sacrum causing neurological symptoms. Clin Orthop 111:201, 1975
10. Hay MC, et al: Aneurysmal bone cysts of the spine. J Bone Joint Surg 60B:406, 1978
11. Reimer RR, et al: Lymphoma presenting in bone. Ann Inter Med 87:50, 1977
12. Blaylock RL, Kempe LG: Chondrosarcoma of the cervical spine: Case report. J Neurosurg 44:500, 1976
13. Whitehouse GH, Griffiths GJ: Roentgenologic aspects of spinal involvement by primary and metastatic Ewing's tumor. J Can Assoc Radiol 27:290, 1976
14. Gilbert RW, et al: Epidural spinal cord compression from metastatic tumor and diagnosis and treatment. Ann Neurol 3:40, 1978
15. Posner JB: Neurological complications of systemic cancer. Med Clin North Am 55:625, 1971
16. Rodriguez M, Dinapoli RP: Spinal cord compression, with special reference with metastatic epidural tumors. Mayo Clin Proc 55:442, 1980
17. Stolinski DC: Emergencies in oncology, current management. West J Med 129:169, 1978

PART III

The Cervical Spine

7

Anatomy

☐ INTRODUCTION

Particularly in the acute setting, the emergency physician must have a working knowledge of the anatomy of the complete spine. The spinal column generally includes 33 vertebrae: 7 cervical, 12 thoracic, and 5 lumbar, which are flexible with multiple articulations (Fig 7–1). The sacrum consists of five fused vertebrae and the coccyx includes four or five irregular ossicles. Although there is a gradual transition throughout its length, resulting in specific regional characteristics to be described in detail later, the vertebrae are sufficiently similar to allow for a general description.

Each vertebra has two major parts, the vertebral body and the vertebral arch. The vertebral bodies consist of cancellous bone, generally in the shape of a cylinder (Fig 7–2). They gradually increase in size in a cranial to caudal direction. The vertebral arch is comprised of multiple segments. It is attached to the posterolateral aspects of the vertebral body by two broad pedicles. These are attached posteriorly to the flat lamina, which are in turn connected posteriorly by the spinous process. In this configuration the vertebral body, bilateral pedicles, bilateral laminae, and the posterior spinous process constitute a ring that forms the spinal canal.

At the most lateral aspect of each vertebra near the junction of the pedicle and the lamina, are the transverse processes, which, depending on their location, articulate with the ribs. Also in this area are the articular processes, which form true synovial facet joints between the vertebrae. Although the specific angle of this joint varies considerably depending on location in the spine, the superior articulating surface is always directed dorsally at an angle complementary to the inferior articular surface that is oriented ventrally.

The height of the pedicles is roughly one-half the height of a vertebral body, as it emanates from the upper part of the posterior aspect of the vertebral body. This creates both a superior and larger inferior notch.

When stacked together, these inferior and superior notches combine to form the intervertebral foramina, through which pass the neural and vascular structures of the spinal column.

☐ VERTEBRAE

The first seven vertebrae in the spinal column constitute the cervical spine. The first two, the atlas and the axis, are quite distinct, whereas the third through the seventh are quite similar and share much the same description. Located at the top of the spinal column, they support the least amount of weight. The vertebral body is relatively small as compared to the vertebral arch and the spinal canal. The superior surface of the vertebral body is concave, although its lateral edges turn upward forming the uncinate processes (Fig 7–2). The inferior surface is convex; it slopes downward from back to front.

The transverse processes in the cervical spine are quite distinct (Fig 7–2). Emanating from the vertebral body and the root of the pedicle is a rudimentary rib forming the anterior tubercle of the transverse process. This is fused to the true transverse process that lies more posterior. Together the vertebral body, the anterior tubercle, two transverse processes, and the costotransverse lamela form a ring, the transverse foramen, through which passes the vertebral artery except at C-7 where it contains the vertebral vein. More laterally the anterior tubercle and the true transverse process, together with the vertebral body, form the lateral walls of a groove, through which passes the ventral ramus of each spinal nerve. As seen throughout the rest of the vertebral column, the inferior and superior components of this groove are formed by the superior and inferior pedicles.

Immediately posterior to the transverse process and the transverse foramen are the articular processes. In the articulating cervical spine, these articular proc-

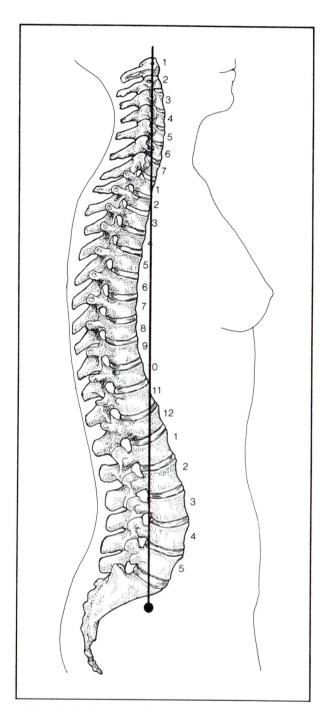

Figure 7–1. Anteroposterior and lateral view of the entire spine.

spinous processes; those of the sixth and seventh vertebrae are singular and progressively longer, the largest being C-7, which is also called the vertebra prominens. The seventh cervical vertebra is a transition vertebra. Although its superior components are more typical of the other cervical vertebrae, the lower seventh cervical vertebra is more like a thoracic vertebra; the body is larger, the articulating facets are more steeply angled, and the anterior tubercle of the transverse process occasionally is more prolonged forming the cervical rib.

The atlantoaxial complex (C-1 and C-2) can also be seen as transitional vertebrae (Fig 7–3). Although appearing grossly quite distinct, they possess all the features of a typical vertebra. The inferior surface of the axis (C-2) is similar to other cervical vertebrae. The laminae are heavy, the spinous processes bifid. The transverse process is heavy as well and includes the tranverse foramen but does not have an anterior tubercle (Fig 7–4).

The upper half of the atlas has a very different morphology (Fig 7–5). The superior facets face upward and outward and are slightly convex. They are relatively large to support the axis and the cranium. Most distinctive, however, is the anterior vertebral body, which projects upward in the form of the odontoid process, the "stolen" body of the first cervical vertebra. The odontoid process or dens has a somewhat narrow base and projects superiorly to the level of the foramen magnum. The dens is faceted anteriorly where it articulates with the posterior aspect of the anterior arch of the atlas.

The atlas, too, has an irregular shape but includes most of the elements of the lower cervical vertebrae, with the exception of a true vertebral body, which it borrows from C-2 in the form of a dens. The overall width of the atlas is greater than the other cervical vertebrae to accommodate articulations with the occiput superiorly. The lateral masses actually include both the pedicles and the articular pillars. The superior articular facets face upward and internally and are concave to accept the occiptal condyles. The inferior facets face downward and internally to articulate with the axis, thus transmitting the weight of the head from the broader base of the occiput focused down to the axis. The larger transverse diameter of the atlas allows for the correspondingly larger diameter of the spinal canal at this level.

Protruding somewhat into the spinal canal are two bony prominences that give rise to the transverse ligament, which maintains the dens in the anterior one-third of the canal. The transverse processes have no costal elements. There is no transverse foramen; the vertebral arteries pass up from C-2 and progress posteriorly around the lateral masses in a groove toward the posterior arches.

esses meet to form posterolateral bony columns. Together with the stacked vertebral bodies, it is apparent that the cervical spine is stacked in the configuration of a bony tripod.

The lamina of the cervical spine are thin and meet posteriorly to form the spinous processes. The third, fourth, and fifth cervical vertebrae usually have bifid

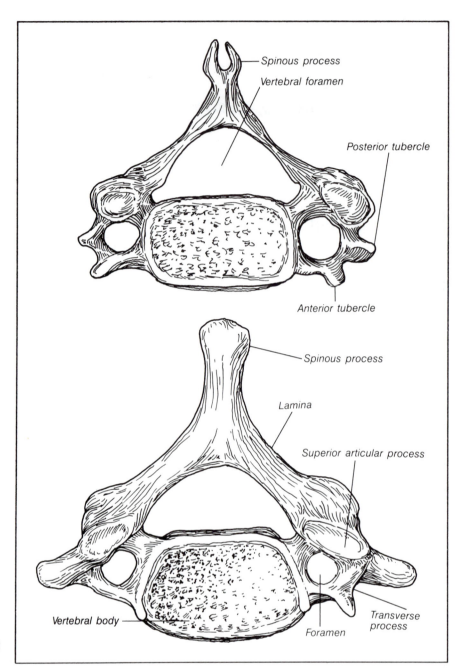

Figure 7–2. Typical lower cervical vertebrae.

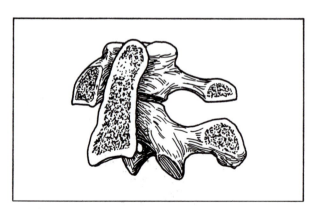

Figure 7–3. Sagittal section of the atlas and the axis.

□ LIGAMENTS AND INTERVERTEBRAL DISCS

Although the vertebrae provide the bony support and protection of the spinal column, the ligaments and intervertebral discs allow for stability and flexibility. The anterior and posterior longitudinal ligaments course the entire length of the spine and are its major stabilizers (Fig 7–6). The anterior longitudinal ligament is comprised of a series of strong fibers that interconnect the anterior surfaces of the vertebral bodies. It is narrowest

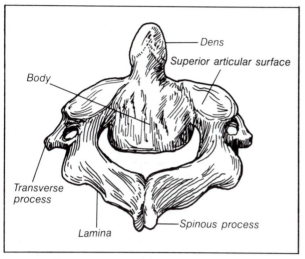

Figure 7–4. The axis as seen from above.

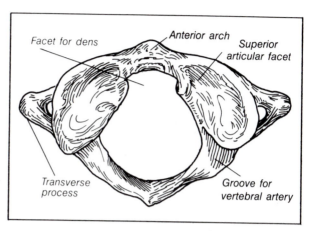

Figure 7–5. The atlas as seen from above.

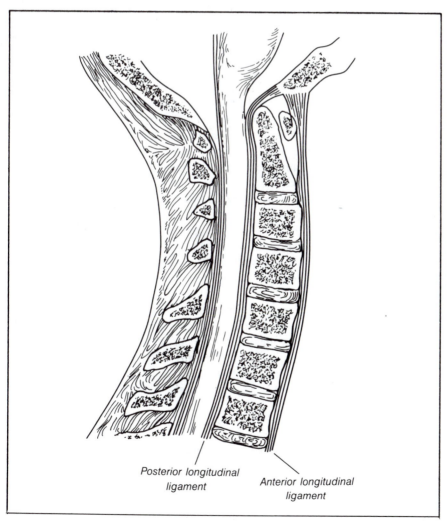

Posterior longitudinal
ligament

Anterior longitudinal
ligament

Figure 7–6. Lateral view of the anterior and posterior longitudinal ligaments of the cervical spine.

at the cervical spine but becomes gradually wider throughout its course. From the level of the axis it extends upward and attaches to the atlas and becomes comingled with the anterior atlanto-occipital membrane. Where it attaches to the vertebral body it forms part of the periosteum, its strongest adherence being at the anterior lip of the body. It is only loosely attached to the intervertebral disc.

The posterior longitudinal ligament, on the other hand, is widest at the level of the cervical spine and narrows as it courses the entire column. This is necessary (as it lies within the spinal canal) to allow relatively more room for the cord and neural elements. It is attached most closely to the lateral aspects of the posterior vertebral body, in a sense strung across the concave posterior body to allow room for vascular elements. At the level of the disc the posterior longitudinal ligament is noted to have two distinct layers. A long superficial layer bridges several vertebral elements. The deeper layer runs across the intervertebral disc and acts as a containing band, restraining the disc from protruding into the spinal canal.

The intervertebral discs are smallest at the level of the cervical spine. They are comprised of four parts: the nucleus pulposus at the center of the disc surrounded by the annulus fibrosus and bounded at the vertebral surfaces by two cartilaginous end-plates. Unlike other levels of the spine, cervical discs appear more closely surrounded by bone (Fig 7–7). The concave superior surface and convex inferior surface of the cervical vertebra appear to hold it closely in place. As well, the upper projection of the superior surface of the vertebra creates a lip, called the uncus, which interfaces with the inferior surface of the superior vertebra called the echancrure. Over time, probably due to degenerative changes, the uncus and the echancrure form

the uncovertebral joints referred to as the joints of Lushka.

In the area of the vertebral arches are numerous ligaments (Fig 7–8). In the level of the cervical spine the supraspinous ligaments are broad and are termed the ligamentum nuchae. They extend from the vertebra prominens at C-7 to the external occipital protuberence and are a major stabilizer of the head and the cervical spine. Deep fibers attach to each of the spinous processes. Deep to the ligamentum nuchae are the intraspinous ligaments that connect adjoining spinous processes. The ligamenta flava are highly elastic and are important stabilizers in flexion. The fibers are highly elastic so as not to cause buckling and compression of the dura when relaxed. The ligamenta flava attach to the anterior surface of the vertebral arch of the superior vertebra and extend to the superior margin of the laminae of the inferior vertebra. They are bilateral and merge with the intraspinous ligaments posteriorly and in the fibrous capsule of the synovial joint anteriorly. The facet joints are true synovial joints with fibrous capsules.

The ligaments of the cervicocranium are quite different and specialized (Figs 7–8 and 7–9). From the level of the axis, the anterior longitudinal ligament runs cranially, attaching to the anterior arch of the atlas, the occipital membrane, and the occiput anterior to the foramen magnum. The posterior longitudinal ligament becomes part of the tectorial membrane, which passes over the odontoid and affixes to the occiput at the level of the hypoglossal canals inside the skull. Deep to the tectorial membrane is the crural ligament, which contains the transverse ligament. The transverse ligament extends across the anterior aspect of the atlantal ring running along the facet on the posterior aspect of the odontoid process. Longitudinal bundles extending from the transverse ligament course the odontoid process inferiorly and superiorly.

Accessory atlantoaxial ligaments fan out from the base of the dens upward to the lateral masses of the atlas. The apical ligament runs from the apex of the dens to the anterior rim of the foramen magnum. The dens is further fixed to the foramen magnum by the alar ligaments coursing from the dens to the lateral margins of the foramen magnum. True synovial joints exist between the dens and the atlas and the occipital condyles and the atlas.

□ STABILITY AND MOBILITY

The spinal column is particularly remarkable in that it provides a bony protective encasement for the spinal

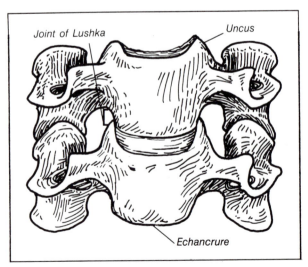

Figure 7–7. Anterior cross-sectional view of a cervical disc.

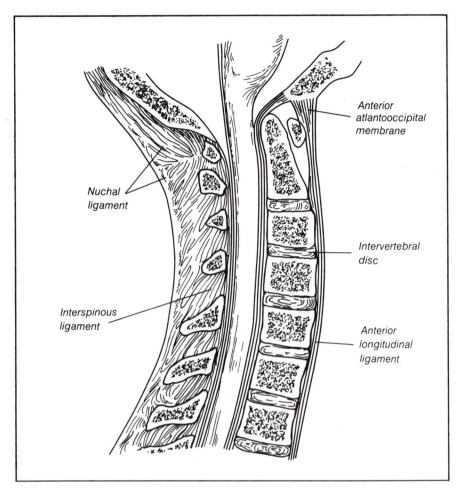

Figure 7–8. Lateral view of the ligament of the upper cervical spine.

Anterior atlantooccipital membrane

Nuchal ligament

Intervertebral disc

Interspinous ligament

Anterior longitudinal ligament

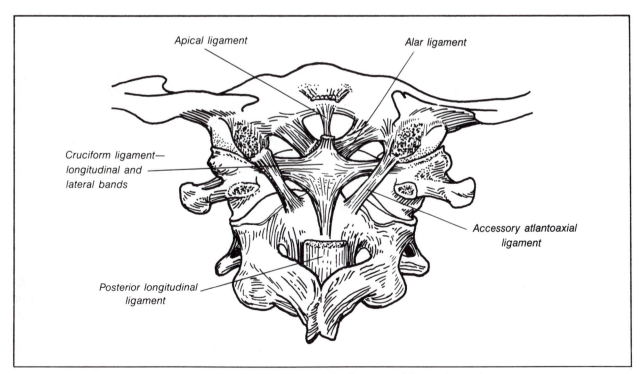

Apical ligament

Alar ligament

Cruciform ligament— longitudinal and lateral bands

Accessory atlantoaxial ligament

Posterior longitudinal ligament

Figure 7–9. Posterior cross-section of the ligaments of the cervicocranium.

cord, while at the same time allows significant flexibility of movement. This is made possible by a series of small stacked vertebrae, each with multiple articulations. Although movement between adjacent vertebrae is limited, some of these movements allow for considerable mobility. Although movement is facilitated by the muscles, stability is facilitated by the ligaments and bony opposition.

The most flexible segment of the spinal column is the cervical spine area. The atlanto-occipital joints provide flexion and extension as well as minimal lateral movement, all of these limited by the atlanto-occipital musculature. These articulations allow for approximately one-half of cervical flexion.

One-half of the rotational mobility of the cervical spine is provided by the atlantoaxial articulations, limited by the alar ligaments and the atlantoaxial facet joints. The lower cervical spine is the most mobile segment of the entire spinal column, made possible by the relatively thick intervertebral discs and the sloping anteroinferior lips of the vertebral bodies, which slide over subjacent vertebrae. Flexion is limited by the posterior ligaments and the muscles, but a firm end point is provided by the chin striking the chest in extreme flexion. Extreme extension, on the other hand, is limited only by anterior structures, the anterior longitudinal ligament and the anterior cervical components. Total flexion extension mobility of the cervical spine is approximately 90 degrees, but without a firm anatomic end point, such as the chin anteriorly, forceful extension can result in severe trauma.

The articular pillars and an intertransverse ligament prevent significant lateral flexion in the cervical spine. The shoulders also provide an anatomic end point of lateral flexion.

Actual movement of the cervical spine is controlled by the surrounding muscles running from the skull and the mandible to the upper thoracic vertebrae and the rib cage with numerous attachments to the cervical spine. Table 7–1 lists those muscles in the cervical area involved in flexion, extension, rotation, and lateral flexion. Figures 7–10 to 7–13 demonstrate their locations.

□ SPINAL CORD AND NERVE ROOTS

At the level of the cervical spine, the spinal cord itself is relatively large to supply nerves to the upper extremities. To accommodate the spinal cord, as well as to allow additional room for flexibility, the cervical canal is correspondingly large and relatively roomy, particularly at the level of the atlas. The cord is covered by

TABLE 7–1. MUSCLES IN THE CERVICAL AREA

Extension
Splenius capitis
Splenius cervicis
Semispinalis capitis
Semispinalis cervicis
Longissimus capitis
Longissimus cervicis
Trapezius
Interspinales
Rectus capitis posterior major
Rectus capitis posterior minor
Obliquus capitis superior
Sternocleidomastoid (posterior fibers)

Flexion
Sternocleidomastoid (anterior fibers)
Longus colli
Longus capitis
Rectus capitis anterior

Rotation and lateral flexion
Sternocleidomastoid
Scalene group
Splenius capitis
Splenius cervicis
Longissimus capitis
Levator scapulae
Longus colli
Iliocostalis cervicis
Multifidi
Intertransversarii
Obliquus capitis inferior
Obliquus capitis superior
Rectus capitis lateralis

Note: Anatomically, these muscles can also be grouped according to their positional relationship.
From Sherk HH, Parke WW: Normal adult anatomy. In Bailey RW (ed): The Cervical Spine. The Cervical Spine Research Society. Philadelphia, JB Llppincott, 1983, pp 14–15.

the dura, arachnoid, and pia mater. The dura runs immediately posterior to the posterior longitudinal ligament and surrounds each of the spinal roots to the level of the intravertebral foramen. The arachnoid is closely applied to the dura, and the arachnoid space contains cerebrospinal fluid to insulate the cord. The pia mater is closely applied to the spinal cord. At its most lateral extent, it is arranged in a fold that runs linearly the length of the spinal medulla, from which arise approximately 20 dentate ligaments on each side (Fig 7–14). The dentate ligaments attach to the dura mater and act as stabilizers; the dura is relatively mobile, but the pia and the spinal medulla remain relatively fixed.

In flexion, the dura is equal to the length of the cervical canal. In extension, the canal shortens and the dura bulges. The cord itself is somewhat stretched, both in flexion and in extension of the neck, but is held relatively fixed by the nerve roots and the dentate ligaments. Overflexion or extension is prevented by the ligaments and bony structure, but these preventive

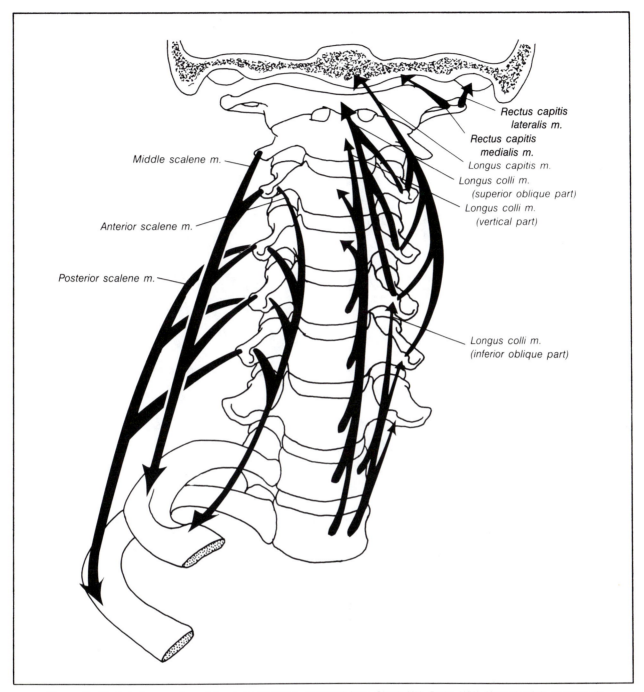

Middle scalene m.

Anterior scalene m.

Posterior scalene m.

Rectus capitis
    lateralis m.
Rectus capitis
    medialis m.
Longus capitis m.
Longus colli m.
    (superior oblique part)
Longus colli m.
    (vertical part)

Longus colli m.
    (inferior oblique part)

Figure 7–10. Anterior muscles of the cervical spine. *Adapted from Sherk HH, Parke WW: Normal adult anatomy. In Bailey RW (ed): The Cervical Spine. The Cervical Spine Research Society. Philadelphia, JB Lippincott, 1983.*

mechanisms cannot withstand the forces of a violent injury.

Unlike the thoracic and lumbar spine, the cervical nerve roots emerge from the spinal canal above their corresponding vertebrae (Fig 7–15). As such their total number is eight. The first two cervical nerves pass behind the corresponding articular masses, whereas all other cervical nerves are in front of the articular masses. The upper three or four cervical nerves become

a part of the cervical plexus; the lower five join the first thoracic nerve to form the brachial plexus. The dermatomes and nerves formed by the corresponding plexus are demonstrated in Figures 7–16 and 7–17. Muscle innervation is usually quite constant; however, sensory distribution can be quite variable. This can occassionally be confusing clinically when sensory and motor findings secondary to injury or space-occupying lesions do not correspond.

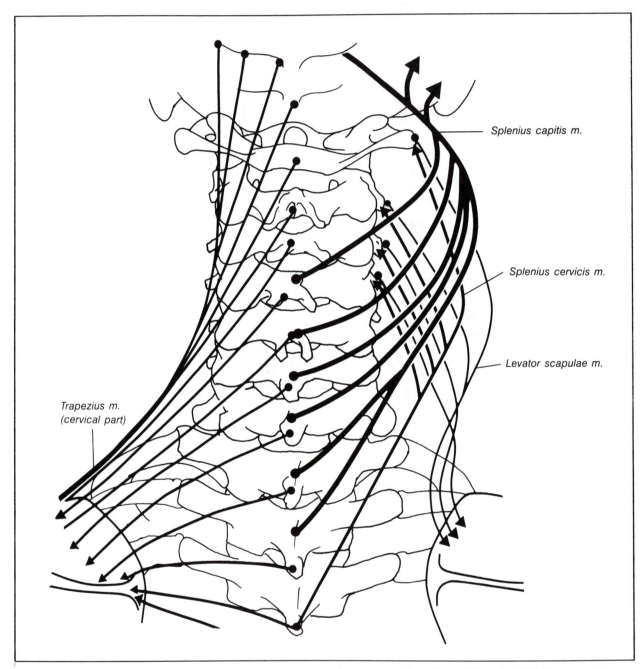

Splenius capitis m.

Splenius cervicis m.

Levator scapulae m.

Trapezius m.
(cervical part)

Figure 7–11. Superficial muscles of the posterior cervical spine. *Adapted from Sherk HH, Parke WW: Normal adult anatomy. In Bailey RW (ed): The Cervical Spine. The Cervical Spine Research Society. Philadelphia, JB Lippincott, 1983.*

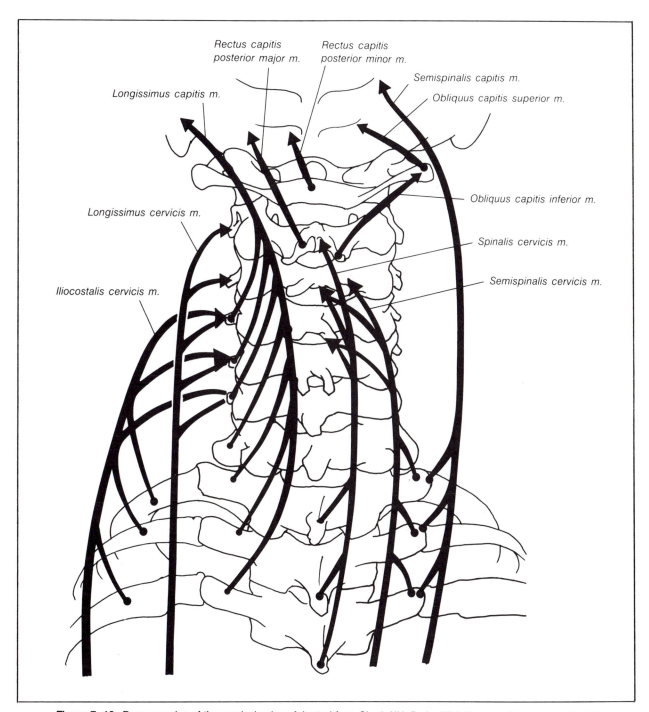

Figure 7–12. Deep muscles of the cervical spine. *Adapted from Sherk HH, Parke WW: Normal adult anatomy. In Bailey RW (ed): The Cervical Spine. The Cervical Spine Research Society. Philadelphia, JB Lippincott, 1983.*

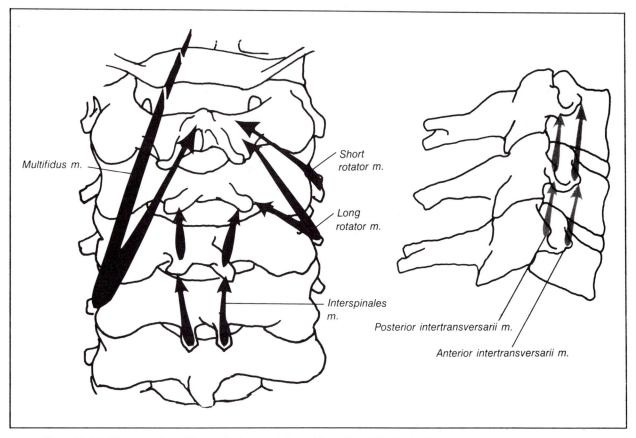

Figure 7–13. Short muscles of the cervical spine. *Adapted from Sherk HH, Parke WW: Normal adult anatomy. In Bailey RW (ed): The Cervical Spine. The Cervical Spine Research Society. Philadelphia, JB Lippincott, 1983.*

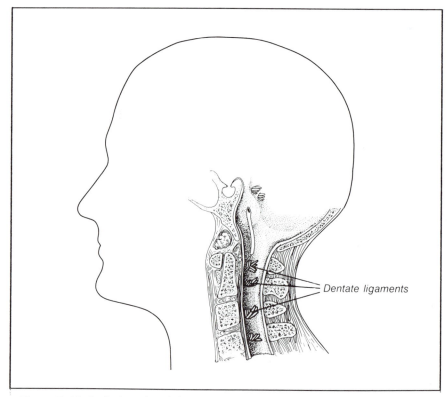

Figure 7–14. Sagittal section of the upper cervical spine including dentate ligaments.

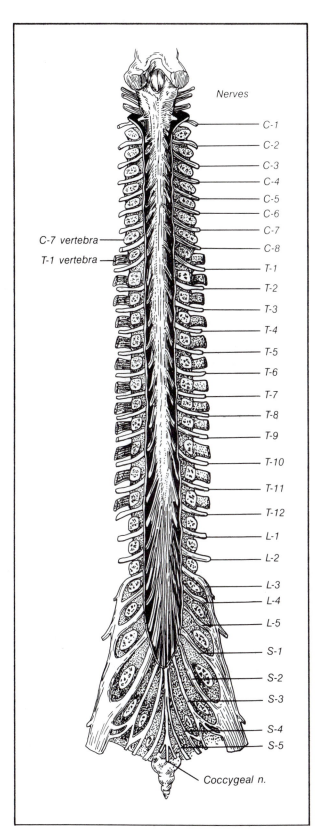

Nerves

C-1
C-2
C-3
C-4
C-5
C-6
C-7
C-8
T-1
T-2
T-3
T-4
T-5
T-6
T-7
T-8
T-9
T-10
T-11
T-12
L-1
L-2
L-3
L-4
L-5
S-1
S-2
S-3
S-4
S-5

C-7 vertebra
T-1 vertebra

Coccygeal n.

Figure 7–15. Dorsal view of the spinal canal and nerve roots.

□ ARTERIES AND VEINS

A major source of blood supply to the cervical spine and cord is the vertebral arteries (Fig 7–18). Arising from the subclavian arteries, the vertebral arteries pass bilaterally through the foramen transversarium and extend to the atlas where they run posteriorly around the lateral masses and over the posterior arch of C-1, passing through the foramen magnum. Just before joining to the basilar artery they give off two branches that fuse and descend anterior to the spinal cord as the anterior spinal artery. At the same level the vertebral arteries yield to posterior spinal arteries that descend the posterior aspect of the spinal cord and yield a series of plexiform channels. The cervical vertebrae are principally supplied by branches from the vertebral arteries. Small segmental branches of the vertebral arteries run superiorly at the level of the axis to supply the dens and anastomose with descending branches from the carotid artery along the alar ligaments.

Of clinical significance is the course of the vertebral arteries through the foramen transversarium and most superiorly the level of the atlas. Degenerative changes of the vertebrae can cause significant compression on the artery resulting in vertebral artery syndrome with dizziness and drop attacks.

Venous blood from the cord returns through fine plexus in the pia by six longitudinal channels: three anterior and three posterior. The veins in the vertebral column are arranged in two plexuses; the external venous plexus is composed of two anastomosing parts, one anterior to the vertebrae, the other posterior, on the posterior surface of the vertebral arches (Fig 7–19). The interior venous plexus is within the vertebral canal between the dura and bone. lt is composed of four main channels, two anterior along the posterior surfaces of the vertebral bodies bilaterally, and two posterior, on either side of the midline, anterior to the vertebral arches. This valveless system runs the length of the spinal cord and interconnects with veins from all parts of the body. This is clinically significant in that it allows for direct hematogenous spread of metastases to the spinal cord and the column.

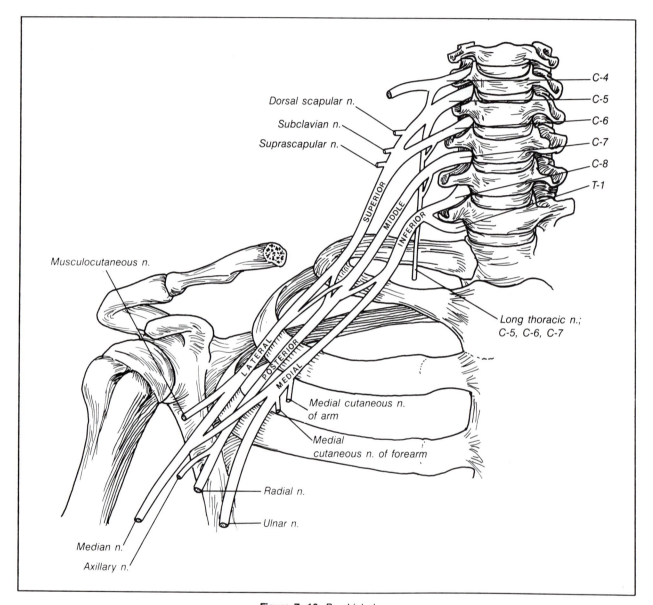

Figure 7–16. Brachial plexus.

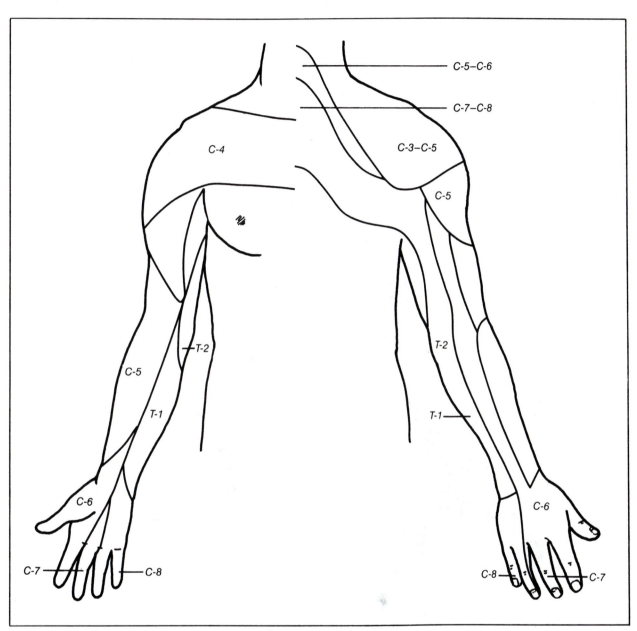

Figure 7–17. Cutaneous dermatomes of the brachial plexus.

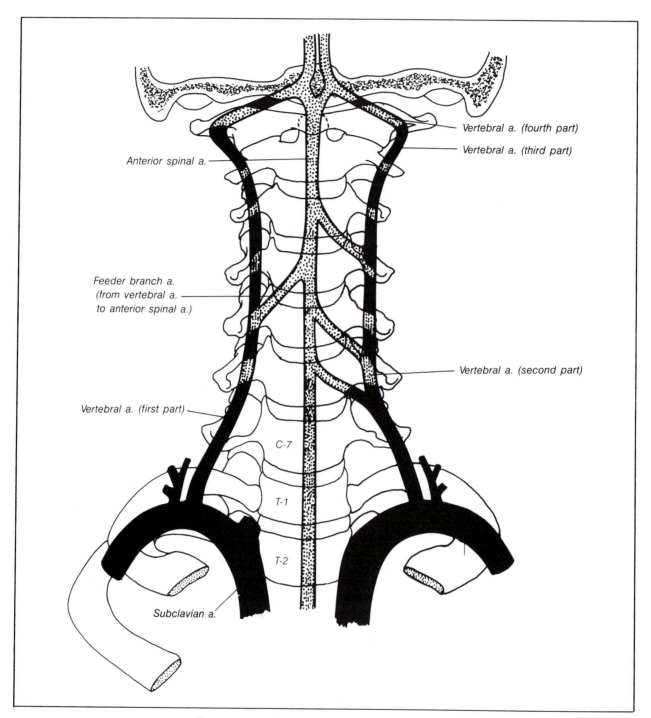

Figure 7–18. The vertebral and anterior spinal arteries.

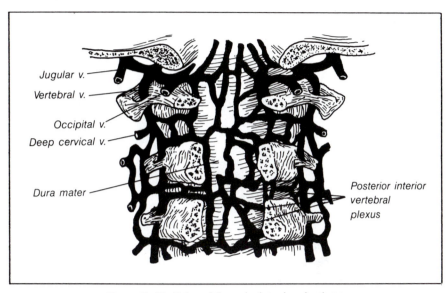

Jugular v.
Vertebral v.
Occipital v.
Deep cervical v.
Dura mater
Posterior interior vertebral plexus

Figure 7–19. Veins of the spinal cord and column.

☐ BIBLIOGRAPHY

Clemente CD: Anatomy, A Regional Atlas of the Human Body. Philadelphia, Lea and Febiger, 1975

Ellis H: Clinical Anatomy. London, Blackwell Scientific Publications, 1976

Goss CM: Gray's Anatomy of the Human Body. Philadelphia, Lea and Febiger, 1975

Jeffreys SE: Disorders of the Cervical Spine. London, Butterworths, 1980

McMinn RMH, Hutching RT: Color Atlas of Human Anatomy. Chicago, Yearbook Medical Publ, 1977

Pansky B, House EL: Review of Gross Anatomy. New York, Macmillan, 1975

Parke WW: Applied anatomy of the spine. In Rothman RH, Simeone FA (eds): The Spine. Philadelphia, WB Saunders, 1982

Sherk HH, Parke WW, Normal adult anatomy. In Bailey RW (ed): The Cervical Spine. The Cervical Spine Research Society. Philadelphia, JB Lippincott, 1983

8

Physical Examination

At the outset, it cannot be stressed too emphatically that in the emergency setting extreme care must be taken in examination of patients with spinal complaints. Particularly, patients with cervical pain, either from severe trauma, trivial strain, or years of discomfort, require cautious handling by the examiner until or unless cervical instability has been ruled out, either clinically or radiographically, or both. Although the examiner's approach may differ for the patient on a long board and full cervical-spine precautions than for the ambulatory patient with a "crick" in the neck, all patients require a thorough examination including inspection, palpation, range of motion, neurologic assessment, and, where appropriate, percussion and auscultation.

What follows is a thorough presentation of the complete physical examination aimed more for the ambulatory patient with cervical complaints. Although still applicable to the multiply traumatized patient, the reader is directed to Chapter 1, which discusses emergency evaluation of acute spinal trauma. Emergency medicine specialists need not be reminded that patients with specific localized complaints also merit a complete and thorough history and physical examination.

☐ INSPECTION

Thorough observation should include examination of posture, movements, and gait. How the patient moves about, rising from a seated position, walking about the examination room, undressing, and climbing onto the examination table can reveal important information. Posture, either sitting, standing, or supine, the presence of increased lordosis, kyphosis, scoliosis, should be noted. Normal head, neck, and arm movements while speaking might betray mild cervical pathology. The gait should be even and flowing and the head held naturally perpendicular to the floor. Observe for the normal cervical lordosis and even carriage of the shoulders.

The supraclavicular area should be carefully examined for asymmetry. Deformity of the clavicle could suggest previous fracture or, more medially, sterno-clavicular joint dislocation or inflammation. Observe the shoulders and the upper extremities for asymmetry. Unilateral muscle wasting can suggest cervical nerve root compression or thoracic outlet syndrome.

Observe the skin for scars or old incisions, ecchymoses, erythema, or nodules. Observe the neck for asymmetry either due to congenital deformation or severe muscle spasm. The chin should be in the midline, but may be deviated either toward or away from the painful side. With severe pain, the patient may support the chin with the hands to relax painful muscles or distract inflamed joints. The patient might also walk delicately so as to avoid painful jarring of the neck. From the back, observe the posterior chest. There should be overall symmetry. Displacement of the scapulae could suggest trapezius muscle spasm from trauma or weakness due to spinal accessory nerve damage. Winging of the scapulae suggests weak serratus anterior muscles.

Cervical spine movements of flexion, extension, lateral bend, and rotation should also be observed, but will be discussed later in this chapter.

☐ PALPATION

Bony Structure
Palpation of the cervical vertebrae is easiest in the thinner patient. This is best accomplished in the supine position, but certain structures, particularly the lower spinous processes and facet joints, are better palpated in the prone or sitting position.

Posterior
Bony palpation of the posterior cervical spine begins at the occiput and the inion, the dome-shaped prominence at the base of the skull on the midline (Fig 8–1). The

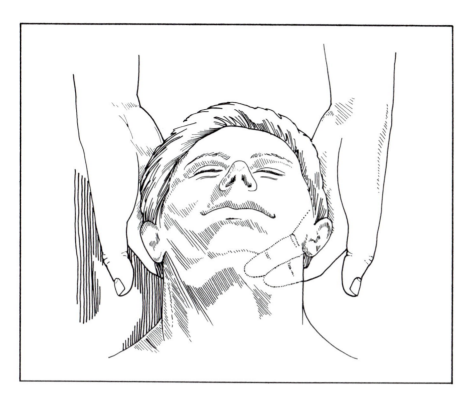

Figure 8–1. Palpation of the base of the skull and the inion. (See Fig 8–4.)

examiner should palpate laterally for tenderness or deformities along the base of the skull toward the mastoid processes (Fig 8–2). Returning to the midline, the examiner should palpate caudally. The next bony prominence will be the spinous process of the axis; the posterior arch of the atlas is generally inaccessible (Fig 8–3). In a stepwise fashion, the examiner can frequently palpate all of the spinous processes from C-2 to C-7, the vertebra prominens, and T-1. In the thin and well-relaxed patient, the bifid nature of the spinous processes C-3 to C-6 can be distinguished.

As can be seen in Figure 8–4, anterior structures can help determine the precise cervical vertebra being palpated. The thyroid cartilage overlies C-4 and C-5, the first cricoid ring aligns with C-6. Size alone frequently distinguishes C-7, but in some individuals, T-1

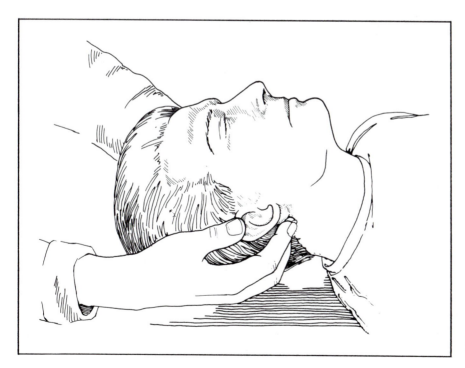

Figure 8–2. Palpation of the mastoid processes.

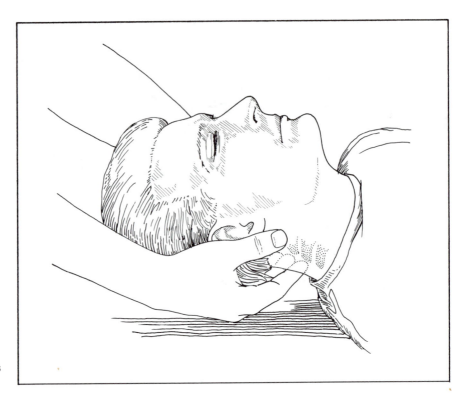

Figure 8–3. Spinous process palpation.

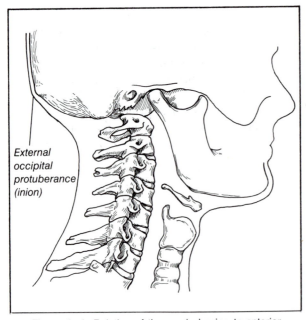

External occipital protuberance (inion)

Figure 8–4. Relation of the cervical spine to anterior structures in the neck.

may be more prominent. As a transitional vertebra between the cervical and thoracic spines, C-7 typically remains stationary with flexion and extension of the neck, whereas C-6 will move forward and backward, respectively.

Pressure on the spinous processes by palpation is transmitted anteriorly to the arches toward the vertebral bodies, eliciting tenderness from inflamed areas.

The facet joints at each cervical level can be palpated approximately 1 to 3 millimeters lateral to and between the spinous processes on each side (Fig 8–5). Tenderness to palpation can be elicited in such conditions as posterior facet syndrome, spondylosis, and facet subluxation or dislocation. Inflammation most typically occurs at the level of greatest cervical mobility between C-5 and C-7. Complete relaxation is required to palpate the joints themselves. If overlying muscles are in severe spasm, an attempt should be made to palpate the facet joints around the involved muscle belly. In the more obese patient, pressure from palpation can be transmitted to the facet joints despite the inability to palpate the structure itself.

Lateral

Although the posterior arch of the atlas is inaccessible to palpation, the transverse processes of C-1 are relatively easy to locate (Fig 8–4). Moving inferiorly from the mastoid processes along the lateral neck, the next bony prominence encountered will be the transverse process of the atlas. It is the broadest transverse process of all the cervical spine, and slight bilateral pressure will cause mild discomfort. Moving further inferiorly and slightly anteriorly, following the cervical lordotic curve, the examiner might be able to appreciate other transverse processes, but only with complete muscle relaxation in the thin patient. Being somewhat more prominent, the anterior tubercule of the transverse process of C-6 can be appreciated at the level of the cricoid

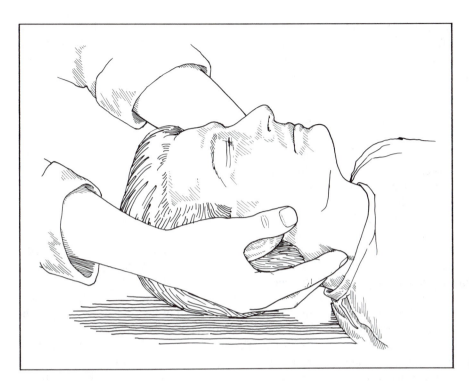

Figure 8–5. Facet joint palpation.

ring. It is recommended that this structure not be palpated simultaneously bilaterally as the carotid arteries pass superficially at this point. Bilateral compression can restrict arterial flow.

Anterior

Palpation of the bony cartilaginous structures of the anterior neck is done at the patient's side. Beneath the mandible and slightly anteriorly, the lateral aspects of the U-shaped hyoid bone are palpable (Fig 8–4). Using the thumb and the index finger, it can be grasped bilaterally, causing slight discomfort to the patient. Movement can be detected as the patient swallows. Inferior to the hyoid bone, the broad thyroid cartilage is easy to palpate. Superiorly, the physician can detect the superior notch and the large prominent Adam's apple. The thyroid cartilage gradually tapers and overlies the C-4 and C-5 vertebrae.

Immediately below the thyroid cartilage is the cricothyroid membrane. Immediately below this level is the cricoid ring that overlies C-6. At this level, the anterior tubercle of the transverse process of C-6 can be appreciated laterally.

Further inferiorly, the examiner can palpate the thyroid gland and cartilaginous rings.

At the level of the superior sternal notch, the physician can palpate the manubrium and extend laterally to palpate the sternoclavicular joint. Further laterally, the examiner can trace the clavicle out to the shoulders.

Superior to the clavicle is a supraclavicular fossa, which should be a smooth depression. Bony irregularities that can be palpated at this level include calculus from a previous fracture of the clavicle or the ribs.

Soft Tissues

After concentrating on the bony structures of the neck, the examiner should now palpate the same areas, this time paying particular attention to the soft tissues. The sternocleidomastoid muscle is used to divide the neck into the anterior and posterior components.

Anterior

Once again, the patient is best examined in the supine position. The sternocleidomastoid muscle is generally quite prominent, but it particularly stands out when a patient is asked to turn the head to the opposite side. Palpation of the muscle belly can reveal significant spasm or focal hematomas due to hyperextension. It is particularly prominent in painfully spastic torticollis. Comparison with the muscle on the other side can help to discern differences in strength and size.

Just medial to the sternocleidomastoid muscle bilaterally is a chain of anterior lymph nodes. In an otherwise healthy individual they might not be palpable, but can be enlarged due to ear, throat, or upper respiratory infection, tumor, or metastatic involvement.

Also medial to the sternocleidomastoid and best palpable at the level of the cricoid cartilage are the carotid pulses. These should be palpated bilaterally, but care should be taken to do one side at a time so as not to restrict flow to the head. This is one area in the examination of the neck where auscultation is helpful to appreciate bruits of the carotid arteries.

Just anterior to the superior insertion of the sternocleidomastoid, the parotid gland is located, running over the angle of the mandible. Although normally not distinctly palpable, patients may complain of discomfort to palpation. The gland does become palpable in pathologic states of obstruction, tumor, Sjögren's syndrome, and mumps.

The inferior insertion of the sternocleidomastoid at the clavicle delineates the anterior aspect of the supraclavicular fossa. When normal, this area should be a smooth depression. Careful examination can reveal abnormal swelling, inflamed supraclavicular lymph nodes, cervical ribs, abnormal fibrous bands, abnormalities of the platysma muscle (which normally is smooth, flat, and unobtrusive unless pathologically involved). Deep to the platysma muscle in the supraclavicular fossa, the scalene muscles can be palpated. With significant ligamentous damage due to hyperextension of the cervical spine, the scalene muscles will be in spasm and painful. The subclavian artery and vein and the brachial plexus pass between the scalene muscles (Fig 8–6). Compression of these structures due to the thoracic outlet syndromes can lead to sensory and vascular abnormalities in the upper extremities, resulting in significant local tenderness of the supraclavicular fossa and the presence of poststenotic arterial

dilatations. Particularly because of the latter, the area should also be auscultated for bruits. A Pancoast tumor arising from the apex of the lung can grow into the space and result in swelling, asymmetry, and pain, and may present as a thoracic outlet syndrome.

Posterior

Palpation of the soft tissues of the posterior aspect of the neck is best accomplished with the patient in the sitting position. Often, however, this is uncomfortable for the patient in acute pain, as it requires active muscular activity to maintain the head erect. In such a case, it is helpful to examine the patient in the prone position.

The trapezius muscle is the most superficial structure in the back of the neck, extending vertically from the inion to T-12 and horizontally to the acromioclavicular joint (Fig 8–7). Examination should begin superiorly, palpating along each of the spinous processes. The muscle is frequently injured due to significant forces of extension, flexion, lateral flexion, and rotation. Indirectly, patients complain of soreness in the trapezius area after hyperextension or whiplash injuries due to rapid reflex straightening of the cervical spine. Simultaneous bilateral palpation will reveal changes in muscle tone, swelling, or asymmetry. The area of maximal tenderness is generally superior, along the broad muscle belly extending from the midline of the cervical spine to the acromioclavicular process.

Deep to the trapezius muscle and just lateral to the spinous processes in the cervical spine are the erector spinae muscles. Although not directly palpable, in the event of significant hyperextension or whiplash injuries associated with ligamentous damage, the erector spinae muscles are a dynamic stablizer of the posterior neck, and with local injury can be quite tender due to muscle spasm. The superior nuchal ligament extends from the inion to C-7 or T-1 and inserts along the spinous processes (Fig 8–8). In significant hyperflexion injury, this ligament can be torn or stretched. Severe injuries will also result in tearing of the interspinous ligaments, typically in the lower cervical region. Tenderness to deep palpation in this area, associated with a widening of the spinous processes, indicates significant injury.

When inflamed, greater occipital nerves will be tender to palpation as they pass superiorly lateral to the inion, extending bilaterally across the occiput and the parieto-occipital area (Fig 8–9). The syndrome of greater occipital neuritis is frequently attributed to migraine headache, but careful examination in this region can avoid an erroneous diagnosis.

In the case of ear, nose, throat, and scalp infections, the posterior lymph node chain running along the anterolateral aspect of the trapezius muscle will be palpable.

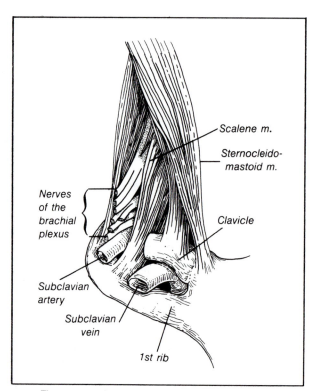

Scalene m.

Sternocleido-mastoid m.

Nerves of the brachial plexus

Clavicle

Subclavian artery

Subclavian vein

1st rib

Figure 8–6. Structures of the supraclavicular area.

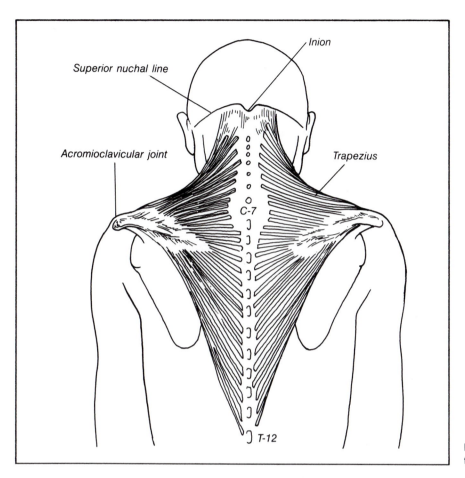

Figure 8–7. Topical landmarks of the posterior cervical spine.

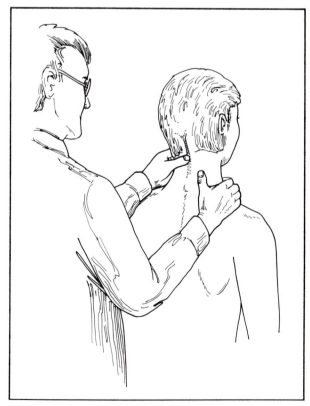

Figure 8–8. The ligamentum nuchae.

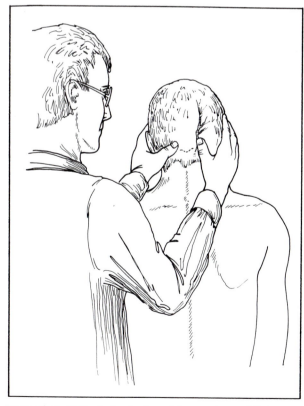

Figure 8–9. Method of palpation of the greater occipital nerve.

TABLE 8–1. MUSCLES OF THE CERVICAL SPINE: THEIR ACTIONS AND NERVE SUPPLY

Action	Muscles Acting	Nerve Supply
Forward flexion of head	1. Rectus capitis anterior	C-1, C-2
	2. Rectus capitis lateralis	C-1, C-2
	3. Longus capitis	C-1, C-2, C-3
	4. Hyoid muscles	Inferior alveolar nerve
		Facial nerve
		Hypoglossal nerve
		Ansa cervicalis
	5. Obliquus capitis superior	C-1
	6. Sternocleidomastoid (if head in neutral or flexion)	Accessory
		C-2
Extension of head	1. Splenius capitis	C-4, C-5, C-6
	2. Semispinalis capitis	C-1–C-8
	3. Longissimus capitis	C-6—C-8
	4. Spinalis capitis	C-6—C-8
	5. Trapezius	Accessory
		C-3, C-4
	6. Rectus capitis posterior minor	C-1
	7. Rectus capitis posterior major	C-1
	8. Obliquus capitis superior	C-1
	9. Obliquus capitis inferior	C-1
	10. Sternocleidomastoid (if head in some extension)	Accessory
		C-2
Rotation of head (Muscles on one side contract)	1. Trapezius (face moves to opposite side)	Accessory
		C-3, C-4
	2. Splenius capitis (face moves to the same side)	C-4–C-6
	3. Longissimus capitis (face moves to same side)	C-6–C-8
	4. Semispinalis capitis (face moves to same side)	C-1–C-8
	5. Obliquus capitis inferior (face moves to same side)	C-1
	6. Sternocleidomastoid (face moves to same side)	Accessory
		C-2
Side flexion of head	1. Trapezius	Accessory
		C-3, C-4
	2. Splenius capitis	C4–C-6
	3. Longissimus capitis	C-6–C-8
	4. Semispinalis capitis	C-1–C-8
	5. Obliquus capitis inferior	C-1
	6. Rectus capitis lateralis	C-1–C-2
	7. Longus capitis	C-1–C-3
Flexion of neck	1. Longus coli	C-2–C-6
	2. Scalenus anterior	C-4–C-6
	3. Scalenus medius	C-3–C-8
	4. Scalenus posterior	C-6–C-8

TABLE 8–1. (*continued*)

Action	Muscles Acting	Nerve Supply
Extension of neck	1. Splenius cervicis	C-6, C-7, C-8
	2. Semispinalis cervicis	C-1–C-6, C-7, C-8
	3. Longissimus cervicis	C-6–C-8
	4. Levator scapulae	C-3–C-4
		Dorsal scapular
	5. Iliocostalis cervicis	C-6, C-7, C-8
	6. Spinalis cervicis	C-6–C-8
	7. Multifidus	C-1–C-6, C-7, C-8
	8. Interspinalis cervicis	C-1–C-8
	9. Trapezius	Accessory
		C-3, C-4
	10. Rectus capitis posterior major	C-1
	11. Rotatores brevis	C-1–C-8
	12. Rotatores longi	C-1–C-8
Side flexion of neck	1. Levator scapulae	C-3–C-4
		Dorsal scapular
	2. Splenius cervicis	C-4–C-6
	3. Iliocostalis cervicis	C-6–C-8
	4. Longissimus cervicis	C-6–C-8
	5. Semispinalis cervicis	C-1–C-8
	6. Multifidus	C-1–C-8
	7. Intertransversarii	C-1–C-8
	8. Scaleni	C-3–C-8
	9. Sternocleidomastoid	Accessory
		C-2
	10. Obliquus capitis inferior	C-1
	11. Rotatores brevis	C-1–C-8
	12. Rotatores longi	C-1–C-8
	13. Longus coli	C-2–C-6
Rotation[a] of neck (Muscles on one side contract)	1. Levator scapulae (face moves to same side)	C-3–C-4
		Dorsal scapular
	2. Splenius cervicis (face moves to same side)	C-4–C-6
	3. Iliocostalis cervicis (face moves to same side)	C-6–C-8
	4. Longissimus cervicis (face moves to same side)	C-6, C-7, C-8
	5. Semispinalis cervicis (face moves to same side)	C-1–C-8
	6. Multifidus (face moves to opposite side)	C-1–C-8
	7. Intertransversarii (face moves to same side)	C-1–C-8
	8. Scaleni (face moves to opposite side)	C-3–C-8
	9. Sternocleidomastoid (face moves to opposite side)	Accessory
		C-2
	10. Obliquus capitis inferior (face moves to same side)	C-1
	11. Rotatores brevis (face moves to same side)	C-1–C-8
	12. Rotatores longi (face moves to same side)	C-1–C-8

[a]Occurs in conjunction with side flexion due to direction of facet joints.
From Magee DJ: Philadelphia, WB Saunders, 1987, pp 28–29.[3]

□ RANGE OF MOTION

There are six basic movements of the neck: flexion, extension, right and left lateral flexion, and right and left rotation. Approximately one-half of the total flexion and extension occurs between the occiput, C-1, and C-2. The remainder of flexion and extension is distributed between the lower cervical vertebrae with proportionately more movement in the extreme lower segments, C-5 through C-7. Lateral flexion is distributed between all of the vertebrae. Rotation occurs in conjunction with lateral movement. Approximately one-half of rotation occurs in the area between the atlas and the axis, the remainder distributed evenly between the lower vertebrae.[1]

Examination of cervical movement entails three aspects: active, passive, and resisted movement. Pathologic processes to the muscles and ligaments of the neck is generally specific, and affects only specific movements. The inability to move the neck at all, therefore, is generally associated with degrees of hysteria. Commonly, at least one or two movements are preserved, although this must be done slowly, with coaxing on the part of the examiner. Although the type of movement limitation will depend on the injury, it is more likely, however, that extension and the combination of rotation with lateral flexion will be disturbed, as these movements more commonly place strain on the facet joint.

Assessing range of motion involves observation and palpation. Observation of muscle symmetry and coordination is primary, but the observer should also regard facial expressions to assess discomfort. All movement should be done with the eyes open, as compression of the vertebral arteries can yield a subtle vertebral artery syndrome associated with nystagmus.

Active neck movement on the part of the patient reveals important clinical information regarding range of motion, motor strength, and the degree of patient compliance. Slight overpressure, that is, maintaining maximal range of motion for several seconds, or increasing the rate and velocity of repeated movements can sometimes reproduce pain not appreciated with single movement. Pain and paresthesias can be reproduced when the examiner slightly overstretches the range of motion with gentle pressure. This should be accomplished with extreme care.

In passive movement, the muscles are completely relaxed allowing the examiner to assess ligaments, tendons, and capsules. When capsules are involved, the patient frequently describes pain throughout passive movement, consistent with inflammation. Ligaments and tendons, however, are painful only when stretched.

In passive movement, the muscles are completely relaxed allowing the examiner to assess ligaments, tendons and capsules. When capsules are involved, the patient frequently describes pain throughout passive movement, consistent with inflammation. Ligaments and tendons, however, are painful only when stretched.

The examiner should pay particular attention to the "end feel," as the firm sensation of bone against bone (as in full extension at the elbow).[2] An "elastic stretch" is a sense of the rubbery end point (as in the

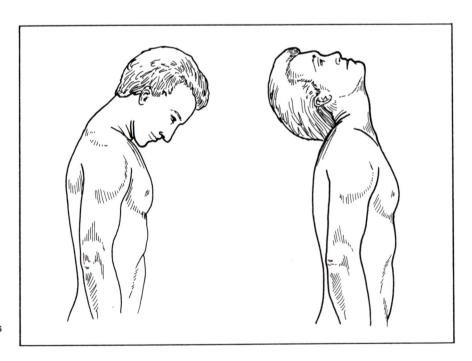

Figure 8–10. Limits of movements of flexion and extension.

arm flexed at the elbow). This is encountered with ligaments and tendons at their full range of motion. The examiner should take note, however, that there is a firm stopping point consistent with ligaments and tendons intact.

Movements against resistance are isometric tests of individual muscle groups, resistance provided by the examiner. Extensive range of movement is pain-free, but movement against resistance causes particular focal pain. By actively participating, the examiner can assess muscle weakness due to a neurologic lesion.

Specific Movements

Range of motion can be assessed in terms of degree of movement. This is more easily assessed when the patient bites down on the tongue depressor, as demonstrated in the figures. Table 8–1 from Macgee[3] depicts the muscles involved in each movement.

Flexion

The neck can be flexed to approximately 90 degrees, the chin coming to within 1 inch of the chest (Fig 8–10). In so doing, the vertebrae shift forward, one over the next, and the intervertebral foramen is enlarged. The primary flexors are the anterior flexors of the neck, the sternocleidomastoids, the scalenus muscles, and the prevertebral muscles. Active movement should be smooth, and normal passive movement should result in the chin touching the chest. Pain on active flexion is generally of muscular or tendinous origin. Passive flexion will distract ligamentous elements and cause pain. Disc lesions might also be painful as flexion anteriorly compresses the vertebral disc.

Extension

The limit of extension is approximately 70 degrees off the vertical plane (Fig 8–10). The principal extensors are the trapezius and the paravertebral extensor muscles (splenius, semispinalis, capitis) and the small intrinsic muscles of the neck. Pain with active motion reflects pathology of these muscles. Extension also distracts the anterior components of the cervical spine, but is particularly sensitive in eliciting pain from the facet joints. The examiner should take care to support the thorax to prevent the patient from leaning backward.

Lateral Flexion

The limits of lateral flexion are approximately 45 degrees to each side, although forced movement can be extended to the shoulder (Fig 8–11). The primary muscles involved include the scalenus group and the small intrinsic muscles of the neck. When examining active range of motion, the examiner should place both hands on the shoulders so as to prevent the patient from elevating the shoulders toward the head rather than truly bending the spine laterally. Injury from true lateral mechanisms is unusual, generally involving the articular masses. Muscle injuries can be assessed by either contracting the involved muscle, or stretching, with movement in the opposite direction.

Rotation

Rotation always involves lateral flexion, the limits of which are approximately 50 degrees to either side (Fig 8–11). The principal muscles involved are the sternocleidomastoid and the small intrinsic muscles of the neck. The examiner should again support the shoulders. Pain to muscles and tendons can be assessed by both contraction and stretching.

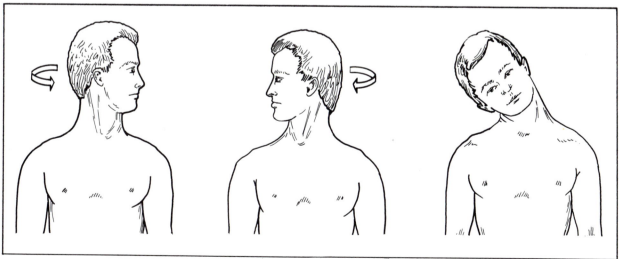

Figure 8–11. Lateral flexion and rotation.

□ NEUROLOGIC EXAMINATION

A complete neurologic examination of the cervical spine includes evaluation of the muscle groups of the cervical spine and specific neurologic levels in the upper extremities. The assessment of range of motion and movements against resistance are outlined in the previous section with particular reference to Table 8–1. The following discussion focuses the examiner's attention to specific motor, sensory, and reflex findings where appropriate, corresponding to cervical nerve roots.

There are eight cervical nerves that exit superior to the vertebral bodies of the cervical spine and the first thoracic vertebra. The first three or four cervical nerves contribute to the cervical plexus, the lower five and the first thoracic nerve roots contribute to the brachial plexus. These plexuses and the nerves that emanate from them are included in the section on anatomy.

C-1 and C-2

Motor Testing

Muscles innervated by roots C-1 and C-2 control neck flexion, principally innervating the muscles of the neck. Refer to Table 8–2,[3] which details all of the specific muscles involved for each of the nerve roots. Testing neck flexion against resistance is done by the examiner applying pressure to the forehead while stabilizing the trunk (Fig 8–12).

Sensory Testing

Sensory evaluation, particularly of C-2, is by the greater occipital nerve that runs laterally to the inion and innervates the occipital scalp.

C-3

Motor Testing

The nerve root of C-3 contributes to the innervation of the trapezius, scalenes, and longus capitis and cervicis muscles. They can be evaluated by testing lateral bending. Against the examiner's resistance and stabilization of the shoulders, the patient is asked to laterally flex the head (Fig 8–13).

Sensory Testing

Sensation of the nerve root to C-3 involves cutaneous testing of the upper neck.

TABLE 8–2. MYOTOMES OF THE UPPER LIMB

Nerve Root	Test Action	Muscles
C-1 and C-2	Neck flexion	Rectus lateralis, rectus capitis anterior, longus capitis, longus coli, longus cervicis, sternocleidomastoid
C-3	Neck side flexion	Longus capitis, longus cervicis, trapezius, scalenus medius
C-4	Shoulder elevations	Diaphragm, trapezius, levator scapulae, scalenus anterior, scalenus medius
C-5	Shoulder abduction	Rhomboid major and minor, deltoid, supraspinatus, infraspinatus, teres minor, biceps, scalenus anterior and medius
C-6	Elbow flexion and wrist extension	Serratus anterior, latissimus dorsi, subscapularis, teres major, pectoralis major (clavicular head), biceps, coracobrachialis, brachialis, brachioradialis, supinator, extensor carpi radialis longus, scalenus anterior, medius and posterior
C-7	Elbow extension and wrist flexion	Serratus anterior, latissimus dorsi, pectoralis major (sternal head), pectoralis minor, triceps, pronator teres, flexor carpi radialis, flexor digitorum superficialis, extensor carpi radialis longus, extensor carpi radialis brevis, extensor digitorum, extensor digiti minimi, scalenus medius and posterior
C-8	Thumb extension and ulnar deviation	Pectoralis major (sternal head), pectoralis minor, triceps, flexor digitorum superficialis, flexor digitorum profundus, flexor pollicis longus, pronator quadratus, flexor carpi ulnaris, abductor pollicis longus, extensor pollicis longus, extensor pollicis brevis, extensor indicis, abductor pollicis brevis, flexor pollicis brevis, opponens pollicis, scalenus medius and posterior
T-1	Hand intrinsics	Flexor digitorum profundus, intrinsic muscles of the hand (except extensor pollicis brevis), flexor pollicis brevis, opponens pollicis

Note: Muscles listed may be supplied by additional nerve roots; only primary nerve root sources are listed.
From Magee DJ: Philadelphia, WB Saunders, 1987, pp 28–29.[3]

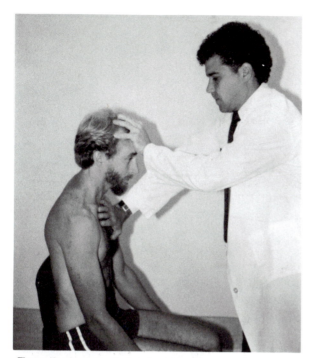

Figure 8–12. Method of motor testing for roots C-1 and C-2.

C-4

Motor Testing

The C-4 nerve root principally involves the trapezius and scapulae muscles as well as the scalenes and the diaphragm. Testing involves shoulder elevation, performed against downward resistance by the examiner on the shoulders bilaterally (Fig 8–14).

Sensory Testing

Cutaneous sensation at C-4 runs along the anterior upper chest in the intraclavicular region.

C-5

Motor Testing

The principal muscles innervated by C-5 are the deltoids and the biceps. Specific evaluation is of shoulder abduction, accomplished by having the patient abduct the arm to 90 degrees with the examiner now applying forceful downward pressure on the arm (Fig 8–15). Innervation to the biceps is from C-5 and C-6 and is, therefore, not a pure testing. Innervation can be assessed by force resistance against flexion of the arm at the elbow.

Sensory Testing

C-5 innervates the lateral aspect of the arm by the axillary nerve for the particular dermatomal distribution.

Reflex Testing

Although not a pure test because it involves both C-5 and C-6, the biceps reflex is used to assess C-5. Percussion over the lower insertion of the biceps is required.

C-6

Motor Testing

Evaluation of the motor component of C-6 is not a pure test (Fig 8–16). Combined testing of the biceps (including C-5 innervation) and wrist extension (involving C-7) should both be done. Wrist extension involves the extensor carpi radialis longus, brevis, and ulnaris. Testing of the biceps (C-5 and C-6) involves resistance of

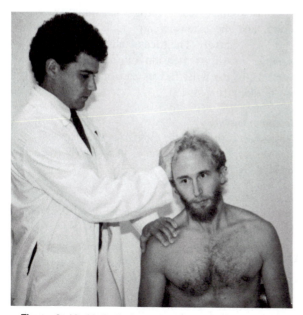

Figure 8–13. Method of motor testing for nerve root C-3.

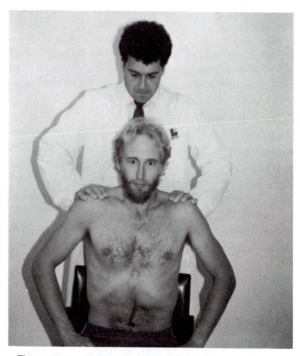

Figure 8–14. Method of motor testing for nerve root C-4.

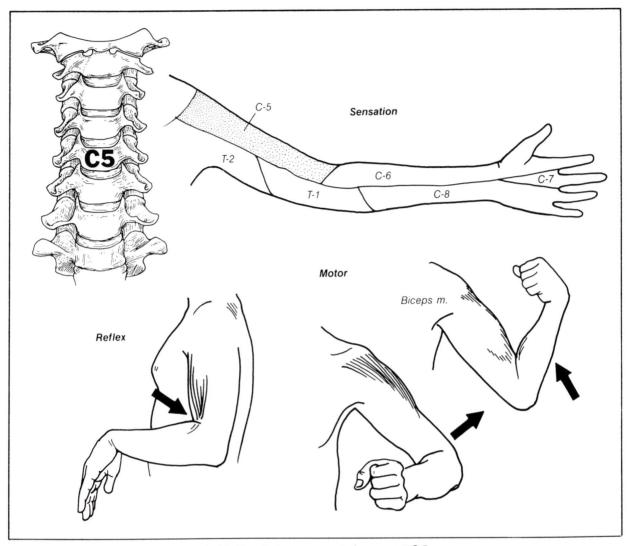

Figure 8–15. Neurologic assessment of nerve root C-5.

flexion at the elbow. Testing of wrist extension (C-6 and C-7) involves supporting the arm at the elbow while applying isometric resistance to the wrist.

Sensory Testing
Distribution of the C-6 nerve root is by the musculocutaneous nerve that innervates the lateral forearm, thumb, index finger, and one-half of the middle finger.

Reflex Testing
Brachioradialis reflex testing is used to test C-6. Percussion of the tendon insertion of the brachioradialis muscle reproduces the reflex.

C-7

Motor Testing
Although it innervates numerous muscles, specific testing for the motor component of C-7 involves extension of the elbow and wrist flexion associated with the tri-

ceps muscle, the extensor carpi radialis muscle (median nerve), and the extensor carpi radialis ulnaris (ulnar nerve), respectively. The triceps muscle is tested by the examiner resisting extension of the forearm. Forced resistance of the wrist flexors and finger extensors can also be done (Fig 8–17).

Sensory Testing
Sensation of the middle finger is used to test C-7; however, sensory innervation at this level is frequently supplied by C-6 or C-8.

Reflex Testing
The triceps reflex, percussion of the distal insertion of the triceps muscle over the elbow, tests C-7.

C-8

Motor Testing
Although innervating a large number of muscles, C-8 can be evaluated by testing the interosseous muscles,

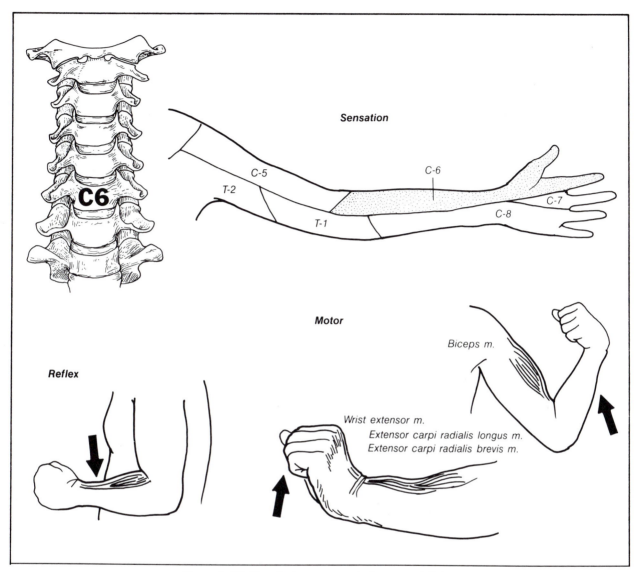

Figure 8–16. Neurologic assessment of nerve root C-6.

finger flexors, thumb extension, and ulnar deviation (Fig 8–18). Opening and closing the fingers, forming a fist, extending the thumb against resistance, and deviating the hand ulnarly will test C-8.

Sensory Testing
C-8 supplies sensation to the ulnar side of the forearm and the little and ring fingers.

Reflex Testing
There is no reflex testing for C-8.

T-1

Motor Testing
T-1 can be principally tested by evaluation of the hand intrinsic muscles, opening and closing the fingers against resistance (Fig 8–19).

Sensory Testing
T-1 is tested through the medial brachiocutaneous nerve that supplies sensation to the medial upper half of the forearm.

Reflex Testing
There is no reflex test specific for T-1.

☐ Major Peripheral Nerves

Table 8–3 lists the major peripheral nerve tests.

Radial Nerve

Motor Testing
The radial nerve can be evaluated by examining wrist extension or thumb extension against resistance.

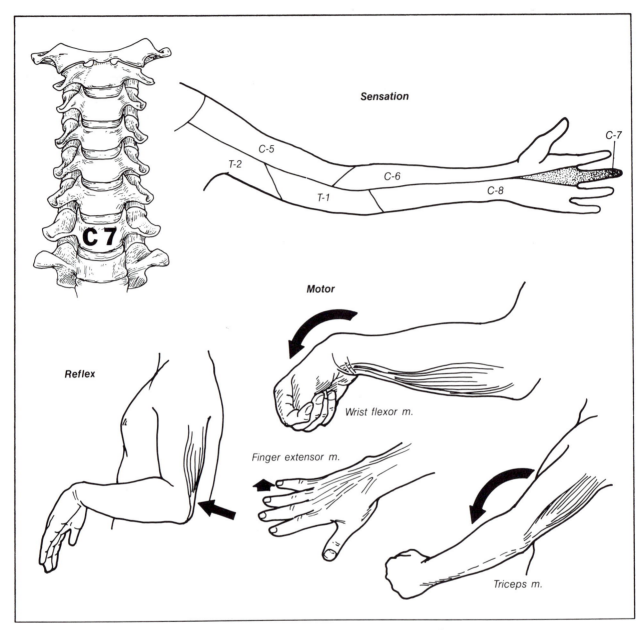

Figure 8–17. Neurologic assessment of nerve root C-7.

Sensory Testing

The most specific area to test the radial nerve is the dorsal web space between the thumb and the index finger.

Ulnar Nerve

Motor Testing

The ulnar nerve can be evaluated by abduction of the little finger.

Sensory Testing

Sensation of the dorsal aspect of the little finger should be done.

Median Nerve

Motor Testing

The median nerve can be evaluated by opposition of the thumb and the little finger, and abduction of the thumb.

Sensory Testing

The distal radial aspect of the index finger is supplied by the median nerve.

Axillary Nerve

Motor Testing

The axillary nerve principally innervates the deltoid muscle. This is evaluated by having the patient raise

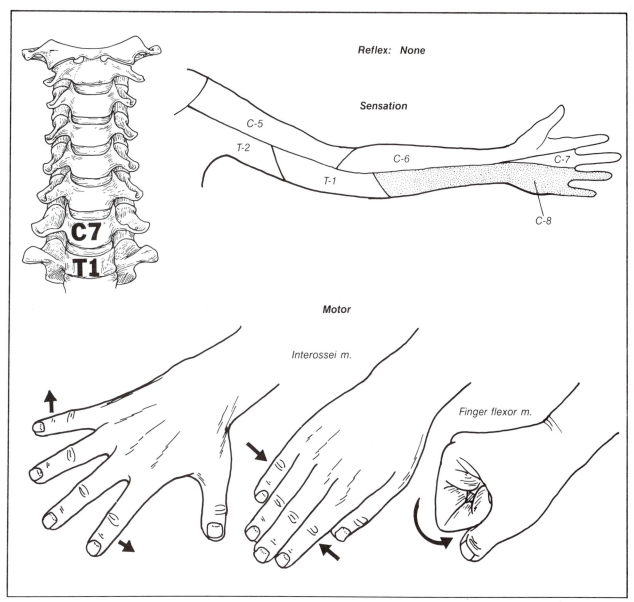

Figure 8–18. Neurologic assessment of nerve root C-8.

TABLE 8–3. MAJOR PERIPHERAL NERVE TESTS

Nerve	Motor Test	Sensory Test
Radial nerve	Wrist extension Thumb extension	Dorsal web space between thumb and index finger
Ulnar nerve	Abduction—little finger	Distal ulnar aspect—little finger
Median nerve	Thumb pinch Opposition of thumb Abduction of thumb	Distal radial aspect—index finger
Axillary nerve	Deltoid	Lateral arm—over deltoid
Musculocutaneous nerve	Biceps	Lateral forearm

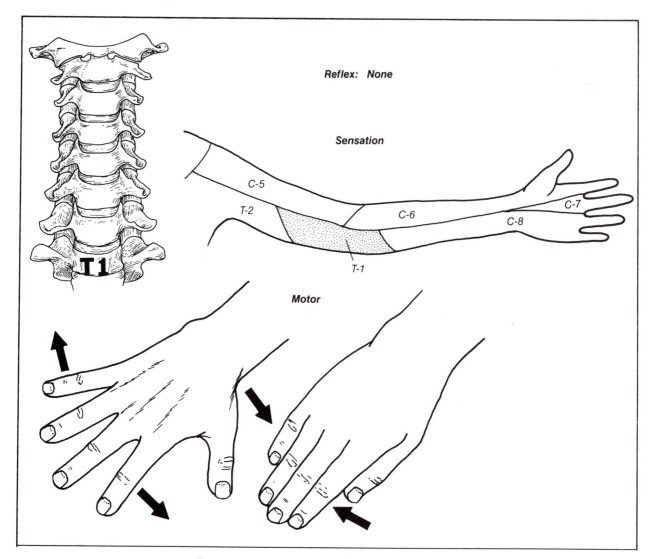

Figure 8–19. Neurologic assessment of nerve root T-1.

the arms in abduction to approximately 90 degrees and applying forceful downward pressure to the arm.

Sensory Testing
Sensory innervation is over the deltoid muscle.

Musculocutaneous Nerve

Motor Testing
The biceps are principally supplied by the musculocutaneous nerve and are evaluated by resistance of flexion of the arm at the elbow.

Sensory Testing
Sensory testing of the musculocutaneous nerve is the lateral aspect of the forearm.

□ SPECIAL TESTS

The discussion that follows describes a number of specific maneuvers used in evaluating specific aspects of the cervical pathology.

Compression Test
The compression test is performed by pressing down on the top of the head of a patient in the seated position. This test is used to evaluate narrowing of the neural foramen or pressure on the facet joints, and will frequently reproduce neurologic pain or symptoms (Fig 8–20).

Distraction Test
The distraction test is done either in the lying or seated position. Grasping the patient's chin and occiput, mild

distraction forces are applied to the cervical spine. This distraction maneuver can reduce neural foramen narrowing, thereby relieving pain due to compression of nerve roots (Fig 8–21).

Foramenal Compression Test

With the patient in the seated position, the head is forcefully flexed to the side. Narrowing of the neural foramen is increased, leading to compression of the nerve root and pain or altered sensation.

Shoulder Depression Test

The examiner pushes down on the shoulder on one side while distracting the head in the opposite direction. Increased pain or changes in sensation are due to nerve root compression (Fig 8–22).

Vertebral Artery Test

The vertebral artery test should be accomplished in the supine position, as a positive test could induce symptoms of vertebral artery insufficiency. The shoulder on the tested side is pushed caudally while the head is laterally rotated to the opposite side. A positive test can induce signs of nerve root compression or vertebral artery insufficiency manifested by dizziness and nystagmus (Fig 8–23).

Intermittent Claudication Test

Both arms are elevated and abducted and externally rotated. The patient rapidly opens and closes the fists. Pain will develop within seconds in states of decreased vascular flow. The healthy person will be able to continue the exercise for 1 minute.

Costoclavicular Maneuver

In the seated position, the patient draws the shoulders downward and backward as if standing at attention. Evidence of a bruit heard inferior to the clavicle at the junction of the lateral two-thirds or decrease in palpation of the radial pulse constitutes a positive test.

Hyperabduction Maneuver

Forced hyperabduction of an upper extremity will diminish distal pulses. It is generally indicative of hyperabduction syndrome, a form of thoracic outlet syndrome.

Adson Maneuver

The patient is instructed to turn the head to the side of the symptoms and take a deep breath with the neck fully extended. A decrease or obliteration of the radial pulse is considered a positive test due to increased entrapment of the scalene muscles. This test is specific for the scalenus anticus syndrome.

Valsalva Maneuver

The patient takes a deep breath and bears down as if moving bowels. A positive test reflects increased intrathecal pressure and results in pain at the level of intrathecal involvement or nerve root compression.

Swallowing Test

Difficulty or pain with swallowing, although more typically involving the esophagus, can reflect cervical spine abnormalities, such as large osteophytes, significant soft tissue swelling, hematomas, infection or tumor, or large bony protuberances.

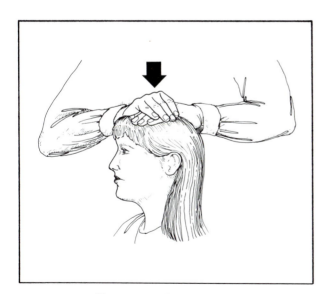

Figure 8–20. Compression test.

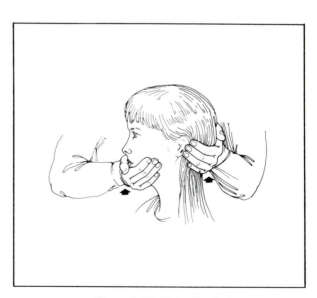

Figure 8–21. Distraction test.

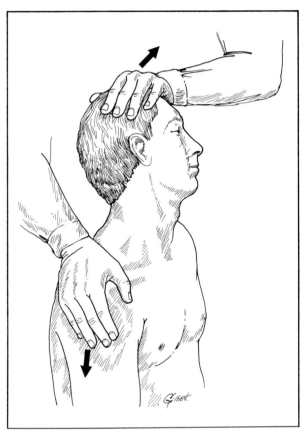

Figure 8–22. Shoulder depression test.

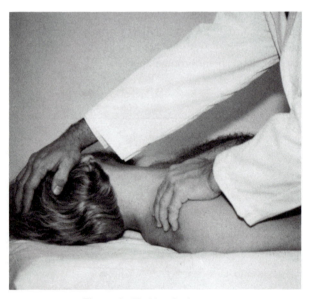

Figure 8–23. Vertebral artery test.

Lhermitte's Sign

The patient is seated on the examining table with the legs extended. Passive flexion of the patient's head and hips simultaneously can produce pain anywhere along the spine where dural irritation exists.

□ REFERENCES

1. Bland JH: Clinical methods. In Disorders of the Cervical Spine. Philadelphia, WB Saunders, 1987, p 79
2. Cyriax J: Diagnosis of soft tissue lesions. Textbook of Orthopedic Medicine, Bailliertindal, 1982
3. Magee DJ: Orthopedic Physical Assessment. Philadelphia, WB Saunders, 1987, p 21

□ BIBLIOGRAPHY

Bland JH: Disorders of the cervical spine. Philadelphia, WB Saunders, 1987

Hohl M: Normal motions in the upper portion of the cervical spine. J Bone Joint Surg 46A:1777, 1964

Hoppenfeld S: Physical Examination of the Spine and Extremities. New York, Appleton-Century-Crofts, 1976

Judge RD, et al: Clinical Diagnosis—A Physiological Approach. Boston, Little, Brown, 1982

Magee DJ: Orthopedic Physical Assessment. Philadelphia, WB Saunders, 1987

McQueen JD, Kahn MI: Evaluation of patients with cervical spine lesions. In Bailey RW (ed): The Cervical Spine. Philadelphia, JB Lippincott, 1983

McRae R: Clinical Orthopedic Examination. Edinburgh, Churchill Livingston, 1976

9

Radiology

□ INTRODUCTION

Although the radiographic anatomy of the cervical spine is extremely complex, the emergency medicine physician now has a number of diagnostic imaging modalities to rely on to make an accurate diagnosis. The purpose of this chapter is to discuss the radiographic approach to cervical pathology.

As acute cervical injury is a frequent problem encountered by the emergency physician, this discussion focuses on the acutely traumatized patient. The indications for each modality are discussed.

This chapter is not intended to describe all of the abnormalities that the emergency physician might encounter. Rather, it presents indications and applications of certain modalities, as well as in some instances an orderly approach to their interpretation. Specific radiographic abnormalities are presented in subsequent chapters.

□ PLAIN RADIOGRAPHY

The principal radiographic tool is the cervical spine series. Given the potential for devastating consequences of a missed diagnosis, the authors recommend both a low threshold for ordering cervical films and a high index of suspicion for potential injury. A cervical spine series is indicated in all patients presenting with localized pain, deformity, crepitus or edema, altered mental status, neurologic dysfunction, head injury, multiple trauma, or patients involved in injuries whose mechanism might suggest cervical spine injury.

Obtaining quality films in the setting of multiple trauma is often difficult. Nevertheless, the importance of optimum technical quality cannot be overemphasized. The emergency physician should not hesitate to have particular views repeated as necessary. Motion artifact, superimposition of shoulders, stabilization equipment, or clothing and jewelry make accurate interpretation impossible. The use of portable x-ray equipment frequently results in suboptimal x-rays.

The cross-table lateral, anteroposterior, open-mouth, and oblique views are considered by most authors to be a complete set. Additional films to be considered are the pillar, swimmer's, and flexion–extension views.

Cross-Table Lateral View

The cross-table lateral view (CTLV) should be the first x-ray in the cervical spine series and in cases of multiple trauma should precede all other films. Although it can reveal much information, numerous studies have demonstrated that even in the best hands, it is accurate in revealing posttraumatic cervical spine abnormalities in only 70 to 79%.[1-3] Additional views, particularly the open-mouth and anteroposterior views, are mandatory before the emergency physician can "clear" the cervical spine.

It is recommended in the setting of acute trauma that an initial CTLV "scout" film be done without applying traction in the albeit unlikely event of atlanto-occipital or altantoaxial dissociation, as even minimal traction can lead to neurologic damage.

Nevertheless, the CTLV should never be considered adequate unless all seven cervical vertebrae are visualized. This generally requires axial traction applied manually by two individuals; one supporting the head, the other at the foot of the table applying traction on the shoulders by pulling down on both arms simultaneously grasped at the wrists (Fig 9–1).

Its limitations notwithstanding, an accurate interpretation of the CTLV is extremely important. An organized approach to reading this film will help the emergency physician avoid misinterpretation. A thorough understanding of the anatomy of the cervical spine is mandatory (refer to Chapter 7). As the radiologist establishes an orderly pattern of reviewing an x-ray, so too the emergency physician must concentrate

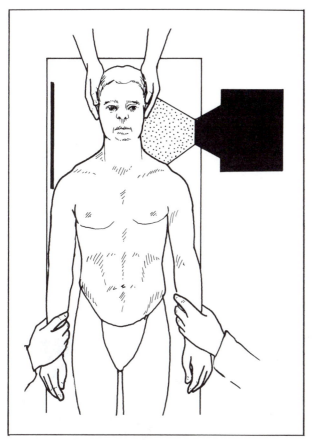

Figure 9–1. Method of cervical stabilization for obtaining lateral cervical spine film with downward traction of the arms.

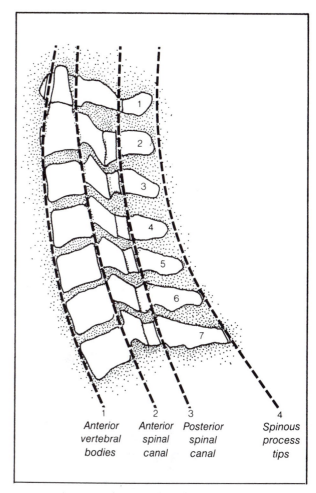

1	2	3	4
Anterior vertebral bodies	Anterior spinal canal	Posterior spinal canal	Spinous process tips

Figure 9–2. Alignment. Four smooth lordotic curves on the lateral cervical spine view. *Adapted from Williams CF et al: Essentiality of the lateral cervical spine radiograph, Ann Emerg Med 10(4), 201, April 1981.*

on all components of anatomy represented on the film. The mnemonic ABCs, proposed by Jackson[4] and later amplified by Williams and colleagues,[5] provides an excellent framework for evaluating not only the CTLV, but all views in the cervical spine series.

Alignment (A)

The cervical spine is composed of seven irregularly shaped vertebrae. Seen in the lateral projection, they are stacked in such a way as to produce four smooth curves as demonstrated in Figure 9–2: (1) the anterior vertebral bodies, (2) the anterior spinal canal, (3) the posterior spinal canal, and (4) the spinous process tips. The first two curves essentially run the course of the anterior and posterior longitudinal ligaments. In particular, these two lines should be essentially parallel. An overlap of less than 2.7 mm is considered normal. A distance 3.5 mm or greater is suggestive of disruption of either or both of the two ligaments and is abnormal (Fig 9–3).[6]

Similarly, angulation between cervical vertebrae of greater than 11 degrees is strongly suggestive of ligamentous disruption or at least dislocation and shows a clear interruption of the smooth lines (Fig 9–4).[6]

The line formed by the spinous process tips is the most irregular of the four, C-2 and C-7 being far more prominent than the other cervical spinous processes.

To properly assess alignment it is imperative that the x-ray be a true lateral. This can easily be assessed by examining the third line or posterior spinal canal. In actuality, it is a double line comprised of superimposed articular masses. If the entire body is slightly rotated these articular masses will create a double line image, which will appear parallel (Fig 9–5A). If only the head is rotated, the articular masses will again not be superimposed, but instead will create a tapering pair of lines (Fig 9–5B).[7] In either case, the x-ray should be repeated.

The second and third curves outline the spinal canal. The spinal cord at this level has a diameter varying between 10 and 13 mm. The canal starts wider at the upper cervical area and tapers in the shape of a funnel to the level of C-7. An anteroposterior distance of less than 10 to 13 mm anywhere along the spinal

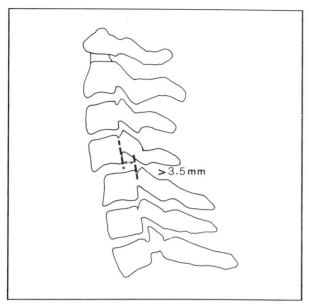

Figure 9–3. Abnormal alignment.

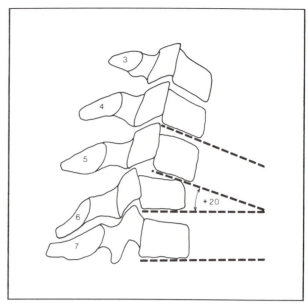

Figure 9–4. Abnormal angulation.

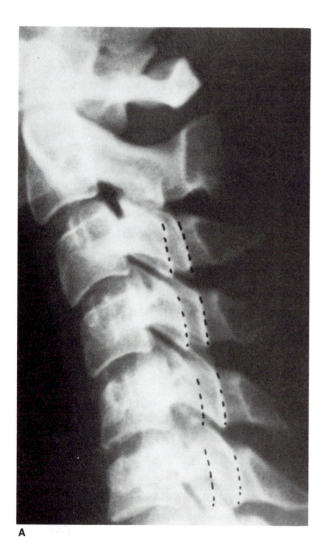

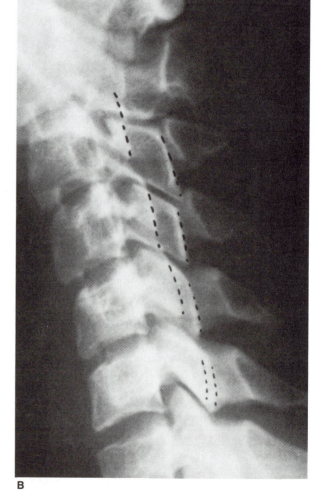

A   **B**

Figure 9–5. Parallel lines of nonsuperimposed articular masses due to entire body rotation. *From Harris JH: The Radiology of Acute Cervical Spine Trauma, 2nd ed. Baltimore, Williams & Wilkins, 1987, pp 32–33.*

canal is strongly suggestive of at least spinal cord impingement.

The normal course of all four lines should outline a smooth lordotic curve. Straightening or reversal of that curve is not necessarily pathologic. Approximately 20% of healthy persons will have a straight cervical spine. Weir[8] found that simply lowering the chin approximately 1 inch increased the percentage of straightened spines to 70%. Particularly in the face of trauma, where there may be significant muscle spasm or with the patient in a recumbent position, loss of the lordotic curve might be insignificant. It is, however, also a pathologic finding in hyperextension injuries. Acute angulation at any point is abnormal.

Bones (B)

Whereas assessing alignment involves smooth, global lines, bony evaluation requires extreme detail. All seven cervical vertebrae must be closely evaluated. Again, an orderly anterorposterior inspection is recommended. The vertebral bodies from C-3 to C-7 are generally uniform rectangles. Degenerative changes in this area would include osteophytes or anterior and posterior ligamentous calcification. A decrease in height of greater than 3 mm is felt consistent with compression fractures.

Fractures of the vertebral bodies are manifest in several ways. Small anterior triangles off the vertebral body are consistent with avulsion fractures associated with anterior longitudinal ligament rupture seen in hyperextension injuries. Larger bony fragments of the anterorinferior portion of the vertebral body are consistent with teardrop fractures due to hyperflexion injuries and are generally associated with a hyperkyphotic angle at the level of the injury. Marked fragmentation of the vertebral body is characteristic of "burst" fractures secondary to vertical compression. These are particularly ominous in that they are frequently associated with fragments of bone being displaced posteriorly into the spinal canal.

The lateral masses lend lateral support around the spinal cord and are superimposed over the spinal canal on the lateral x-ray. They are comprised of the pedicles, laminae, facets, and transverse processes. This is a particularly complex region of the cervical spine due to superimposition of shadows. Fractures and dislocations may appear quite subtle, but are usually associated with abnormal alignment. The entire complex should slope downward, anterior to posterior, overriding one another like stacked shingles. Distances between each of the lateral masses should be relatively uniform. Widening or improper alignment is abnormal and seen with facet dislocations, either unilateral or bilateral, as occurs with hyperflexion–rotation injuries. Fractures through the pedicles and laminae usually run vertically, but can

be severely disruptive in the case of hyperextension fracture–dislocations.

The most posterior structures are the spinous processes. They are relatively easily evaluated due to the lack of superimposing structures. Fractures are most commonly due to avulsions of supraspinous and interspinous ligaments, usually involving C-7, C-6, and T-1 in that order.

Evaluation of the cervicocranium, the occiput, C-1, and C-2 is most difficult, particularly anteriorly due to superimposition of shadows. Pedicle and spinous process injuries at this level are more easily seen as vertical fractures or avulsions. The relationship between the anterior arch of C-1 and the dens is key for adults. The distance between these two structures should be less than 3 mm. A distance of 3 to 5 mm is consistent with transverse ligament disruption.

Fractures of the odontoid are difficult to see on this view. Type 1 fractures of the superior portion of the dens may be visualized, but in general the odontoid is best seen on the open-mouth view. Refer to Chapter 10 for a detailed discussion of odontoid fractures

Cartilage (C)

Evaluation of cartilage on the CTLV principally concerns the disc spaces. In the normal patient, the intervertebral disc space is uniform, more narrow in the upper cervical spine but widening caudally. Acute disc rupture in the cervical area is often a subtle finding. In hyperflexion injuries the disc tends to rupture posteriorly and will show increased widening anterior to posterior. Anterior widening of the intervertebral space is more commonly seen with vertebral compression fractures. In general, abnormal disc findings are quite subtle, and definitive diagnosis is dependent on further radiographic studies including discography, myelography, and computed tomography (CT) scanning.

Soft Tissue Space (S)

Soft tissue injuries may be quite subtle but might be the only indication of serious injury. The examiners should direct their attention to the retropharyngeal and retrotracheal spaces, the soft tissue space outlined anteriorly by the air column and posteriorly by the vertebral body. Widening of this space can be attributed to hemorrhage, abscess, infection, tumor, foreign body, or air. In the setting of trauma it must be assumed that widening of the soft tissue space is due to hemorrhage and associated with fracture or ligamentous rupture. In some cases, it might be the only indication of significant injury, particularly in the case of hyperextension injuries and fractures of the odontoid process without displacement. Table 9–1 and Figure 9–6[9] show the limits of normal measurements for the widths of prevertebral soft tissue at each cervical vertebra. Note that the pres-

TABLE 9–1. NORMAL PREVERTEBRAL SOFT TISSUE WIDTH

Level	Flexion (mm)	Midposition (mm)	Extension (mm)
C-1	5.6 (2–11)	4.6 (1–10)	3.6 (1– 8)
C-2	4.1 (2– 6)	3.2 (1– 5)	3.8 (2– 6)
C-3	4.2 (3– 7)	3.4 (2– 7)	4.1 (3– 6)
C-4	5.8 (4– 7)	5.1 (2– 7)	6.1 (4– 8)
C-5	17.1 (11–22)	14.9 (8–20)	15.2 (10–20)
C-6	16.3 (12–20)	15.1 (11–20)	13.9 (7–19)
C-7	14.7 (9–20)	13.9 (9–20)	11.9 (7–21)

The midposition widths were measured on lateral radiographs of 50 noninjured patients, normal except for varying degrees of cervical spondylosis in some; their average age was 46 years, with a spread of 15 to 78 years. Widths in flexion and extension were measured in 20 patients with normal prevertebral widths in midposition; their average age was 31 years, with a spread of 16 to 67 years. No correction has been made for radiologic magnification (about 1.3).

From Penning L: Prevertebral hematoma in cervical spine injury: Incidence and etiological significance. Am J Neuroradiology 1:557–565, 1980.

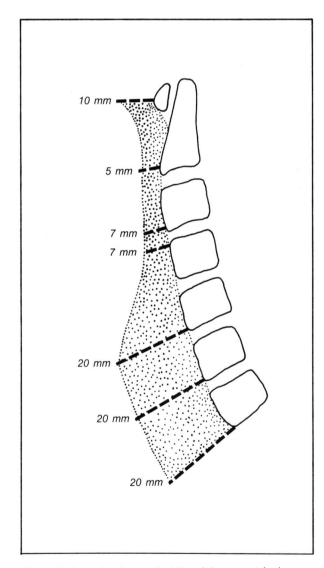

Figure 9–6. Limits of normal widths of the prevertebral space.

ence of a nasogastric or endotracheal tube can compress the edematous tissue and invalidate the measurement.

A second soft tissue finding on the CTLV is the prevertebral fat stripe. A thin band of fatty tissue runs from the upper regions of the cervical spine to the level of C-6, parallel to the anterior longitudinal ligament. Displacement of the fat stripe is suggestive of significant injury, even if there is no overall widening of the prevertebral soft tissue space.

Posteriorly, the distances between the spinous processes should be examined. Significant widening between the spinous processes is suggestive of rupture of the interspinous and supraspinous ligaments, generally due to a flexion injury and may be associated with fractures or dislocations anteriorly.

Anteroposterior View

The anteroposterior (AP) film can provide useful information but is limited by the superimposition superiorly of the mandible and the occiput. As such, the extreme upper cervical spine cannot be visualized, and only the lower five cervical and upper thoracic segments can be seen. The superior and inferior end-plates, uncinate processes, joints of Luschka, and the lateral cortical margins can be seen well. Due to superimposition of lateral masses, interfacetal joint spaces cannot be seen. This superimposition on the AP projection, however, presents the lateral cortical margins of the articular masses as a continuous, smoothly undulating density. Traumatic tilting of the articular process is abnormal, as is a scoliotic angulation seen in unilateral compression fracture or interlocking facets.

The spinous processes are seen in the midline, arranged in a vertical row approximately equally spaced. A widening of any two spinous processes by approximately 1½ times the normal distance is considered abnormal, consistent with hyperflexion sprain or interlocking facets.

The trachea is demonstrated by an air shadow in the midline, tapering superiorly in the subglottic area. Lateral displacement of the tracheal air shadow is generally secondary to hemorrhage or edema due to trauma.

Open-Mouth View

The open-mouth view is an AP projection of the upper cervical spine. By opening the patient's mouth, the mandible is no longer superimposed over C-1 and C-2 as is seen in the AP view. There are five key observations to be made on this view, and the ABCs of interpretation once again apply.

Alignment (A)

The atlas should sit on top of the axis with the dens equidistant from the lateral masses of the atlas. The lateral margin of the atlantoaxial surfaces should be perfectly aligned and symmetrical, with no overriding of the edges.

Bones (B)

Both vertebrae should be carefully observed for fractures, particularly the dens, which may be fractured superiorly, at its base, where it meets the vertebral body of C-2, or inferiorly, cracked through the vertebral body. The spinous process of the axis is bifid and should be in the midline.

Cartilage (C)

The lateral atlantoaxial joint space should be open and the surfaces parallel.

Oblique View

The oblique views are particularly important for visualizing the intervertebral foraminae, the uncinate process of the vertebral bodies, the articular masses, and the laminae. To be effective, it is imperative that the entire patient be rotated 45 degrees on the longitudinal axis, rather than simply rotating the head and the neck. Sometimes less rotation at an angle of 15 degrees offers a better view of the articular processes. When the patient is in a cervical spine traction or otherwise cannot be moved due to spinal immobilization, a portable C-arch may be required.

In particular, the normal relationship of the facets is well demonstrated. The superior facet lies above and posterior to the inferior facet. Lines extending through the axis of the laminae reveal a configuration similar to shingles on a roof. Abnormalities in this configuration suggest interlocking facets.

Because the articular masses and interfacetal joints of the opposite side cannot be seen due to superimposition of the vertebral bodies, oblique radiographs are required from each side.

Pillar View

The pillar view provides direct visualization of individual lateral masses and is generally used only when fractures in this area are suspected. With the patient lying supine, the head facing to the side to eliminate superimposition of the mandible, the x-ray is angled from a position 35 degrees caudad with the central beam off-centered 2 cm from the midline in the opposite direction to which the head is rotated. It is, of course, imperative that upper cervical segments have been "cleared" for the patient to be allowed to rotate the head to this extent.

Swimmer's View

The swimmer's (Twining's) view is used to reveal the lower cervical spine segments. When pulling on the shoulders is inadequate to assess C-6 and C-7 on the lateral view, one arm is abducted 180 degrees, extended over the head and the other extremity extended posterocaudally, the patient thus being rotated slightly. In the severely injured patient this position is difficult or impossible and is contraindicated if a low cervicothoracic spine injury is suspected.

Flexion–Extension View

Actual flexion–extension of the cervical spine occurs in a gradual fashion. In flexion, the upper portion of the column moves to the greatest extent, each segment gliding foward and pivoting on its anterorinferior corner. The posterior vertebral line, therefore, becomes a smooth, convex curve. Intervertebral discs become slightly narrowed anteriorly and widened posteriorly. The articular masses glide upward and forward uniformly. Interspinous spaces increase in width. The reverse is true in extension.

Axiom: *Flexion–extension views should be done only when stability of a certain region is in doubt. These views are absolutely contraindicated when instability is obvious or in the presence of neurologic deficit. The physician should be in attendance at all times.*

Pitfalls

Due to the complexity of interpreting cervical spine films and the gravity of missing potentially dangerous fractures, it is easy to see why both false-positive and false-negative readings can be made. Remember that it is the emergency physician who has primary responsibility for the care of the patient in the emergency department. If there is any doubt about a given aspect of any view, it must be repeated until you, the responsible physician, are satisfied that an injury does or does not exist. As needed, other modalities, such as tomography and CT, should be used.

Axiom: *Pursue all doubts about x-ray interpretation of the cervical spine until you, the responsible physician, are completely satisfied.*

Although in certain instances false-negative interpretations of cervical spine films can lead to disastrous results, false-positive interpretations can lead to unnecessary hospitalizations and inappropriate application of traction devices. Familiarity with certain difficult portions of the cervical spine series as well as certain conditions that lend themselves to misinterpretation is desirable.

A description follows of the more common conditions from Kim and colleagues[10] and Penning[9] that lend themselves to complicated interpretation.

Degenerative Disease

Degenerative disease has been found to be the most common cause of misinterpretation of acute traumatic subluxation or fracture. With degenerative disease, motion is limited at the level of a narrowed disc space. Increased stresses lend toward stretching of ligaments, which sublux corresponding vertebrae forward. This can be differentiated from traumatic subluxation by the fact that there is no fracture evident, but diffuse disc space narrowing, facet arthrosis, and other accompanying degenerative changes, such as spur formation and vacuum disc phenomenon, are seen.

When significant disc space narrowing is present, the backward subluxation of vertebrae may be seen, as the upper vertebral body is pulled backward by the posteroinferior tilt of the facet joint surfaces. This is most common in the mid-cervical region. Backward subluxation can be misinterpreted as traumatic hyperextension injuries, but again can be differentiated by the absence of fractures and the presence of numerous other degenerative changes.

Degenerative fattening of the vertebral body should not be confused with compression fractures. The former is usually associated with other degenerative changes and is generally diffuse.

Calcification of the anterior longitudinal ligament is a degenerative change that should not be confused with an avulsion fracture. The presence of other degenerative changes, as well as the absence of soft tissue swelling or anterior widening of the disc space, helps differentiate this from an avulsion or acute traumatic injury.

Remember that acute trauma can coexist with degenerative changes. Carefully examine the chronically changed cervical spine for acute injuries.

Preexisting Congenital Anomaly

A common anomaly of the cervical spine is congenital block vertebrae, which causes stresses above and below the block and may lead toward early spondylosis and subluxation. It is generally not associated with facet abnormalities or intervertebral disc space narrowing, but can be seen with spur formation. This should not be misinterpreted as acute injury.

Atlanto-occipital fusion is the most common congenital anomaly of the upper cervical spine and it is frequently associated with congenital fusion of C-2 and C-3. It commonly causes atlantoaxial laxity due to greater stresses at this area resulting from the block

formations above and below. Atlantoaxial joint space widening can be noted but is not necessarily unstable.

Congenital abnormalities in the development of the dens are not common, but may be difficult to distinguish from acute fracture. Os odontoideum has previously been felt to be a congenital anomaly, but more recently is seen to be a nonunion fracture of the dens. It is differentiated from acute fractures in that the os is rounded and does not necessarily "fit" with the remainder of the body of the dens.

Physiologic Subluxation

The underdeveloped cervical spine in children and young adults commonly leads to physiologic subluxation of the upper cervical spine. This is generally attributed to laxity of the transverse ligament, which allows a greater degree of motion between the atlas and the axis. Consequently, the atlantodental interval ranges between 3 and 5 mm. Pseudosubluxation can also occur between C-3 and C-4, but to lesser extents.

Prominent Uncinate Process of C-3

The uncinate process is that part of the vertebral body that is most lateral and posterior. Particularly in the C-3 vertebra it can project beyond the cortex of the rest of the vertebral body and give the appearance of impinging on the cervical canal or resemble a double density suggesting fracture. In actuality, it circles the canal and should not be included as a component of the posterior vertebral line in the examination of the smooth curves of alignment in the lateral radiograph.

Mach Effect

Mach bands are optical phenomena in which dark and light lines appear at the borders of structures of differing radiodensity in x-rays. They may produce the illusion of fractures, but, if carefully observed, will generally be noted to continue beyond the suspected bony structure. In particular, superimposition of the teeth or air of the vocal fissure can suggest odontoid fractures.

Normal Anatomic Variants

Kim and coworkers[10] describe numerous anatomic variants that were misinterpreted as acute injury.

- "Normal" wedging of the vertebral bodies
- "Normal" backward displacement of the spinolaminar line at C-2
- Superior end-plate irregularities due to Schmorl's nodes
- Slight increases in disc spaces
- Pseudospread of the atlas suggesting a Jefferson fracture

Artifactual Lines

Artifacts can occur from a variety of sources but more commonly in the setting of trauma, with a patient in spinal precautionary equipment, surrounded by tape, bands, sandbags, saline bags, spinal boards, and oxygen and intravenous lines.

☐ OTHER IMAGING MODALITIES

Although the plain film spinal series is required as the initial x-ray evaluation, numerous other imaging modalities are available. No other single method is universally applicable, however, and an understanding of their relative utility in the emergency setting is necessary.

Tomography

Tomography is that technique in which radiographic slices are employed to better visualize specific parts of the anatomy. In the case of the cervical spine, it has the advantage of honing in on complex radiographic areas frequently obstructed by other superimposed structures. The two most commonly used techniques are plain film tomography and computed tomography.

Plain Film Tomography

Plain film tomography has several advantages including low cost and wide availability. The images are presented in a vertical orientation, either coronal or sagittal sectioning of multiple segments simultaneously. It is particularly useful in evaluation of the cervicocranium, an area that is difficult to evaluate on the plain film spinal series. Specifically, it is of value in visualizing the dens, horizontally oriented fractures (particularly of the atlas), and Jefferson fractures.

Unfortunately, in the setting of trauma, it frequently requires that the patient be moved. In addition, although horizontal fractures are better picked up through vertical slicing, vertical fractures are relatively poorly seen as the imaging is in the same plane.

Computed Tomography

Computed tomography (CT) has established itself as the tomographic procedure of choice in trauma, and is also very useful in the evaluation of other cervical pathology including tumors, inflammation, infection, and disc herniation.

The radiation dose is less than with plain film tomography and projections are recorded in the horizontal (axial) plane and reconstructed to form sagittal, coronal, or oblique images. The axial views are particularly useful in evaluating vertebral bodies and posterior elements. The size and configuration of the spinal canal is seen well, including impingement from bony fragments in trauma, degenerative changes, or masses. Improved resolution over plain film tomography allows for evaluation of the paravertebral soft tissue. Other pathologic lesions involving the spinal canal that show significant attenuation differences from bone, the cerebrospinal fluid, and fat are also well seen, including calcified meningiomas, lipomas, osteoblastomas, neurofibromas, highly vascularized intramedullary tumors, herniated discs, epidural hematomas, demographic states, and certain cases of syringomyelia.

Unfortunately, the procedure is relatively expensive and not available at all institutions. Although resolution is better than plain film tomography, it is not detailed enough to provide a precise evaluation of the spinal canal and resolution is significantly worse in reformatted images.

The axial plane is suboptimal in evaluating horizontal fractures, vertebral subluxation, or dislocation. Individual thin axial cuts do not allow for evaluation of curvatures of the spine, and the fact that the spine is naturally curved often results in images of tilted fragments of vertebral bodies, making interpretation difficult. Large cuts can often miss subtle fractures entirely.

Myelography

Although plain film and computed tomography allow improved visualization, particularly of the spinal canal, soft tissue contents are poorly evaluated and require contrast material. Myelography using either iophendylate (oil-based) or metrizamide (water-soluble) contrast material is the imaging technique used to assess the soft tissue contents of the spinal canal.

Standard Myelography

Myelography affords imaging of the contents of the spinal column, including spinal cord and nerve roots, by means of plain radiography after the intrathecal injection of contrast material. Multiple levels can be visualized simultaneously and spot radiography limits artifact. The procedure is invasive, however, and complete obstructions must be evaluated using two punctures, both above and below an obstructing lesion, to define its extent. As only the outline of an image is visualized, the actual extent of paravertebral lesions cannot be seen. Obstructions due to trauma can be visualized, but the patient must be moved to inject the contrast material.

Computer Assisted Myelography (CAM)

Computed tomography of the cervical spine after injection of metrizamide as contrast material markedly improves the ability to evaluate the contents of the spinal column. Transverse views better demonstrate impingement on the cord than does myelography. As smaller amounts of metrizamide are detected by CT, what appears to be a complete block on routine myelography is often shown to be incomplete with CAM, thus obviating the need for a second puncture above the lesion. The greater sensitivity of CT also allows for the use of smaller doses of metrizamide, particularly important in evaluating upper cord lesions that have the added risk of seizures due to contrast material.

Still, the procedure is invasive, requires contrast, and exposes the patient to ionizing radiation. Transverse projection limits evaluation of the spinal column to small cuts.

Nevertheless, this technique is extremely useful in detection, localization, and diagnosis of pathologic states of the cervical spine, including herniated cervical discs, spondylosis, syringomyelia, arachnoiditis, and tumors. Its use in trauma, however, is limited and controversial as it requires patient movement.

Magnetic Resonance Imaging

Magnetic resonance imaging (MRI) provides direct, multiplanar images without ionizing radiation. Although cortical bone is poorly visualized, evaluation of the tissues in and around the spinal canal are well seen without contrast. As such, it is becoming the procedure of choice in certain pathologic states including syringomyelia, Chiari malformation, disc space infection, multiple sclerosis, degenerative diseases of the spine, tumors of the spinal axis, and congenital abnormalities.

In its present form, however, slice thickness is still quite large as compared with CT, the procedure is lengthy, and patient handling is more difficult in the confined spaces of MRI. Patients requiring advanced life support equipment and cardiac pacemakers cannot be studied. Thus, its use in evaluation of trauma of the cervical spine is still quite limited.

☐ REFERENCES

1. Lahd WH, et al: Efficacy of the post-traumatic cross table lateral view of the cervical spine. Emerg Med 2:243, 1985
2. More SE: Emergency evaluation of cervical spine injuries: CT versus radiographs. Ann Emerg Med 14(10):973, 1985
3. Streitweiser DR, et al: Accuracy of standard radiographic views in detecting cervical spine fractures. Ann Emerg Med 12(9):538, 1983
4. Jackson NE: The Achilles' neck and other vulnerable vertebrae. Emerg Med 9:22, 1977
5. Williams CF: Essentiality of the lateral cervical spine radiograph. Ann Emerg Med 10(4):198, 1981
6. White AA, et al: Biochemical analysis of clinical stability in the cervical spine. Clin Orthop 109:85, 1975
7. Harris JH: Radiology of Acute Cervical Spine Trauma. Baltimore, Williams & Wilkins, 1978
8. Weir DC: Roentgenographlc signs of cervical injury. Clin Orthop 109:9, 1975
9. Penning L: Obtaining and interpreting plain films in the cervical injury. In The Cervical Spine Research Society. Bailey RW (ed): The Cervical Spine. Philadelphia, JB Lippincott, 1983, p 62
10. Kim KS, et al: Pitfalls in plain film diagnosis of the cervical spine injury: Positive interpretation. Surg Neurol 25:381, 1986

☐ BIBLOGRAPHY

Barrow DL, et al: Clinical indications for computer-assisted myelography. Neurosurgery 12(1):47, 1983

Brant-Zawadzki M, et al: CT in the evaluation of spine trauma. AJR 136(2):369, 1981

Cacayorin ED, Kieffer SA: Applications and limitations of computed tomography of the spine. Radiol Clin North Am 20(1):185, 1982

Clark WM, et al: Twelve significant signs of cervical spine trauma. Skeletal Radiol 3:201, 1979

Post MJD, et al: The value of computed tomography in spinal trauma. Spine 7 (5):417, 1982

Maravilla KR, et al: The influence of thin section tomography of the treatment of cervical spine injuries. Radiology 127(4):131, 1978

McAfee PC, et al: Comparison of nuclear magnetic resonance imaging and computed tomography in the diagnosis of upper cervical spinal cord compression. Spine 11(4):295, 1986

Paushter DN, et al: Magnetic resonance imaging of the spine: Applications and limitations. Radiol Clin North Am 23(3):551, 1985

Roub LW, Drayer BP: Spinal computer tomography: Limitations and applications. AJR 133:267, 1979

Schaffer MA, Doris PE: Limitation of the cross-table lateral view in detecting cervical spine injuries: A retrospective analysis. Ann Emerg Med 10(10):508, 1981

Stratemeier PH: Evaluation of the lumbar spine: A comparison between computed tomography and myelography. Radiol Clin North Am 21(2):221, 1983

Wang A, et al: Spinal cord or nerve root compression in patients with malignant disease: CT evaluation. J Computer Assist Tomogr 8(3):420, 1984

10

Fractures, Dislocations, and Subluxations

To evaluate appropriately cervical spine trauma, it is essential that the emergency physician have an organized and complete understanding of acute spinal injuries. As the patient's initial physician and primary diagnostician, the emergency physician must have a working knowledge of factors specific to cervical spine trauma, including mechanism of injury and forces applied, the concept of stability, associated injuries, and primary treatment. A discussion of these important concepts and the authors' philosophy of the approach to cervical spine trauma are given initially. The remainder of the chapter consists of detailed descriptions of each injury likely to be encountered, including discussions of mechanism, clinical features, specific x-ray findings, complicating factors, and treatment designed to provide a quick reference for the emergency physician. The final section addresses specific considerations of the pediatric population.

☐ CLASSIFICATION

On both a conceptual and clinical basis, the authors find a classification in terms of mechanism of injury to be the most practical in the emergency room. Laboratory experiments applying hyperflexion, hyperextension, vertical compression, lateral flexion, and rotation produce specific injuries depending on the force applied. Accident victims present with similar injuries although often a combination of the above mechanisms produces a complex injury. On the basis of history, clinical presentation, and x-ray data, the emergency

physician can, therefore, reasonably reconstruct the probable mechanism involved.

The basic pathophysiology of spinal injury is straightforward. Application of forces to the spine is analogous to a tree being blown by the wind. In a severe storm, the trunk of the tree will be bent in the direction of the force applied by the wind. The side of the tree exposed to the wind will be stretched, potentially to the point of breaking. The opposite side of the trunk is compressed and buckles. So, too, in the cervical spine, a construct of bones and ligaments, the side of the spine receiving the force will be stretched, the opposite side compressed.

More specifically, numerous authors have described the spine as a two-column construct.[1,2] Anterior elements include the anterior longitudinal ligament, vertebral body, intervertebral disc, and posterior longitudinal ligament. The posterior column is composed of all bones and ligaments posterior to, but not including, the posterior longitudinal ligament. A force directed from behind would result in hyperflexion. The elements of the posterior column directly receiving the force will be stretched or distracted, resulting in damage to the supraspinous and interspinous ligaments, the facet capsules, and the ligamenta flava, generally leaving the bony elements intact. At the same time, elements of the anterior column will be compressed, generally involving compression of the vertebral body and the intervertebral disc, while sparing ligamentous structures. Pathophysiologically, it is easy to extrapolate that forces from other directions will have similar effects, i.e., hyperextension, vertical compression, lateral flexion, and rotation.

The extent of damage incurred will be dependent on the amount of force applied. A mild breeze will bend the tree but leave no damage, whereas gale force winds tear the bark or break the trunk. So, too, forces applied to the cervical spine might serially only stretch the outermost ligaments, tear outer ligaments, tear inner ligaments, and cause enough compression on the opposite side to crush bone and disc. Hence, with more force there is greater injury.

Although several classifications have been proposed, the authors find the one presented by Harris and co-workers[3] to be the most complete and clinically useful to the emergency physician. Table 10–1 lists the essential scheme, categorized by major force or vector, and within each group, the type of lesions attributable to that force.

Hyperflexion is caused by forceful forward rotation of the head. Forward movement generally stops when the chin strikes the chest wall. Such forceful movement will apply distracting forces to the most posterior elements and compression forces to the anterior elements. Depending on the degree of force, there will be ligamentous damage, bone involvement, including compression or avulsion fractures, or both (Fig 10–1).

Simultaneous flexion and rotation usually involves a predominant flexion force with the head being slightly rotated at the outset or resulting in rotation secondary to an eccentric vector. The principle lesion caused by the combination of these forces is a unilateral facet dislocation (Fig 10–2).

In simultaneous extension and rotation, the principle force is hyperextension with the head already rotated or being rotated due to the eccentric force, resulting in a pillar fracture (Fig 10–3).

Vertical compression or axial loading is that force applied to the top of the head with the cervical spine in a neutral position, neither flexed, extended, nor rotated. The forces are transmitted through the skull onto the cervical spine resulting in burst type fractures. In the atlas this includes the Jefferson fracture and, in the lower cervical spine, bursting of the vertebral body (Fig 10–4).

Hyperextension involves a force vector applied to the forehead or the face, the head being rotated backward. Unlike hyperflexion where motion is limited by the chin striking the chest, the head is able to rotate to a far greater extent in hyperextension, resulting in increased stresses on the cervical spine. As in hyperflexion, hyperextension can result in ligamentous damage, bone fractures, or both (Fig 10–5).

Lateral flexion occurs with forces applied to the side of the head. This is rarely seen as a principle vector and is usually in combination with other predominant forces.

Atlanto-occipital and atlantoaxial disassociation and odontoid fractures result from combinations of forces as well as mechanisms not well understood. Although distraction is a force applied to the cervical spine, it does not generally manifest in specific types of injuries that are reliably reproducible.

TABLE 10–1. CERVICAL SPINE INJURIES: MECHANISM OF INJURY

Flexion
    Anterior subluxation (hyperflexion sprain)
    Bilateral interfacetal dislocation
    Simple wedge (compression) fracture
    Clay-shoveler (coal-shoveler) fracture
    Flexion teardrop fracture
Flexion-rotation
    Unilateral interfacetal dislocation
Extension-rotation
    Pillar fracture
Vertical compression
    Jefferson bursting fracture of atlas
    Burst (bursting, dispersion, axial loading) fracture
Hyperextension
    Hyperextension dislocation
    Avulsion fracture of anterior arch of atlas
    Extension teardrop fracture of axis
    Fracture of posterior arch of atlas
    Laminar fracture
    Traumatic spondylolisthesis (hangman's fracture)
    Hyperextension fracture–dislocation
Lateral flexion
    Uncinate process fracture
Diverse or imprecisely understood mechanisms
    Atlanto-occipital disassociation
    Odontoid fractures

From Harris JH, Edeikin-Monroe B, Lopaniky DR: A practical classification of acute spine injuries. Orthop Clin North Am 17(1):17, 1986.

☐ STABILITY

The bones and the ligaments that comprise the spinal column are designed to allow motion in the neck while, at the same time, protecting the spinal cord from injury. If a given part of this bone and ligament construct is damaged by trauma, this protective mechanism breaks down. Neurologic damage can occur either at the time of the injury or, if bones and ligaments are damaged, abnormal motion can result, leading to neurologic injury at a later time. Clinical instability has been defined as the loss of the ability of the spine under physiologic loads to maintain relationships between vertebrae in such a way that there is neither damage nor subsequent irritation to the spinal cord or nerve roots and, in addition, no development of deformity with excessive pain.[2]

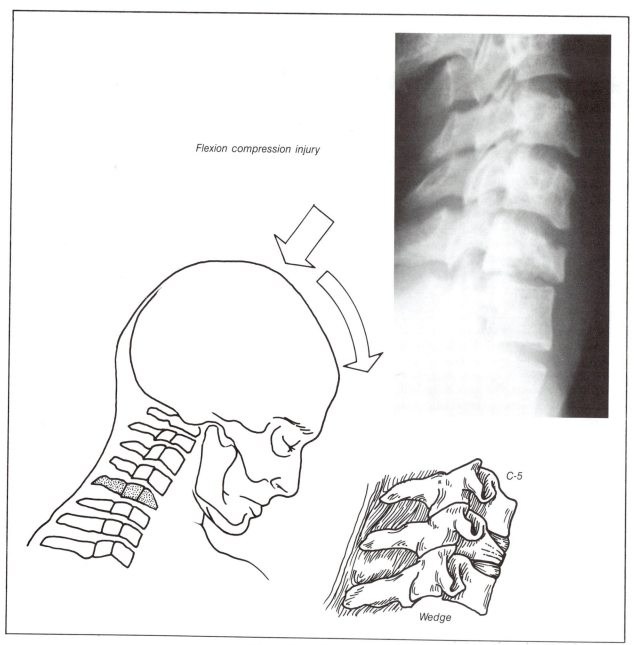

Flexion compression injury

C-5

Wedge

Figure 10–1. Hyperflexion.

Assessing stability is particularly important to the emergency physician involved in early care. It is essential to know the types of injuries likely to cause or eventually result in additional neurologic damage. The stability of specific injuries is outlined elsewhere in this chapter. It is critical, however, to know the types of injuries and findings in spinal trauma that are associated with instability. One should consider the cervical spine as having two distinct sections, the upper and the lower cervical spine.

Upper Cervical Spine

Potential instability due to injuries that involve the upper cervical spine must be evaluated by specific injury. Fractures of the ring of the atlas (C-1) can be stable or unstable depending on the integrity of the transverse and alar ligaments (Fig 10–6). The emergency physician can make that assessment on the basis of the open-mouth view of the cervical spine x-ray series. Simple fractures of C-1 will exhibit minimal lateral displacement of the lateral masses of the atlas. Displacement of

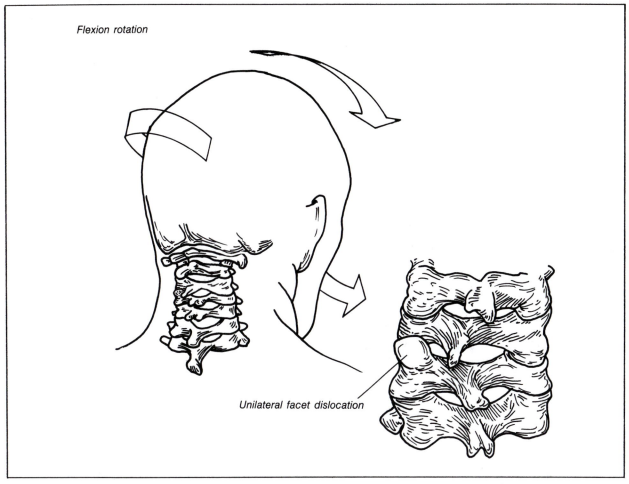

Flexion rotation

Unilateral facet dislocation

Figure 10–2. Simultaneous flexion and rotation.

the lateral masses of the atlas. Displacement of the lateral masses overriding C-2 by a distance less than 5.7 mm indicates that the transverse ligament is intact (Fig 10–7, top).[4] A distance of 7 mm or greater is evidence of a ruptured transverse ligament (Fig 10-7, bottom).[5,6] This constitues an unstable injury, allowing the odontoid process to compress the cord and potentially cause neurologic damage. Similarly, fractures of the odontoid process at its base or, occasionally through the body of C-2, are unstable.[4,7]

Fractures, however, are not a requirement of instability at the C-1 and C-2 level. Atlantoaxial instability occurs with rupture of the transverse ligament alone. The emergency physician can diagnose this injury on the lateral cervical spine film. The normal distance between the dens and the anterior ring of the atlas should be between 0 and 3 mm (Fig 10–8). A distance of 3 to 5 mm suggests rupture of the transverse ligament.[6,8] A distance greater than 5 mm strongly suggests that the transverse and alar ligaments are ruptured. If there is any suspicion of injury at this level, flexion-extension views may be contraindicated as these are

precisely the mechanisms that will lead to neurologic damage.

Axiom: *Suspicion of rupture of transverse ligament contraindicates doing flexion–extension views. Patients with greater than 3 to 5 mm separation between the dens and the anterior ring of the atlas should be suspect of a transverse rupture until proven otherwise.*

Patients with advanced rheumatoid arthritis may normally have a distance of 3 mm between the atlas and the dens and there is controversy as to what distinguishes instability in these patients. The decision to surgically stabilize is controversial. It is recommended that these patients be emergently referred.

Traumatic spondylolisthesis of the axis (hangman's fracture) is manifested by a fracture through the posterior neural arch (Fig 10–9). If only the fracture is

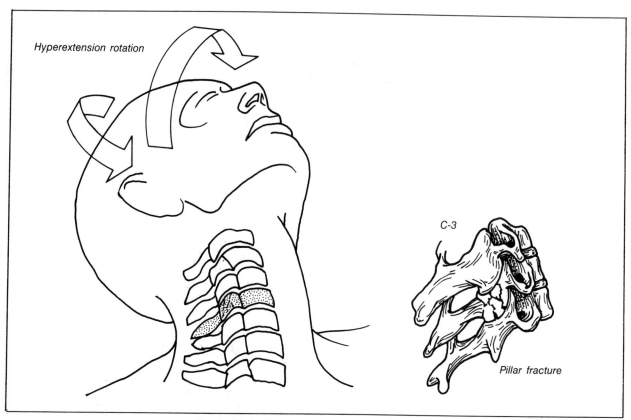

Figure 10–3. Simultaneous extension and rotation.

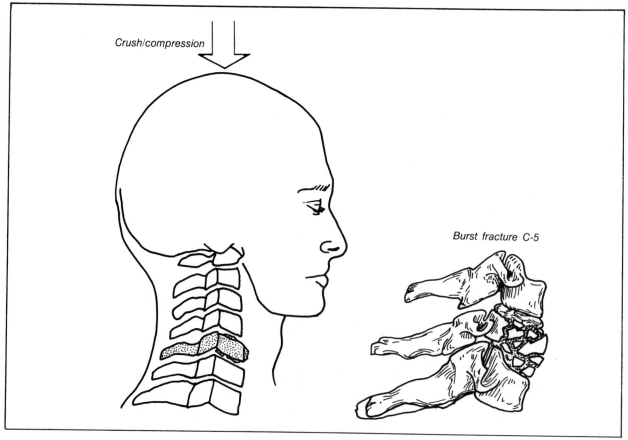

Figure 10–4. Axial compression.

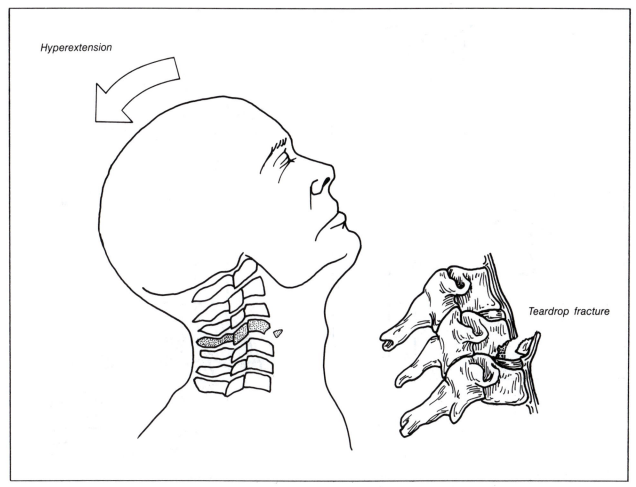

Figure 10–5. Hyperextension.

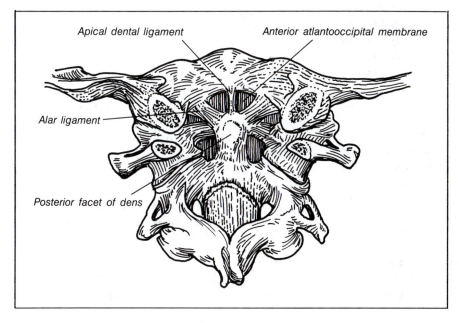

Figure 10–6. Posterior view of transverse and alar ligaments of the ring of the atlas.

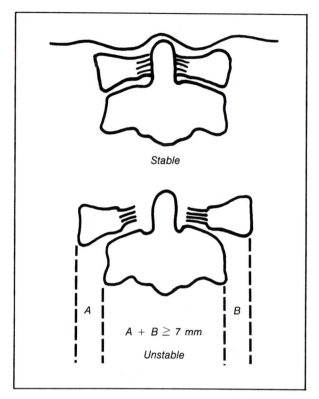

Figure 10–7. Displacement of the left lateral masses of C-1 overriding C-2.

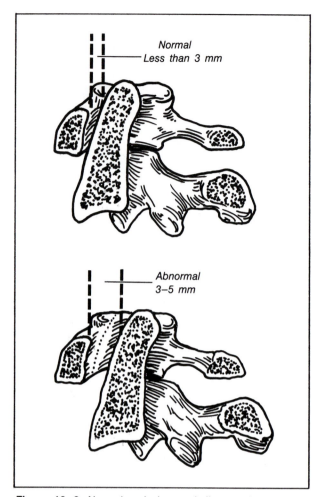

Figure 10–8. Normal and abnormal distance between the dens and the anterior ring of the atlas.

present, the injury is stable, as supporting ligaments prevent abnormal motion. It is not uncommon that anterior and posterior longitudinal ligaments and the intervertebral disc can rupture. This is extremely unstable. In this instance, very cautious flexion views can assist in the diagnosis.

Lower Cervical Spine

Biomechanical studies have shown that ligamentous support allows very little motion between vertebrae and that horizontal motion of one vertebral body over the subjacent vertebra never exceeds 3.5 mm and that angular motion between vertebrae was always calculated to be 11 degrees or less.[2]

Clinically the emergency physician can use this information to assess instability in the lower cervical spine. Faced with an overriding vertebra, a measurement between the posterior–inferior corner of the upper vertebral body and the posterior–superior corner of the inferior vertebral body should be less than 3.5 mm in healthy adults (Fig 10–10). Instability should be suspected with measurements greater than 3.5 mm. Bilateral facet dislocation, for instance, is generally associated with a displacement of 7 mm or greater. Anteriorly, this is seen as an overriding of the superior vertebral body by a distance equal to or greater than one-half of its anteroposterior diameter (Fig 10–11).

Axiom: *Instability should be suspected when there is greater than a 3.5-mm distance between the adjacent vertebral bodies as shown in Figure 10–10.*

Angular measurements can also be determined from the lateral cervical spine x-ray. By drawing lines extending from the inferior aspects of the vertebral body, the intersecting angle should be less than 11 degrees. An angle greater than 11 degrees strongly suggests instability (Fig 10–12).

Axiom: *Instability should be suspected when angular measurement between vertebrae is greater than 11 degrees.*

In the face of acute trauma, a cervical spine x-ray series in the emergency room is generally undertaken

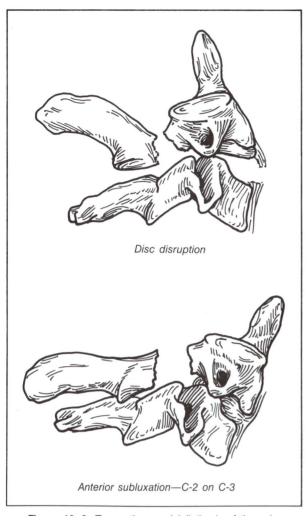

Disc disruption

Anterior subluxation—C-2 on C-3

Figure 10–9. Traumatic spondylolisthesis of the axis (hangman's fracture).

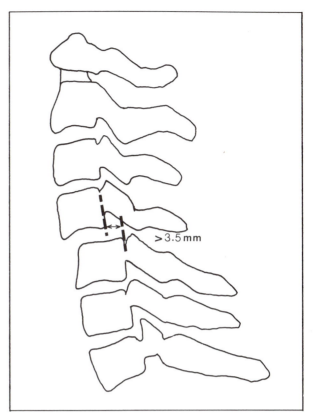

Figure 10–10. Limits of normal overriding of cervical vertebrae.

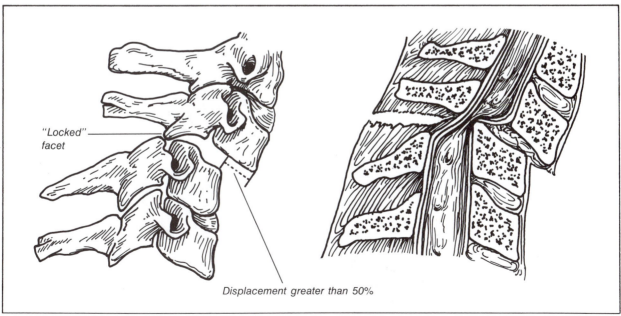

"Locked" facet

Displacement greater than 50%

Figure 10–11. Bilateral facet dislocation 50% overriding of the superior vertebral body.

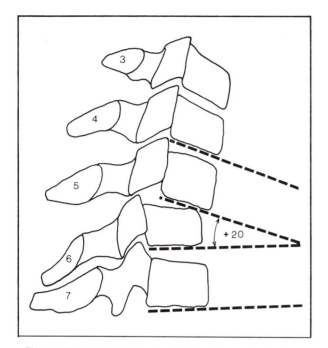

Figure 10–12. Excessive angulation of the cervical spine.

with the spine at rest. If there is no associated neurologic damage, the emergency physician can supervise flexion–extension views to assess instability. In the setting of injury, however, there is frequently significant paraspinal muscle spasm that may limit motion. It is the recommendation of the authors that if the index of suspicion is great enough, the patient should be treated as having an unstable injury. If neurologic deficit is already present or the question of instability is not in doubt, flexion–extension views are contraindicated. It should be assumed that if either all of the anterior elements or posterior elements are destroyed, the injury is unstable.

Axiom: *Injury to both anterior and posterior elements should be presumed unstable.*

☐ NEUROLOGIC INJURY

Injury to the cord occurs due to stretching, crushing, vascular compromise, or compression. Certain types of injury mechanisms are more likely to be associated with specific neurologic damage (Fig 10–13).[9] Spinal injury with flexion injuries is due to retropulsed disc material compressing the cord. Bilateral facet dislocation causes an impingement on the spinal cord.

Anterior cord syndrome occurs after vertical compression or hyperflexion injuries (Fig 10–14). Motor and sensory loss are evident in the presence of an intact posterior column.[10] Anterior dislocations and hyperextension injuries can cause a central cord syndrome evidenced by motor more than sensory loss in the upper extremities (Fig 10–15). With incomplete cord lesions, posterior cord lesions are associated with the best prognosis, anterior cord lesions with the worst.[11]

Many patients may present with normal appearing cervical spine films in the face of significant neurologic damage. This is generally due to marked deformation of the cervical spine at the instant of injury, thus crushing the cord, the spine returning to its normal position immediately after the injury, as is frequently the case in hyperextension injuries. Conversely, a markedly abnormal cervical spine film may be associated with no neurologic damage. This is more likely the case in upper cervical lesions due to the increased width of the cervical canal at that level.

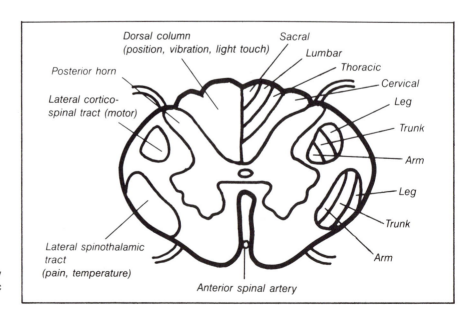

Figure 10–13. Types of injury mechanisms resulting in specific neurologic damage.

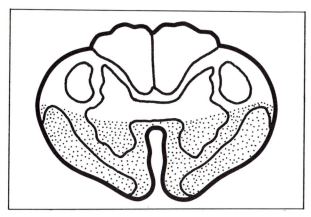

Figure 10–14. The anterior cord syndrome.

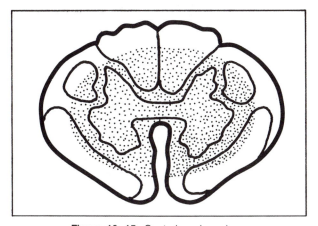

Figure 10–15. Central cord syndrome.

□ TREATMENT

Definitive treatment of fractures and dislocation is to relocate the bony fragments and reduce joint dislocations. In the face of neurologic damage, this should be done as rapidly as possible.[12] A patient manifesting no neurologic damage requires no such urgency. In the emergency center, axial traction is generally the procedure of choice for cervical injuries with neurologic deficit or instability and the potential of deficit. Application of Gardner-Wells tongs with the addition of weights should be done in the emergency room.

The tongs consist of a rigid semicircle that follows the coronal contour of the calvaria. A threaded hole, which accommodates a screw for the advancement of the cone-shaped points, is retractable by an enclosed spring that is calibrated to indicate when a squeeze pressure of 30 lb is reached. The instrument is designed for emergency bedside application under antiseptic, rather than aseptic, conditions.

Hair should be shaved around the site where the tong is to be applied. This will decrease the chance of osteomyelitis of the skull. The scalp is then prepped with an antiseptic solution. Lidocaine is injected at the site where the points of the tongs will be applied, above the ears and below the "equator" (Fig 10-16). Flexion and extension of the head is obtained by adjusting the height of the pulley.

The tapered points are advanced into the skin.

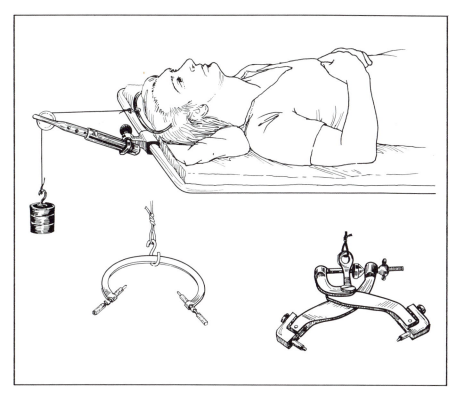

Figure 10–16. Application of Gardner-Wells tongs.

Because the points are directed upward as they advance, the skin is stretched about them. This seals the point of entry and prevents bleeding. When bone is encountered, the stiff spring yields until the posterior end of the spring-loaded point just protrudes out of the casing. This indicates that the spring is fully compressed and is exerting 30 lb of pressure between the points. The tongs are then tilted back and forth to insure proper seating, after which they are retightened if the posterior end of the spring-loaded point has recessed. The total excursion of the spring is approximately 5 mm, thus avoiding the possibility of penetrating too deeply and resultant pressure atrophy. The points of the tongs, when applied properly, rarely pull out due to their angle. The points should be just below the temporal ridges.

Weights are attached to the tongs to provide the appropriate amount of traction. Ten pounds of traction is needed to overcome the weight of the head and approximately 5 lb of traction can be added for each interspace above the lesion. The tongs will easily tolerate a traction of 65 lb. Rotation of the head is prevented by placing a sandbag under each projecting end of the points. This is especially important when dealing with fractures of the odontoid.

Muscle spasm can make reduction significantly more difficult, but can be treated with muscle relaxants and sedation. X-ray guidance is imperative with the use of traction and each additional increment of weight. Even minimal axial traction in the face of gross ligamentous instability can lead to overdistraction. In general, the more ligamentous the disruption, the easier the reduction.

☐ FLEXION

Hyperflexion Sprain

Stable Injury

Mechanism. Simple severe flexion. Only moderate forces applied to the posterior ligamentous structures resulting in incomplete tearing of interspinous and supraspinous ligaments. In passive hyperflexion, range of motion is limited as the chin strikes the anterior chest wall (Fig 10–17).

Clinical Features. The patient is generally able to describe a pure flexion injury. This sprain is rarely associated with other injuries. Complaints are of posterior neck pain attributed to the areas of interspinous or supraspinous ligament disruption or sprain. Pain may be noted at the base of the neck, shoulders, trapezius and deltoid muscles, and interscapular region. If nerve

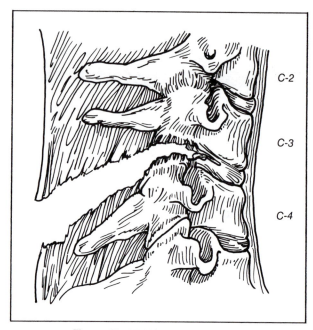

Figure 10–17. Hyperflexion sprain.

roots were impinged at the time of hyperflexion, patients may complain of radiating pain to the occiput or arms and fingers. Occasionally hoarseness, dysphagia, dizziness, and vertigo may be present.[13]

Radiographs. May be normal or show a slight kyphotic angulation at the area of injury without anterior–posterior vertebral displacement. Severe forms of injury may demonstrate slightly increased space between spinous processes.

Complications. Disruption of the posterior ligament complex has been associated with a 30 to 50% incidence of delayed instability due to poor ligamentous healing.[7]

Emergency Management and Referral. An initial trial of conservative therapy is recommended, including rest, nonsteroidal anti-inflammatory medications, analgesics, and cold and heat treatments. The use of a soft collar is controversial; if the patient feels more comfortable, use one. Early referral is recommended.

Simple Wedge (Compression) Fracture

Potentially Unstable Injury

Mechanism. Forceful flexion generally associated with mild anterior compressive forces sufficient to cause impaction of one vertebra by adjacent vertebrae (Fig 10–18).

Clinical Features. Variable depending on the degree of injury. Initial injury may have included sufficient compressive forces accounting for skull injuries. Neurologic sequelae are uncommon and limited only to nerve

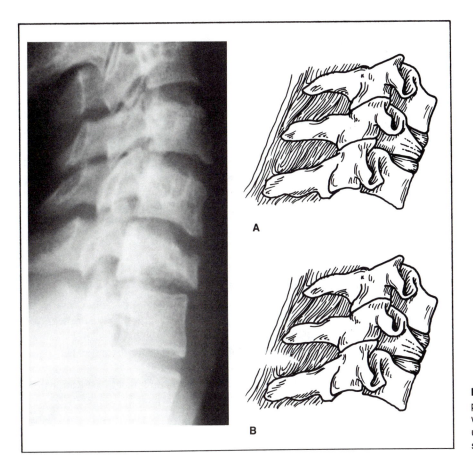

Figure 10–18. Simple wedge (compression) fracture. **A.** Stable injury with ligaments intact. **B.** Potentially unstable injury with ruptured supraspinous and interspinous ligaments.

root involvement. Pain is described in the neck, shoulders, trapezius and deltoid muscles, and interscapular regions, occasionally radiating pain to the arms and fingers depending on nerve root involvement. Hoarseness, dysphagia, dizziness, vertigo, and tinnitus may be present. The intervertebral disc may be disrupted or detached. Posterior elements (supraspinous and inter-

spinous ligaments, liagmentum flavum, and capsular ligaments) are generally intact. Only if the posterior elements are involved is this injury potentially unstable.

Radiographs. Vertical height of the involved vertebral body is flattened. The superior end-plate is impacted. Depending on the degree of posterior ligamentous involvement, widening of the spinous processes may be seen.

Complications. If separation of the spinous process is present, the posterior ligamentous apparatus is disrupted. If significantly so, this injury is potentially unstable.

Emergency Management and Referral. As in hyperflexion injury. Early referral. If posterior involvement is present, immediate referral.

Clay-Shoveler Fracture

Stable Injury

Mechanism. As suggested by the name, this injury occurs when the head and the upper cervical segments are forced into flexion against the action of the interspinous and supraspinous ligaments. It may also occur with blunt trauma (Fig 10–19).

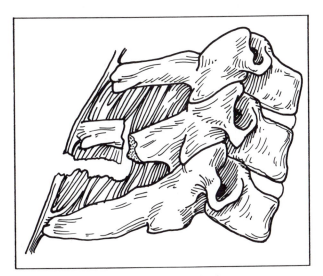

Figure 10–19. Clay-shoveler fracture.

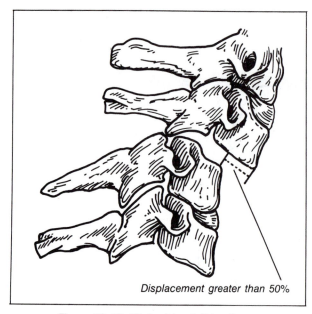

Displacement greater than 50%

Figure 10–20. Bilateral facet dislocation.

Clinical Features. Patient complains of focal pain over the affected spinous processes and neck stiffness. Point tenderness is noted on physical examination.

Radiographs. Avulsion fracture of one or more of the spinous processes of C-7, C-6, and T-1, in that order.[3,25]

Complications. None.

Emergency Management and Referral. Supportive, ice, analgesics, rest, early referral.

Bilateral Facet Dislocation

Very Unstable Injury

Mechanism. Marked hyperflexion without rotation. There is complete disruption of the posterior ligament complex, including the posterior longitudinal ligament and the annulus. With anterior dislocation, the superior facets pass upward and forward over the inferior facets and become entrapped ("locked") in the intervertebral foramina (Figs 10–11 and 10–20).

Clinical Features. Presentation is variable. Patients complain of neck pain, stiffness, and inability to rotate the head. The chin is in the midline and there is often a slight prominence of the spinous process of the inferior vertebra. This lesion is often associated with nerve root and cord compression, including quadriplegia.

Radiographs. The lateral x-ray is quite dramatic. Bilateral facet dislocation is characterized by anterior displacement of the involved vertebral body by at least 50% of its anteroposterior (AP) diameter (Fig 10–11).

The facets of the involved vertebra lie anterior to the facets of the subjacent vertebra. Impaction fractures of the involved facets are common. They are small and generally clinically insignificant. Incomplete bilateral dislocation is called *perched* facets, where the inferior aspect of the superior facets come to rest on the superior aspect of the inferior facets without complete override.

As the dislocation of the facets is bilateral, the entire upper cervical spine is pushed forward but appears almost unremarkable on the AP film. Oblique radiographs clearly show the bilaterality of the defect.

Complications. As evidenced by the marked distortion on the lateral radiograph, bilateral facet dislocation results in significant narrowing of the spinal foramen. The majority of these lesions occur between C-5, C-6, and C-7, where the cervical spinal foramen is most narrow. Cord compression resulting in quadriplegia frequently occurs. Emergent reduction can potentially result in significant recovery. Due to the extent of the ligamentous damage, bilateral facet dislocations are easier to reduce than unilateral facet dislocations. As such, they are markedly unstable.

Emergency Management and Referral. Immediate referral. Emergent reduction is imperative. Axial traction either manually or, more effectively, with Gardner-Wells tongs and weights can lead to closed reduction. (See Chapter 1 for application.) Open reduction may be necessary. Incidence of chronic instability is quite high.

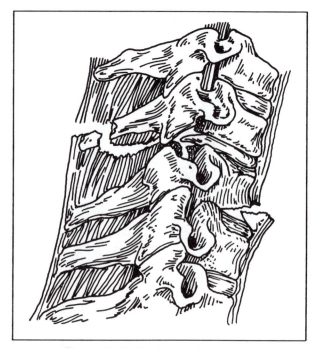

Figure 10–21. Flexion teardrop fracture.

Flexion Teardrop Fracture

Extremely Unstable Injury

Mechanism. This lesion is produced by severe hyperflexion associated with marked compressive forces resulting in complete disruption of all ligaments as well as the intervertebral disc. Disruptions of the facetal joints and a comminuted fracture of the vertebral body occur, including the characteristic large triangular fragment off the anterior portion of the vertebral body. Large fragments of the posterior aspect of the vertebral body are pushed into the spinal canal (Fig 10–21).

Clinical Features. The most frequent cause of this type of injury is a diving accident, the patient striking his or her head on a rock, sand, or pool bottom with the cervical spine in flexion (Fig 10–22). This produces the worst possible flexion injury, resulting in a comminuted burst-type fracture. The vertebral body fragments are pushed forward, resulting in anterior longitudinal ligament rupture, and backward, displaced fragments into the spinal cord resulting in cord compression. The patient, therefore, presents with an anterior cord syndrome, sparing the posterior columns, resulting in paralysis, loss of pain and temperature, with preservation of vibration, motion, touch, and position. It is not uncommon, however, to find the cord completely crushed at the level of the lesion.

Radiographs. The lateral radiograph will show the upper cervical spine in a state of flexion. The involved vertebra shows a fracture of the anterior–inferior corner, triangular in shape, hence the name, teardrop fracture. The involved vertebra appears displaced and rotated anteriorly. An associated injury might well be fracture or dislocation of the facet joints. Further impingement on the spinal cord is caused by a large fragment of the vertebral body that has been displaced posteriorly.

Complications. As this injury is often associated with diving accidents, the emergency physician is frequently

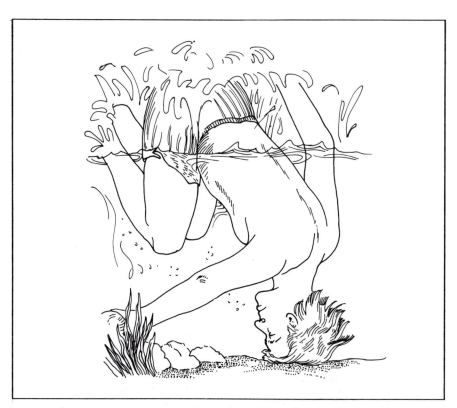

Figure 10–22. Mechanism of injury resulting in flexion teardrop fracture.

presented with a patient described as a drowning or near-drowning victim. If the involved vertebra is in the C-4 and C-5 area, paralysis might include respiratory muscles and the patient will be apneic. While primary cardiorespiratory resuscitative measures are paramount, institution and preservation of spinal precautions will prevent further neurologic compromise.

Emergency Management and Referral. Immediate referral. The flexion teardrop fracture results from a combination of compressive and flexion forces. Thus, compressive forces result in a comminuted vertebral body with displacement of fragments posteriorly, impinging on the cord. Hyperflexion, however, results in major ligamentous disruption, both posteriorly and, potentially, anteriorly and is extremely unstable. Axial traction with Gardner-Wells tongs can potentially reduce fragments in the spinal cord. This should be done under radiographic guidance. In the emergency center, complete immobilization of the spine is essential, as discussed in Chapter 1. Immediate referral is recommended for definitive emergent care.

☐ FLEXION–ROTATION

Unilateral Facet Dislocation

Generally Stable Injury—Potentially Unstable If Chronic

Mechanism. Combination of flexion and rotation forces. The interfacetal joint on the side of the direction of the rotation acts as a pivot. The opposite joint becomes dislocated when the superior facet moves an-

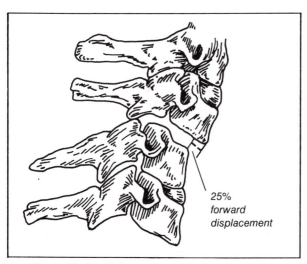

25%
forward
displacement

Figure 10–23. Unilateral facet dislocation rotation of vertebrae in unilateral facet dislocation.

teriorly and superiorly above the inferior facet. The capsule of the involved facet joint is disrupted. The anterior and posterior longitudinal ligaments on the involved side may be partially disrupted. The pivotal facet joint on the contralateral side is still completely intact, providing significant stability. The involved joint is "locked" (Fig 10–23).

Clinical Features. The patient complains of neck pain, usually isolated to one side. The head is rotated away from the side of the lesion, the chin pointing to the opposite shoulder. Nerve root impingement is not uncommon. The spinal cord is rarely involved, however, as the injury is manifested by rotating the upper portion of the cervical spine around an intact cord without encroaching on the spinal foramen.

Radiographs. The cross-table lateral cervical radiograph shows the involved vertebral body anteriorly displaced by a distance of approximately 25% of the AP diameter of the vertebral body. It is extremely important to obtain a true lateral view of the cervical spine as there is a significant rotational component to this injury. The portion of the cervical spine inferior to the injury will be shown in its true lateral position. The cervical spine superior to the injury, however, will demonstrate a degree of obliquity, as the anterior displacement of the involved "locked" facet will rotate the upper cervical spine.

The posterior–inferior margin of the dislocated superior facet is displaced anterior to the superior tip of the inferior facet, coming to rest in the intervertebral foramen. The dislocated superior facet may sustain a small, clinically insignificant injury.

Oblique views of the dislocated superior facet clearly show the anterior displacement. In the AP view, the spinous process is deviated toward the side of the dislocation, and the typical undulating lines of the lateral masses will appear distorted.

Complications. A chronic pain syndrome can result from an unreduced facet dislocation.

Emergency Management and Referral. Reduction of the dislocation is favored. If only the capsule has been disrupted, the injury is truly a "locked" facet and difficult to reduce with traction. The greater the amount of ligamentous damage, i.e., involvement of the posterior longitudinal ligament, the easier the reduction. Without reduction and with posterior longitudinal ligament involvement, the incidence of chronic instability and pain leads most authors to recommend open reduction and repair. As such, immediate referral is recommended. Unilateral facet dislocation without rupture of the posterior longitudinal ligament is very difficult to reduce

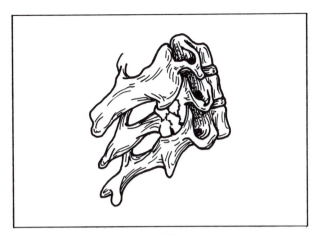

Figure 10–24. Pillar fracture.

with traction. If there is no evidence of neurologic damage, the injury is quite stable and can be left to heal in the dislocated position. This can, however, result in limitation of rotation and a chronic pain syndrome.

☐ EXTENSION–ROTATION

Pillar Fracture

Mechanism. Hyperextension and rotation. Hyperextension brings the articular pillars into contact. With simultaneous rotation of the head, range of motion is compromised and the force of hyperextension is directed toward a single pillar (Fig 10–24).

A pillar fracture results with tear in the anterior longitudinal ligament as well. The patient usually has a vertical fracture line through the articular pillar.

☐ VERTICAL COMPRESSION

Jefferson Burst Fracture

Stable, Rarely Unstable Injury

Mechanism. Vertical compression or axial loading. The injury occurs with a significant vertical compression at a time when the cervical spine is perfectly straight with neither flexion nor extension. The force is transmitted to the spine through the occipital condyles. This results in one of two fracture configurations: (1) lateral mass fracture if the force is slightly eccentric. Therefore, it is often on one side, the fracture line passing either through the articular surface just anterior or posterior to the lateral mass. Lateral mass

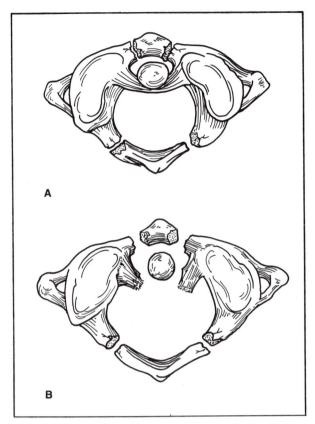

Figure 10–25. Jefferson burst fracture. **A.** Transverse ligament intact. **B.** Transverse ligament disrupted.

displacement is asymmetric. (2) The burst injury or true Jefferson fracture, consisting of four fractures, two in the posterior arch and two in the anterior arch. There is generally no cord damage. Anterior and posterior ligaments are intact. These are generally stable fractures (Fig 10–25).

Clinical Features. The patient presents with pain in the upper part of the neck and the vertex of the skull. Often there is a contusion, hematoma, or laceration on the top of the head.

Radiographs. Fractures of the lateral masses and Jefferson fractures are difficult to appreciate on the lateral cervical film. Prevertebral soft tissue swelling can be significant. The open-mouth view demonstrates displacement of the lateral masses of C-1 in relation to the articular surface of C-2. Measurement of this displacement on each side should be added. A total distance of less than 5.7 mm is considered stable, the transverse ligament being intact. Some authors believe a distance greater than 7 mm strongly suggests that the transverse ligament is ruptured, making this lesion potentially unstable.[14,15] Others believe that in the setting of axial loading alone, the alar ligaments and portions of the facet capsules remain intact, thus preventing gross instability even in the setting of transverse ligament rupture (Fig 10–7).[6]

Complications. Up to 50% association with concomitant cervical fractures, most commonly traumatic spondylolisthesis of the axis and posteriorly displaced type II and III dens fractures. If a Jefferson fracture is found, therefore, the emergency physician should be wary of other cervical spine fractures. Conversely, in the setting of cervical spine fractures due to hyperextension with significant axial compression, a C-1 fracture should be ruled out.

Axiom: *Jefferson fractures have a 50% incidence of concomitant cervical-spine fractures.*

Emergency Management and Referral. The vast majority of C-1 burst fractures are stable and treated with halo traction. The possibility of instability due to transverse ligament disruption significantly alters this approach. Immobilize the cervical spine as described in Chapter 1 and the patient needs urgent referral.

Burst Fracture

Potentially Unstable Injury

Mechanism. Vertical compression or axial loading. This force results in an explosive comminuted fracture of the vertebral body. Most typically, it occurs at the level of C-5. The anterior 25% of the body is displaced anteriorly, often resembling a teardrop fracture. The posterior portion of the vertebral body is fragmented and displaced posterolaterally, the inferior margin being pushed into the spinal canal with the inferior disc. Dor-

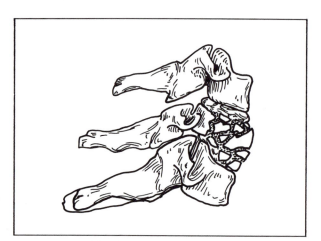

Figure 10–26. Burst fracture.

sal spine elements are generally not fractured but forces displaced posteriorly can disrupt the facet capsules, further posteriorly subluxing the vertebral body. The posterior ligament complex, however, generally remains intact, providing the only remaining stability (Fig 10–26).

Clinical Features. There is a significant incidence of neurologic damage, secondary to impingement of bone and disc on the cord. Patients complain of pain at the vertex of the skull as well as neck pain at the level of the lesion. Evidence of cord compression and neurologic compromise localize the lesion.

Radiographs. The lateral cervical radiograph demonstrates comminution of the vertebral body. The anterior portion may be thrust forward similar to the teardrop fracture seen in hyperflexion, but is usually much larger. There is decrease of the disc space below. The spinous processes are generally not spread apart. The posterior portion of the vertebral body may be displaced posteriorly into the spinal canal. The cervical spine is generally straight. The alignment of the posterior elements is normal. The AP view will demonstrate a vertical vertebral body fracture. The advent of computed tomography has demonstrated a posterior arch fracture usually involving the laminae. Although rarely seen with conventional x-ray, it is almost always present.

Complications. Neurologic sequelae quite common. Closed head injuries.

Emergency Management and Referral. Immediate referral. Although many consider the burst fracture of the lower cervical spine and the flexion teardrop fracture to be degrees of the same injury, differences in the lateral x-ray, neurologic findings, and pathologic characteristics of the involved vertebra strongly suggest these to be two separate entities.

☐ EXTENSION

Hyperextension Sprain

Stable, Potentially Unstable Injury

Mechanism. A direct posteriorly directed force applied to the face or forehead, or, as more commonly seen, in rear-ended automobile accidents. Posterior elements act as a fulcrum, but unlike flexion injuries where the forward movement is limited by the chin hitting the chest wall, there is no stopping point posteriorly. There

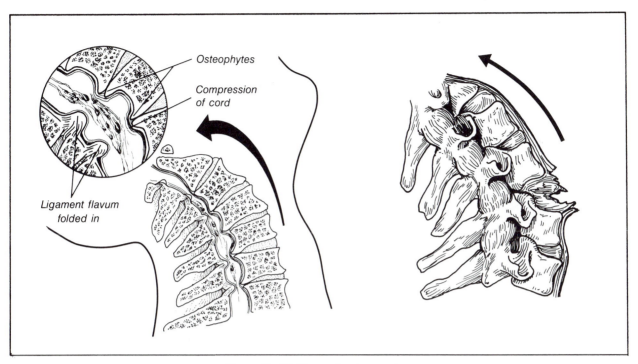

Figure 10–27. Hyperextension sprain.

is thus the possibility of significant soft tissue injury, including torn anterior muscles, chiefly sternocleidomastoid, scalene, and longus colli muscles, distraction of the esophagus and trachea, possible disruption of the anterior longitudinal ligament, and rupture of intervertebral discs. Fractures caused by this mechanism are described in the hyperextension fracture–dislocation section. If the anterior longitudinal ligament is torn, the vertebra superior to the tear will be forced posteriorly. The spinal cord then becomes compressed between the posteriorly displaced vertebra anteriorly and the posterior neural arch and ligamentum flavum posteriorly (Fig 10–27).

Clinical Features. The patient will describe a hyperextension mechanism of injury as in a blow to the head or rear-end auto accident without appropriate neck support (i.e., head rests improperly positioned). Complaints are of pain in the neck, particularly anteriorly, with tenderness and spasm of the sternocleidomastoid, scalene, and longus colli muscles, dysphagia, or hoarseness. Neurologic findings are those of posterior cord syndrome characterized by motor loss distal to the lesion or even complete quadriplegia.[28]

Radiographs. The lateral cervical film may appear normal with only varying degrees of prevertebral soft tissue swelling. A small avulsion fracture may be noted from the anterior aspect of the inferior end-plate of the involved vertebral body. A vacuum defect or widened disc space at the level of the injury is sometimes seen. Carefully supervised flexion–extension views may reveal significant instability. It is important to note that the patient presenting with quadriplegia or significant neurologic deficit at the level of the cervical spine may have a "normal" film. Although little radiographic abnormality may exist, spinal cord damage is due to a pinching of the cord at the time of hyperextension.

Axiom: *Posttraumatic quadriplegia with "normal" cervical spine radiographs should be assumed due to severe hyperextenion injury.*

Complications. Variable depending on the degree of hyperextension. Although x-rays may appear normal and outward signs of trauma may appear minimal, patients may complain of severe neck pain and other symptoms consistent with a whiplash syndrome. Varying degrees of neurologic deficit including quadriplegia or posterior cord syndrome may be present.

Emergency Management and Referral. Patients who on physical examination are neurologically intact and whose injury is limited to soft tissue with a stable cervical spine can be treated conservatively with rest, analgesics, cold and heat therapy, and early referral. X-rays suggesting possible instability (i.e., abnormal flexion–extension laxity or avulsion fracture and disc

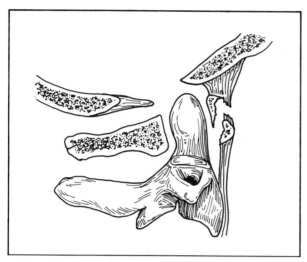

Figure 10–28. Avulsion fracture of the anterior arch of the atlas.

space abnormality) or neurologic symptoms require immediate referral.

Avulsion Fracture of the Anterior Arch of the Atlas

Potentially Unstable Injury

Mechanism. Hyperextension against intact longus colli muscle and atlantoaxial ligament, both of which insert on or inferior to the anterior tubercle of the atlas (Fig 10–28).[29]

Clinical Features. Patient presents with a history of injury consistent with hyperextension. Complains of pain in the upper, anterior neck.

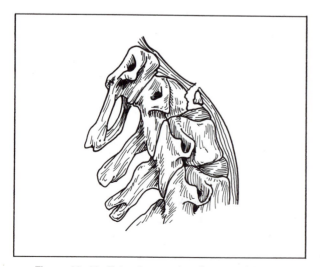

Figure 10–29. Extension teardrop fracture of the axis.

Radiographs. On the lateral cervical radiograph there is a horizontal fracture along the anterior arch of C-1. Prevertebral soft tissue swelling.

Emergency Management and Referral. Immobilize the spine and refer this patient. If the avulsion involves the complete anterior arch, the fracture is unstable; if only a fragment, this is a stable injury.

Extension Teardrop Fracture of the Axis

Potentially Unstable Injury

Mechanism. Pathognomonic injury of hyperextension. Avulsion of the anterior–inferior corner of the axis secondary to rupture of the anterior longitudinal ligament. As such, in extension this injury becomes potentially unstable, particularly if accompanied by significant disruption of the disc. As the posterior ligament complex and facet joints are intact, it is stable in flexion (Fig 10–29).

Clinical Features. Generally seen in elderly patients with osteopenia or preexistent degenerative osteoarthritis of the cervical spine. Patient complains of neck pain and describes an injury consistent with pure hyperflexion.

Radiographs. The lateral cervical film reveals a triangular fragment off the anterior–inferior corner of the axis.

Emergency Management and Referral. Immobilize and admit this patient. These patients probably require computed axial tomography scan to evaluate if there is any compromise to the neural canal.

Fracture of the Posterior Arch of the Atlas

Stable Injury

Mechanism. Hyperextension with compression transmitted through the posterior arch between the occiput and the spinous process of the axis. Unlike other C-1

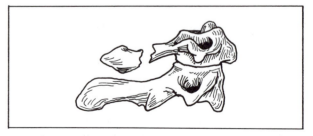

Figure 10–30. Fracture of the posterior arch of the atlas.

fractures, i.e., Jefferson fracture, the major vector in this injury is hyperflexion. The fracture occurs at the junction of the posterior arch and the lateral mass (Fig 10–30).

Clinical Features. Patient describes injury consistent with hyperextension. Injuries to the forehead may be present. Complains of posterior upper neck pain. No neurologic symptoms.

Radiographs. Isolated posterior arch fractures are best demonstrated in the lateral cervical film. It is seen as a vertical fracture of the posterior arch with little or no displacement. There is typically no prevertebral soft tissue swelling. The open-mouth view shows no lateral displacement of the C-1 articular masses.

Complications. Frequently associated with other cervical spine fractures, particularly posteriorly displaced type II dens fractures and type I traumatic spondylolisthesis of the axis. See Jefferson fracture.

Emergency Management and Referral. In the absence of associated cervical injury, collar immobilization. Early referral.

Laminar Fracture

Stable Injury

Mechanism. Hyperextension with compression resulting in fracture of the posterior arch of the lower cervical vertebra between the articular mass and the spinous process (Fig 10–31).

Clinical Features. Older patients with cervical spondylosis sustaining hyperextension injuries.[29]

Radiographs. On the lateral film, a vertical fracture is seen through the lamina. It is best seen on computed tomography.

Emergency Management and Referral. This stable injury requires cervical immobilization and referral.

Traumatic Spondylolisthesis of the Axis (Hangman's Fracture)

Potentially Unstable Injury

Mechanism. Hyperextension with axial compression. Forced hyperextension applied to the lower limits of the cervicocranium (occiput, C-1, C-2) leads to fracture at the weakest point, the pars interarticularis of C-2. Historically described as the ideal lesion of judicial hanging, it is more commonly seen as a result of motor vehicle accidents where the patient is thrust forward, striking the forehead against the windshield, the head violently hyperextended.

When only a bilateral pedicle fracture is seen, little displacement occurs and no instability is present (type I). Greater than 3 mm anterior translation and angulation of C-2 is termed type II. If further force is applied, disruption of the anterior and posterior longitudinal ligaments can occur, as well as disruption of the disc between C-2 and C-3; thus is type III. In this injury, there is true instability. It is this injury that occurs in judicial hanging, resulting in severing of the cord and instant death. As seen in automobile accidents, however, the trauma is often less severe, and neurologic sequelae are seldom seen because (1) hyperextension forces are less dramatic and (2) the disruption occurs where the cervical canal is at its widest point (Fig 10–32).

Clinical Features. The patient complains of diffuse pain and stiffness. The pain may radiate along the course of the occipital nerve from C-2, so-called occip-

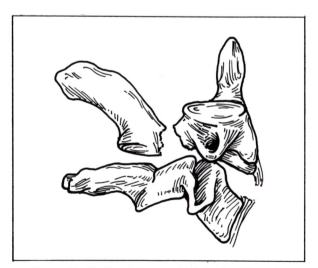

Figure 10–32. Traumatic spondylolisthesis of the axis (hangman's fracture).

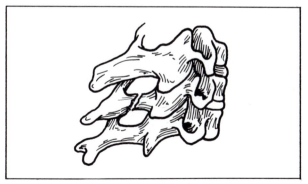

Figure 10–31. Laminar fracture.

ital neuralgia. There is evidence of trauma on the forehead, secondary to striking the windshield, and may be associated with facial or skull fractures. In hanging injuries, evidence of strangulation is present. If instantaneous death does not occur, neurologic compromise is rare.[30]

Radiographs. The lateral cervical film may be variable depending on the extent of the lesion. This can be limited to vertical fractures of the pedicles of C-2 without displacement or may show marked anterior displacement and angulation of the C-1 and C-2 complex, suggestive of a flexion mechanism. A wedge fracture of the vertebral body of C-3 may be present. Marked prevertebral hemorrhage is invariably present.

Complications. Associated fractures of the lower cervical spine are not uncommon, including burst or spinous process fractures. Fracture of the posterior arch of the atlas may also be seen.

Emergency Management and Referral. Immediate referral. Treatment depends on stability. Marked anterior displacement of C-2 on C-3 notes marked instability. Flexion–extension views are contraindicated. If only pedicle fractures are seen, carefully supervised flexion–extension views will help determine stability.

Hyperextension Fracture–Dislocation

Unstable Injury

Mechanism. Marked hyperextension with an axial compressive component, perhaps with eccentrically di-

rected force or the head rotated, resulting in force being driven through the lateral masses and the posterior elements. The articular mass becomes comminuted and fractures can occur in the pedicle and the lamina. As such, the vertebral body can be displaced anteriorly and the anterior longitudinal ligament can be disrupted, allowing for this injury to be mistaken as a flexion injury (Fig 10–33).

Clinical Features. Trauma may be present on the forehead and the face, potentially causing facial and skull fractures. Neurologic lesions are not uncommon. Patients present with severe neck pain in the midcervical region often radiating to the head.

Radiographs. The lateral cervical film reveals a severely comminuted fracture of the articular masses frequently with many small fragments. The involved vertebral body will be anteriorly displaced. Fractures may involve the lamina, the pedicle, and the spinous process, as well as the superior articulating facet of the subjacent vertebra. As the forces may be eccentrically applied, one side may be involved with contralateral facet joint dislocation.

The AP view will show marked disruption of the lateral margin of the involved articular mass.

The oblique view of the involved side shows the inferior articulating facet to be compressed and displaced upward, resulting in the "horizontal facet."

Complications. Neurologic compromise is common.

Emergency Management and Referral. Spine stabilization as described in Chapter 1. Immediate referral.

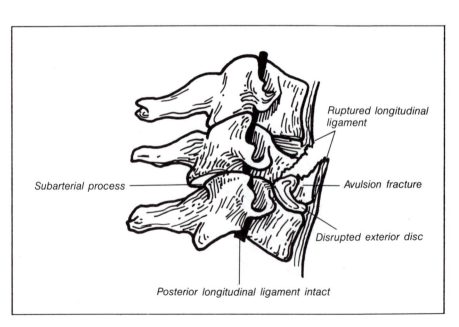

Figure 10–33. Hyperextension fracture–dislocation.

☐ LATERAL FLEXION

Uncinate Process Fracture

Stable Injury

Mechanism. This is the only fracture known to be caused purely by lateral flexion. In general, lateral flexion is an additional vector associated with other predominant mechanisms, offsetting the primary vector. Isolated injuries due to lateral flexion are rare. Injuries are limited as the head strikes the shoulder reducing the ligamentous damage.

Clinical Features. Neck pain on the involved side of the level of the injury. Contralateral soft tissue strain and spasm. Neurologic sequelae are uncommon.

Radiographs. The fracture is most readily seen on the AP view or as a double shadow on the lateral view.

Emergency Management and Referral. Immobilize the spine and refer the patient.

☐ DIVERSE MECHANISMS

Atlanto-Occipital Disruption

Extremely Unstable Injury

Mechanism. Violent thrusting of the head, tearing all ligamentous connections between the occiput and C-1. Nearly always fatal (Fig 10–34).

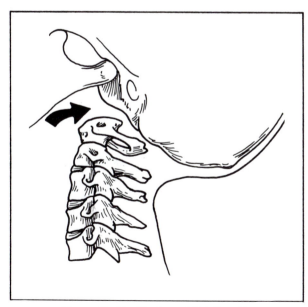

Figure 10–34. Atlanto-occipital disruption.

Clinical Features. The patient is frequently comatose due to concomitant severe cranial trauma. If awake, complaints of upper cervical or low occipital pain are present. Hemiparesis has been described but it is possible to have no distal neurologic sequelae due to the wide spinal foramen at this level. Case reports document potential resolution of neurologic deficits. Aggressive resuscitation is mandatory.

Radiographs. The lateral cervical spine film may show retropharyngeal soft tissue swelling. Displacement of the occipital condyles from the superior articulating facets of C-1 is obvious in severe cases. In more subtle dislocations, careful observation of the distances between the occiput, the atlas, and the dens is required. A horizontal distance of 1 mm or more between the basion (tip of the clivus) and tip of the dens or a vertical distance greater than 5 mm suggests instability. Calculation of the Powers ratio (the distance between the tip of the basion to the anterior aspect of the posterior arch of C-1 over the distance between the opisthion of the occiput and the posterior aspect of the anterior arch of C-1) is considered more reliable in determining true dislocation. A ratio less than 1.0 is normal, greater than or equal to 1.0 is abnormal.[31]

Flexion–extension views are extremely hazardous.

Complications. Atlantoaxial dislocation is frequently associated with atlanto-occipital dissociation. Other cervical spine trauma and closed head injuries are also associated with this injury. As this is an extremely unstable injury, treatment with axial traction may increase displacement.

Emergency Management and Referral. Immediate referral. Skeletal immobilization with careful application of traction under x-ray guidance.

Atlantoaxial Disruption, C-1 and C-2

Potentially Unstable Injury

Mechanism. Four varieties of this lesion have been described, each with a different mechanism (Fig 10–35).[32]

1. Anterior dislocation with rupture of the transverse ligament—this injury is extremely unstable and usually fatal due to a high level of cord compression between the posteriorly displaced, intact odontoid process and the posterior neural arch of C-1.
2. Anterior dislocation with fracture through the base of the odontoid. Depending on the extent of the force, this injury is less likely to be associated with neurologic damage.
3. Posterior dislocation—The mechanism of this un-

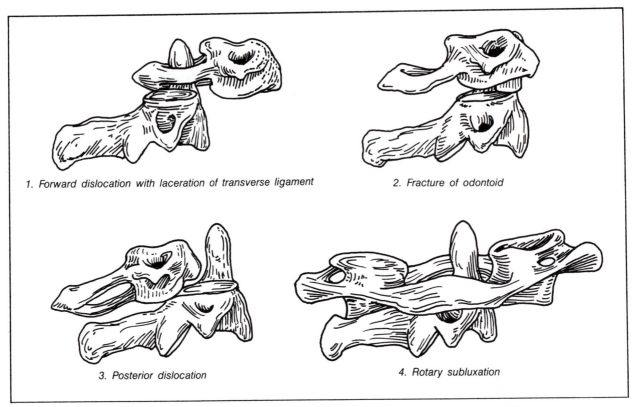

1. *Forward dislocation with laceration of transverse ligament*

2. *Fracture of odontoid*

3. *Posterior dislocation*

4. *Rotary subluxation*

Figure 10–35. Atlantoaxial disruption. See description that begins on page 127.

common lesion is believed to be sudden hyperextension with significant distraction generally due to a blow in the submental area. This results in a posterior displacement of C-1 over the top of the odontoid process, which remains intact and anterior to the anterior arch of C-1. The transverse ligament remains intact.

4. Rotary subluxation—This injury is rarely seen in adults. It is generally associated with motor vehicle accidents. The dislocation is due to a primary rotary vector and may not be associated with ligamentous disruption. Stability depends on intact ligaments.

Clinical Features. Presentation of this injury is highly variable. Death is frequently immediate. Rotary subluxation is more likely to present with pain in the neck, worse with movement. Significant muscle spasm is present in all cases. The deformity may be palpated at the back of the mouth. The extent of neurologic damage is variable.

Radiographs. The lateral cervical film will be helpful in distinguishing each of these lesions. The relationship of C-1 to C-2 will appear abnormal in all cases. Careful examination of the C-1 odontoid relationship is important in evaluating stability. The normal distance between the posterior aspect of the anterior arch of C-1 and the odontoid process should be between 0 and 3

mm. A distance between 3 and 5 mm strongly suggests transverse ligament disruption; greater than 5 mm is consistent with rupture of transverse and alar ligaments and is extremely unstable. Posterior C-1 to C-2 dislocation will reveal the odontoid process in front of the anterior arch of C-1.

The open-mouth view will demonstrate odontoid fractures and is most helpful in evaluating rotary subluxation. Overriding of C-1 on C-2 on one side will present as a narrowing of the joint space, the so-called wink sign.

Complications. Neurologic sequelae. Rupture of the transverse and alar ligaments can lead to immediate or potentially chronic instability.

Emergency Management and Referral. Immediate referral. Spinal stabilization and reduction of the dislocation. Axial traction under careful x-ray guidance is usually required for anterior (with or without odontoid fracture) and posterior dislocations. As all of these lesions are associated with chronic instability, open reduction and fusion may be necessary. Once the direction of rotation has been definitely determined, rotary dislocation can be reduced with gentle axial traction and rotation. Reduction is frequently associated with an audible pop. This injury is a true dislocation; all ligamentous structures may remain intact. Open reduction or fusion may not be necessary.

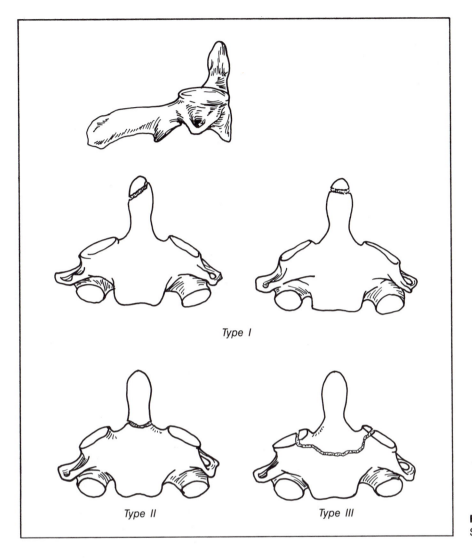

Figure 10–36. Odontoid fractures. See text for description.

Odontoid Fracture

Pontentially Unstable Injury

Mechanism. There are three types of odontoid fractures.[33] The precise mechanism for any or all of them is not known. Horizontal translation, hyperflexion, hyperextension, lateral hyperflexion, and combinations of each have all been implicated (Fig 10–36).[3]

1. Type I—Avulsion fracture of the tip of the dens at the site of attachment of the alar ligament. This is an uncommon injury felt more to be associated with occipitoatlantal dissociation. It is considered stable.
2. Type II—Transverse fracture at the base of the odontoid. This fracture may be anteriorly or posteriorly displaced and is unstable.
3. Type III—Fracture through the body of C-2, generally involving one or both of the superior articulating facets. The fragment may be displaced or nondisplaced. The latter are stable and generally

involve no neurologic deficit. Displaced fractures may be unstable.

Clinical Features. This injury is more frequent in men than in women. Patients complain of occipital or suboccipital pain and are unable or unwilling to sit up without supporting their head with their hands. Scalp lacerations, concussion, and mandible fractures are seen. Other cervical spine fractures may be present. Neurologic findings are rare; when present they vary from mild upper extremity weakness to decreased occipital sensation or Brown-Séquard syndrome. Most neurologic symptoms resolve.

Radiographs. The open-mouth view best shows the fractured odontoid process. In combination with the lateral cervical film, one can determine the degree and direction of displacement. Occasionally only retropharyngeal soft tissue swelling is present. Fractures may be difficult to appreciate and false-positive readings may be interpreted of congenital nonfusion of the odontoid and the body of C-2, os odontoideum, or rack effect at the junction of the odontoid and the body of C-2 caused by superimposition of the anterior arch of the atlas. Flexion–extension views are contraindicated if a dens fracture is suspected. Displacement may be potentially fatal. Conventional tomography is the optimal radiographic study. Computed tomography is not as effective, as the transverse fracture is generally in the same plane.

Complications. Posteriorly displaced fractures are associated with other cervical spine fractures and generally involve less neurologic damage. Anteriorly displaced fractures more commonly have associated neurologic findings. There is a high rate of nonunion. Several factors are involved including displacement (more than 5 mm is associated with a greater nonunion rate), adequacy of initial reduction, age and type of immobilization. Associated injuries also include scalp lacerations, inaudible fractures, concussion, and extremity fracture.

Emergency Management and Referral. Type I requires early referral. This is a stable injury occurring above the level of the transverse ligament. Nonunion is of no consequence. The patient is treated symptomatically. Types II and III require immediate referral. Spine stabilization and traction.

☐ PEDIATRIC CERVICAL SPINE

The evaluation of the pediatric patient always presents a special challenge to the emergency physician. Interpretation of cervical spine injuries is no exception. Fortunately, significant fractures and dislocations of the spine in children are quite rare, most studies quoting an incidence of approximately 1 to 3%.[16–18] This is largely attributable to the greater mobility of the pediatric cervical spine relative to adults.

Confounding evaluation of cervical injuries is the difficulty in interpreting x-rays in the skeletally immature. By age 8 or 9 significant ossification occurs, such that the radiographic configuration of the cervical spine in older children is similar to that of adults. It is particularly important, therefore, that the emergency physician be familiar with characteristics of injury and radiographic evaluation of the infant and the young child.

Clinical Evaluation

Primary assessment of the young child is similar to that of adults in that a thorough history and physical exami-

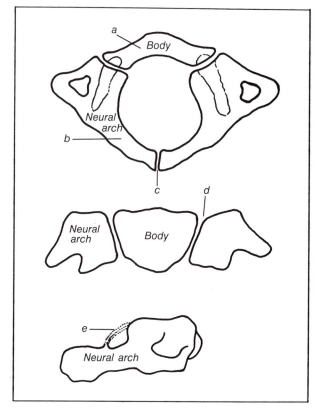

Figure 10–37. First cervical vertebra: *a,* Body. Not ossified at birth. Center appears on x-ray during the first year after birth. Although the body may fail to develop, forward extension of the neural arches takes its place. *b,* Neural arches. Appear bilaterally at the seventh fetal week. *c,* Synchondrosis of spinous processes. Unite by the third year. Rarely, union may be preceded by the appearance of a secondary center within the synchondrosis. *d,* Neurocentral synchondrosis. Fuses about the seventh year. *e,* Ligament surrounding the superior vertebral notch. May ossify, especially later in life. *From Bailey DK: Normal cervical spine in infants and children. Radiology 59: 713, 1952.*

nation should be done including a complete neurologic evaluation. Obtaining this data, however, may be more difficult. If there is suggestion of significant injury, including a history of a mechanism of considerable force, head injury, local tenderness, or neurologic impairment, complete cervical immobilization is mandatory until adequate radiographic evaluation is completed.

X-ray Evaluation

As in the adult the plain film cervical spine series should include at least lateral, anteroposterior, and open-mouth views. Obtaining an adequate series might be difficult. If plain radiography does not specifically rule out cervical spine injury, computed tomography scanning is recommended.

Interpretation of the plain cervical spine series in infants and young children is complicated by two fac-

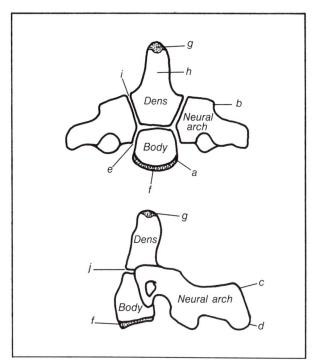

Figure 10–38. Second cervical vertebra: *a*, Body. Center appears by fifth fetal month. *b*, Neural arches. Appear bilaterally by the seventh fetal month. *c*, Neural arches. Fused posteriorly by the second or third year. *d*, Bifid tip of spinous process. May have secondary center in each tip. *e*, Neurocentral synchondrosis. Fuses at 3 to 6 years of age. *f*, Inferior epiphyseal ring. Appears at puberty and fused at about 25 years. *g*, "Summit" ossification center of the odontoid. Appears at 3 to 6 years and fuses with the odontoid by 12 years. *h*, Odontoid. Two separate centers appear by the fifth fetal month and fuse by the seventh fetal month. *i*, Synchondrosis between odontoid and neural arch. Fuses at 3 to 6 years. *j*, Synchondrosis between odontoid and body. Fuses at 3 to 6 years. *From Bailey DK: Normal cervical spine in infants and children. Radiology 59: 713, 1952.*

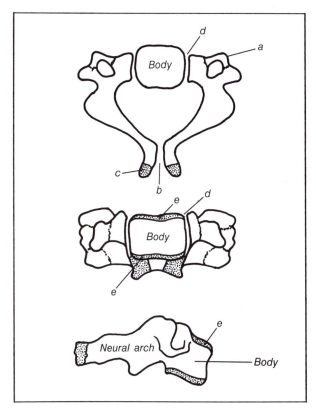

Figure 10–39. Third cervical vertebra.

tors: (1) ossification patterns and (2) mobility of the immature spine. Although variable depending on the individual, ossification patterns of the immature spine are fairly predictable. Figures 10–37, 10–38, and 10–39 demonstrate the patterns of ossification for the atlas, the axis, and the lower cervical segments.[19] It is important to remember that normal ossification junctions between bone and cartilage will be represented on the plain film as smooth, often rounded margins. Fractures, however, are generally irregular and sharp. In particular, areas that require specific attention include the base of the odontoid, where a large synchondrosis can persist until age 7 or 8, normal anterior wedging of the vertebral body that can be confused with compression fractures, spinous process centers that appear as avulsion fractures, and the apical epiphysis of the odontoid process that should not be confused with a fracture.[20]

Hypermobility and ligamentous laxity, particularly of the upper cervical segments, can give the appearance of pseudosubluxation. At the level of C-1 and C-2, mobility of the atlas can result in a predental space of up to 4 mm in flexion and in extension the anterior arch of the atlas can override the dens.

Ligamentous laxity, horizontal configuration of the facet joints, and underdevelopment of the joint of Luschka are believed responsible for the phenomenon of pseudosubluxation of C-2 on C-3. As much as a 3- to 4-mm excursion of the vertebral body of C-2 on C-3 can occur in flexion. Figure 10–40 demonstrates that the anterior aspect of the vertebral arches of C-1 through C-3 will be in alignment in the case of physiologic displacement. If the posterior vertebral arch of C-2 does not fall in line, a pathologic etiology is suggested.

Ligament laxity and lack of complete cooperation during radiography are also responsible for frequent absences in what is considered a normal cervical lordosis in adults. The characteristic smooth lines of the adult cervical spine may also be absent.

Specific Injuries

Newborn

Cervical muscles of the neck of the newborn are too weak to provide adequate support of the cervical spine.

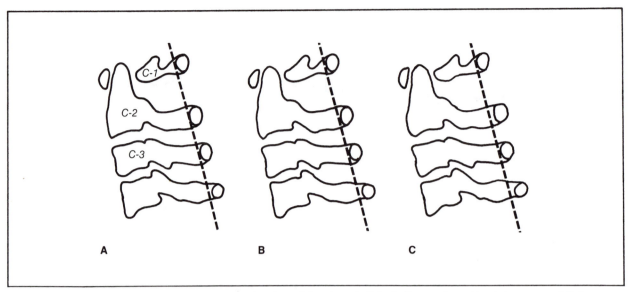

Figure 10–40. Anterior aspect of the vertebral arches of C-1 through C-3. **A.** Passes through anterior cortex of C-2. **B.** Touches anterior aspect of C-2 cortex. **C.** Comes within 1 mm of anterior aspect of C-2 cortex.

Obstetric trauma from traction occasionally in cephalad presentations or, more typically in breech presentations, can cause significant neurologic injury. Radiographically there may be no evidence of cervical spine damage, probably due to the large proportion of cartilage. At this age the cervical spine might be more elastic than the cervical cord resulting in neurologic damage. Autopsy results of perinatal specimens include longitudinal damage to the cord nerve roots, brain, and vertebral arteries.

Caffey[21] and Swischuck[22] first described a form of child abuse called "whiplash shaken infant syndrome." With repeated violent shaking, the relatively heavy head atop the weak musculature of the cervical spine is violently shaken to and fro. The emergency physician should take careful note on examination of children with no outward appearance of trauma but findings of unexplained convulsions, hyperirritability, bulging fontanelle, intraocular hemorrhage, paralysis, and vomiting that infant abuse may be present. Intracranial and intraocular hemorrhages, cerebral injury, retardation, visual and hearing defects, and fractures of the spine and skull have been reported.

Upper Cervical Spine Injuries

Although cervical fracture–dislocations are more rare in children than in adults, the majority occur in the upper cervical segments, particularly of the atlas and the axis.[16,23] The most common of these are odontoid fractures, transverse ligament disruption, and atlantoaxial dislocation.

Odontoid Fracture. In actuality the fracture of the odontoid process is seen at the level of the subdental synchondrosis within the body of the axis. The fragment frequently angulates forward anteriorly with respect to the body. Significant displacement is rare. Almost all cases are treated with conservative therapy. Referral to an orthopedist is required immediately. As the injury occurs through the cartilaginous growth plate, growth disturbances should be observed but are rarely noted. Although there is evidence that this lesion is the cause of os odontoideum, there is no definitive proof at this time. Apical fractures of the odontoid process are extremely rare.

Ligament Disruption. Due to ligamentous dislaxity the normal predental space in children is acceptable up to 4 mm. A distance of 5 mm or more suggests transverse ligament compromise, generally associated with trauma. Aid to evaluating this area on the lateral cervical x-ray is Steel's rule of thirds.[35] The canal of the atlas should be equally occupied in thirds by the spinal cord, the dens, and an empty space. If the atlas is displaced by a distance exceeding the thickness of the odontoid, potential risk to the spinal cord exists. All patients should be immediately referred. Therapy is usually conservative with a halo or Minerva device.

Atlantoaxial Dislocation or Subluxation (Grisel's syndrome). Laxity of the transverse, apical, alar, and facet joint ligaments at the C-1 and C-2 level are factors associated with this entity. It is suggested that local edema secondary to local inflammation or infection (pharyngitis, otitis, tonsillar abscesses, or other local infections) permits additional stretching of the ligaments resulting in an atlantoaxial displacement. Displacement of the atlas on the axis may be anterior, posterior, right or left lateral, or right or left rotary.[24] Lateral x-rays are notable for an enlarged predental space. AP views may show deviation of the spinous process of C-2 toward the side to which the chin may be rotated. All patients should be referred immediately. Reduction may be spontaneous or require traction or neck extension followed by a Minerva jacket or halo device.

Other Injuries

Fracture of the pedicles of C-2 is not an uncommon fracture of the cervical spine in children. These are generally isolated lesions. Differentiation from pseudo-subluxation of C-2 on C-3 may be difficult. Evaluation of the posterior vertebral arches as described in the radiology section is helpful, as well as physical examination and history. All patients should be referred immediately. Treatment consists of immobilization for 6 to 8 weeks.

Jefferson fractures, burst fractures of the atlas, can be seen in the pediatric population. Identification and management are similar to that of adults. All patients should be immediately referred.

Lower Cervical Spine Injuries

Bony injuries of the lower cervical spine are quite rare in children. It is speculated that this is due to the increased mobility of the pediatric spine and the relative increased proportion of cartilage to bone in children. Typically patients will present with neurologic injury and a relative sparing of the cervical spine. X-rays may only be notable for small fissures in the vertebral body or widening of an intervertebral space. Particular attention should be paid to prevertebral soft tissue swelling. All patients require immediate referral. Most patients are treated conservatively and surgical stabilization is rarely necessary.

□ REFERENCES

1. Holdsworth F: Review article: Fractures, dislocations and fracture–dislocations of the spine. J Bone Joint Surg 52:1534, 1970
2. White AA, Southwick WO, Panjab MM: Clinical instability in the lower cervical spine: A review of past and current concepts. Spine 1 (1):15, 1976
3. Harris JH, Edeikin-Monroe B, Lopaniky DR: A practical classification of acute cervical spine injuries. Orthop Clin North Am 17(1):15, 1986
4. Eisenfeld US, Wiesel SW: The spine. In Eisenfeld US (ed): Emergency Orthopedic Radiology. Edinburgh, Churchill Livingstone, 1985, pp 11–34
5. Bohlman HH, et al: Spine and spinal cord injuries. In Rothman RH, Simeone FA (eds): The Spine. Philadelphia, WB Saunders, 1982, pp 661–756
6. Levine AM, Edwards CC: Treatment of injuries in the C1-C2 complex. Orthop Clin North Am 17(1):31, 1986
7. Anderson LD: Fractures of the odontoid process of the axis. In The Cervical Spine. The Cervical Spine Research Society. Philadelphia, JB Lippincott, 1983, pp 206–222
8. Schneider RC, et al: Hangman's fracture of the cervical spine. Neurosurg 22:141, 1981
9. Penning L: Obtaining and interpreting plain films in cervical spine injury. In Bailey RW (ed): The Cervical Spine. The Cervical Spine Research Society. Philadelphia, JB Lippincott, 1983, pp 62–95
10. McQueen JD, Khan MI: Evaluation of patients with cervical spine lesions. In Bailey RW (ed): The Cervical Spine. The Cervical Spine Research Society. Philadelphia, JB Lippincott, 1983, pp 128–140
11. Jacobs B: Cervical fractures and dislocations (C3-7). Clin Orthop 109:20, 1975
12. Bohlman HH, Boada E: Fractures and dislocations of the lower cervical spine. In Bailey RW (ed): The Cervical Spine. Philadelphia, JB Lippincott, 1983, pp 231–267
13. Anderson DK, et al: Spinal cord injury and protection. Ann Emerg Med 14(8):147, 1985
14. Johnson RM, Wolf JW Jr: Stability. In Bailey RW (ed): The Cervical Spine. The Cervical Spine Research Society. Philadelphia, JB Lippincott, 1983, pp 35–53
15. Pierce DS, Barr JS: Fractures and dislocations of the base of the skull and upper cervical spine. In Bailey RW (ed): The Cervical Spine. Philadelphia, JB Lippincott, 1983, pp 196–206
16. Hasue M, et al: Cervical spine injuries in children. Fukushima, J Med Sci 20:111, 1971
17. Rang M: Children's Fractures. Philadelphia, JB Lippincott, 1974
18. Bohlman HH: Acute fractures and dislocations of the cervical spine. J Bone Joint Surg 61A:1119, 1979
19. Bailey DK: Normal cervical spine in infants and children. Radiology 59:713, 1952
20. Sherk HH, et al: Fractures and dislocations of the cervical spine in children. Symposium on Fractures and Other Injuries in Children. Orthop Clin North Am 7(3): 1976.
21. Caffey J: The whiplash shaken infant syndrome: Manual shaking by the extremities with whiplash-induced intracranial and intraocular bleedings, linked with residual permanent brain damage and mental retardation. Ped 54 (4): 396–403, 1974
22. Swischuck LE: Spine and spinal cord trauma in the battered child syndrome. Radiology 92:733, 1969
23. Hubbard DD: Injuries in the spine in children and adolescents. Clin Orthop 100:56, 1974
24. Marar BC, Balachandran N: Non-traumatic atlantoaxial dislocation in children. Clin Orthop 92:220, 1973
25. Cancelmo JJ: Clay shoveler's fracture: A helpful diagnostic sign. AJR 115:540–541, 1972
26. Harris JH, et al. A practical classification of acute clinical spine injuries. Orthop Clin North Am 17(1):19, 1986.
27. Swischuck LE: Spine and spinal cord trauma in the battered child syndrome. Radiology 92:733, 1969
28. McNab I. Acceleration injuries of the cervical spine. In Rothman RH, Simeone FA (eds): The Spine. Philadelphia, WB Saunders, 1982, p 651

29. Harris JH, et al: A practical classification of acute clinical spine injuries. Orthop Clin North Am 17(1):24, 1986

30. Garfin SR, Rothman RH. Traumatic spondylolisthesis of the axis (hangman's fracture). In Bailey RN (ed): The Cervical Spine, Philadelphia, JB Lippincott, 1983, p 228

31. Powers B, et al: Traumatic anterior atlanto-occipital dislocation. Neurosurgery 4:12-17, 1979

32. Stauffer ES, Kaufer H: Fractures and dislocation of the spine. In Rockwood CA, Green OP (eds): Fractures in Adults, 2nd ed. Philadelphia, JB Lippincott, 1984, pp 987–1035.

33. Anderson LD, D'Alonzo RT: Fracture of the odontoid process of the axis. J Bone Joint Surg 56:1663–1674, 1974

34. Swischuk LE: Anterior displacement of C-2 in children: Physiologic or pathologic? Radiology 122:759–763, 1977

35. Steel HH: Anatomical and mechanical consideration of the antlantoaxial articulation. Proceedings of the American Orthopaedic Association. J Bone Joint Surg 50A:1481, 1968

☐ BIBLIOGRAPHY

Babcock JL: Cervical spine injuries, diagnosis and classification. Arch Surg 111:646, 1976

Cattel HS, et al: Pseudosubluxation and other normal variations in the cervical spine in children. J Bone Joint Surg 47A (7):1295, 1965

Cloward RB: Acute cervical spine injuries. Clin Symp, CIBA, 32:1, 1980

Dorr L, et al: Clinical review of the early stability of spine injuries. Spine 7(6):545, 1982

Ducker TB, et al: Timing of operative care in cervical spinal cord injury. Spine 9(5):525, 1984

Fever H: Management of acute spine and spinal cord injuries, Symposium on cervical spine injuries. Arch Surg 111:638, 1976

Fielding JW: Cervical spine injuries in children. In Bailey RW (ed): The Cervical Spine. The Cervical Spine Research Society. Philadelphia, JB Lippincott, 1983, pp 268–281

Garfin SR, Rothman RH: Traumatic spondylolisthesis of the axis (hangman's fracture). In Bailey RW (ed): The Cervical Spine. Philadelphia, JB Lippincott, 1983, pp 223–231

Harris JH: Radiographic evaluation of spinal trauma. Orthop Clin North Am 17(1):75, 1986

Harris JH: The Radiology of Acute Cervical Spine Trauma. Baltimore, Williams and Wilkins, 1978

Henrys P, et al: Clinical review of cervical spine injuries in children. Clin Orthop 129:172, 1977

Hockberger RS: Spinal cord injury. In Callahan BC (ed): Current Therapy in Emergency Medicine. New York, Decker, 1987, pp 109–114

Hohl M: Soft tissue neck injuries. In Bailey RW (ed): The Cervical Spine. The Cervical Spine Research Society. Philadelphia, JB Lippincott, 1983, pp 282–287

Hubbard DD: Injuries of the spine in children and adolescents. Clin Orthop 100:56, 1974

Hunter GA: Non-traumatic displacement of atlanto-axial joint. J Bone Joint Surg 50B (1):44, 1968

Iserson KV: Strangulation and hanging. In Callaham, M (ed): Current Therapy Emergency Medicine. New York, Decker, 1987, pp 114–116

Jackson DW, et al: Cervical spine injuries. Clin Sports Med 5(2):373, 1986

Jacobs B: Cervical fractures and dislocations (C3-7). Clin Orthop 109:18, 1975

Kiwerski J, Weiss M: Neurological improvement in traumatic injuries of cervical spinal cord. Paraplegia 19:31, 1981

Knopp RK: Cervical spine trauma. In Callaham M (ed): Current Therapy in Emergency Medicine. New York, Decker, 1987, pp 98–101

Levine AM, Edwards CC: Complications in the treatment of acute spinal injury. Orthop Clin North Am 17(1):183, 1986

Maull KI, Sachatello CR: Avoiding a pitfall in resuscitation: The painless cervical fracture. South Med J 70(4):477, 1977

McNab I: Acceleration extension injuries of the cervical spine. The Spine. In Rothman RH, Simeone FA (eds): Philadelphia, WB Saunders, 1982, pp 647–660

Miller MD, et al: Significant new observations of cervical spine trauma. Am J Roentgenology 130:654, 1978

Morse SD: Acute central cervical spinal cord syndrome. Ann Emerg Med 11(8):436, 1982

Powers B, et al: Traumatic anterior atlanto-occipital dislocation. Neurosurg 4(1):12, 1979

Riggins ER, Kraus JF: The risk of neurologic damage with fractures of the vertebrae. J Trauma 17(2):126, 1977

Roda JM, et al: Hangman's fracture with complete dislocation of C2 on C3. J Neurosurg 60:663, 1984

Scher AT: Unrecognized fractures and dislocations of the cervical spine. Paraplegia 19:25, 1981

Sherk HH: Lesions of the atlas and axis. Clin Orthop 109:33, 1975

Stauffer ES: Management of spine fractures C3 to C7. Orthop Clin North Am 17(1):45, 1986

Stauffer ES, Rhoades ME: Surgical stabilization of the cervical spine after trauma. Arch Surg 111:652, 1976

Stauffer ES, Kaufer H: Fractures and dislocations of the spine. In Rockwood CA, Green DP (eds): Fractures in Adults, 2nd ed. Philadelphia, JB Lippincott, 1984, pp 987–1035

Steel HH: Anatomical and mechanical considerations of the atlanto-axial articulations. J Bone Joint Surg 50:1481, 1968

Sullivan CR, et al: Hypermobility of the cervical spine in children: A pitfall in the diagnosis of cervical dislocation. Am J Surg 95:2636, 1958

White AA, et al: Biomechanical analysis of clinical stability in the cervical spine. Clin Orthop 109:85, 1975

Williams CF, et al: Essentiality of the lateral cervical spine radiograph. Ann Emerg Med 10(4):198, 1981

11

Strains and Sprains

The previous chapter dealt with fractures and dislocations of the cervical spine due to a variety of mechanisms of injury of considerable force. The same mechanisms, with lesser forces, result in injuries to the soft tissue that are commonly seen by the emergency department physician.

☐ CERVICAL SPRAIN

Cervical sprain is injury to the soft tissues of the cervical spine as a result of acceleration forces to the head and the neck. Injury occurs to muscles, ligaments, discs, nerves, vessels, and other viscera of the neck, the degree of which is dependent on the amount of force applied. The most common presenting syndrome to the emergency department is one of hyperextension and is presented in the most detail. Accelerating forces resulting in hyperflexion or extreme lateral bend are less common and are described later.

☐ HYPEREXTENSION INJURY

Commonly referred to as whiplash, soft tissue injury to the neck due to forced hyperextension was first recognized in airline pilots catapulted from aircraft carriers.[1] The causes most commonly seen, however, are the result of rear-end automobile collisions. When the car is rear-ended, the seat support pushes the patient's trunk forward relative to the head, which is forcefully hyperextended (Fig 11–1). The head snaps backward, the mouth snaps open, the anterior cervical muscles are stretched, as well as the anterior longitudinal ligament and fibers of the annulus. If the automobile is not equipped with safety head rests, there is nothing to stop the head from hyperextension except the back of the seat.

Acceleration depends on the amount of force applied (a fully loaded truck or bus vs. subcompact automobile) and the inertia of the vehicle being struck (moving vehicle vs. stationary with brakes applied, dry road conditions vs. ice).[2] Head rests limit the degree of hyperextension but only if properly adjusted (Fig 11–2).

It is important to note that the events described occur in milliseconds. As such, it is impossible for reflex protective mechanisms to take place. Because it is rare for victims to require acute surgery, few pathologic specimens in humans have ever been obtained. Numerous experimental hyperextension injuries in primates, however, have revealed anterior cervical injuries including muscle ruptures and hemorrhages, anterior longitudinal ligament tears, intervertebral disc ruptures, esophageal hemorrhages, and brain hemorrhages.[3,4]

Clinical Features

By history, the patient is typically the front seat passenger who may remember being jolted by the injury or is described by witnesses as being unconscious or confused around the time of the incident. Initially, the victim may be asymptomatic but as events become clear, will complain of discomfort and pain in the neck, nausea, and increasing neck stiffness. More severe symptoms may take hours or even a few days to develop.

Complaints and physical findings will vary depending on the degree of injury.[5] The most common scenario is one of a mild sprain, usually involving muscles, and is manifested by muscle tenderness, spasm, and restricted motion. The patient is relatively asymptomatic when the neck is at rest. Symptoms can be expected to resolve within days with conservative therapy.

A moderate sprain includes more severe damage not only to muscles, but ligaments are also involved. Physical examination will reveal significant spasm of

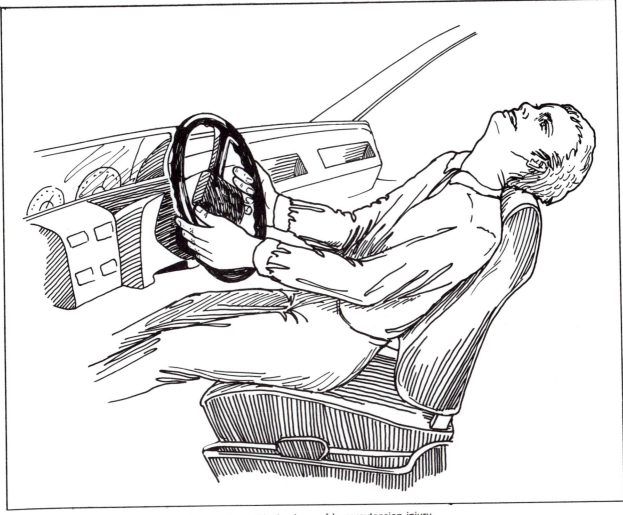

Figure 11–1. Mechanisms of hyperextension injury.

the scalene muscles. Pain in the neck is generalized and can be referred to the occiput, scapula, upper extremities, and anterior chest. Patients complain of severe pain with any movement of the head and even an inability to maintain the head upright. Severe pain or muscle spasm can last for several days. Symptoms gradually resolve between 3 and 6 weeks as ligaments repair.

Severe cervical sprain includes injury to muscles and disruption of ligaments. Symptoms as seen with moderate sprain are present as well as headache, nausea, vertigo, and occasionally blurred vision and tenderness. Muscle pain and spasm are intense, the patient complains of weakness in the neck and inability to control the position of the head due to muscle and ligament tears. The emergency physician should be acutely aware that this can be an unstable injury. Symptoms also include pain, paresthesias, and weakness of the upper extremities, shoulder and interscapular area.

Particularly in moderate and severe sprains it is not uncommon for the patient to complain of a number of unusual symptoms, including headache, dizziness, visual disturbances, tenderness, dysphagia, hoarseness, and pain extending down the arms and in the interscapular regions. Although the pathophysiology of these symptoms is difficult to explain, they have been repeatedly described and should not necessarily be perceived as an hysterical reaction.[6]

Associated Injuries

Although a wide variety of unexplained symptoms have been described and attributed to referred pain, complaints of tenderness, dysphagia, and hoarseness should be carefully investigated. Experimental injuries have revealed brain damage, esophageal and tracheal tears and hemorrhages.

Radiographs

Cervical spine films are usually negative. Loss of the typically lordotic curve is difficult to interpret. Al-

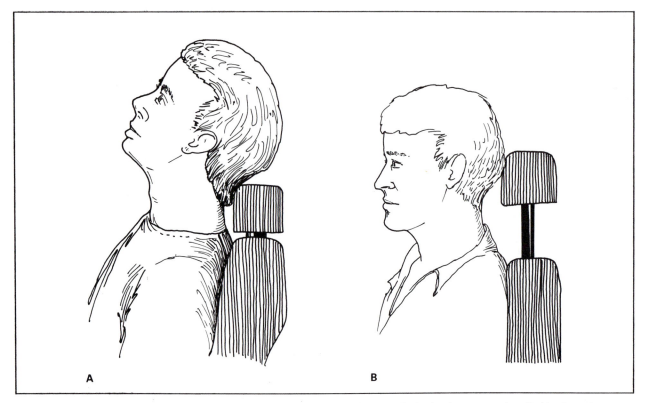

Figure 11–2 A. Head rest is inappropriately set too low. This allows for a cervical spine hyperextension. **B.** Head rest is correctly positioned. This prevents a cervical hyperextension.

though it was previously felt to be consistent with significant muscle spasm, it has been shown that simply lowering the chin 1 inch reverses the normal curvature of the spine.[7] A sharp reversal on the cervical curve, however, over a span of one or two verterbrae, is significant for soft tissue damage. Avulsion fractures and retropharyngeal soft tissue swelling can be seen. Flexion and extension views should be done with caution. Except for retropharyngeal soft tissue swelling, x-rays might appear normal despite complete rupture of the anterior longitudinal ligament and disruption of the intervertebral disc due to in hyperextension injuries, resulting in complete instability.

Emergency Management and Referral

Emergency management of severe cervical sprain includes cervical immobilization until stability is assured. In the event of significant ligamentous disrupture, immediate referral is required. Numerous modalities have been shown to be effective for moderate and severely symptomatic patients including soft collars, heat, and bedrest.[1,2,5] In the acute setting, traction is discouraged. Medications to relieve pain and spasm are recommended including anti-inflammatories, analgesics, and antispasmotics. Early range of motion and isometric exercises have been shown to be beneficial, but only

after acute symptoms of severe pain and spasm resolve.[8] Early referral is suggested for all patients.

☐ HYPERFLEXION INJURY

The primary mechanism for hyperflexion cervical sprain is an automobile accident, but it is also frequently seen in diving, football, and other sporting injuries. The most superficial posterior structures are the trapezius muscles and the ligamentum nuchae, both of which run from the base of the occiput inferiorly down the length of the cervical spine and attaching in the upper thoracic area. In extreme hyperflexion, the ligamentum nuchae can be torn generally at the most flexible level of the cervical spine between C-5 and T-1 (Fig 11–3). If completely torn, it is likely that the interspinous ligaments at that level will also be ruptured. In the event of significant injury capsular ligaments might as well be involved and the nerve roots compressed. The disc can be compressed anteriorly but actual disc protrusion is rare. Damage to bone is most likely seen as the ligamentum nuchae tears away from the spinous processes posteriorly, resulting in avulsion

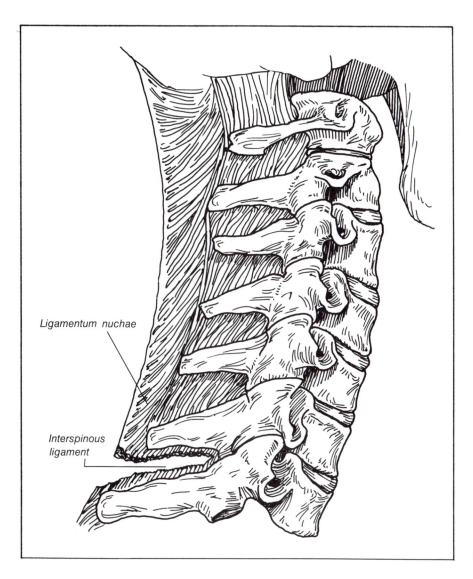

Ligamentum nuchae

Interspinous ligament

Figure 11–3. Hyperflexion injury.

chip fractures. In extreme hyperflexion, the vertebral bodies may undergo compression anteriorly.

Clinical Features

Hyperflexion sprain can present clinically as mild, moderate, and severe injuries.[5] As in hyperextension sprain, mild sprain is most commonly seen involving primarily muscles in the posterior neck. Initially pain is only minimal, but over a period of hours it becomes more intense and associated with muscular spasm.

Moderate sprain involves the muscles and the ligamentum nuchae. The patient complains of significant pain and spasm in the posterior aspect of the neck running to the occiput and the scapular area. There is significant tenderness on palpation at the level of the nuchal and interspinous ligaments involved. As all of the muscles of the neck come to play in keeping the head in the neutral position, the patient complains of inability to keep the head upright, particularly when bending over at the waist.

A severe sprain involves a complete tear of ligaments. The nuchal ligament is the first to be disrupted and is commonly associated with disruption of the interspinous ligament at that same level. The patient complains of severe pain, similar to that in moderate sprain, only more intense. Acute pain and muscle spasm can be associated with headache, nausea, tenderness, and blurred vision. As multiple stabilizing ligaments can be disrupted, it is imperative that the emergency physician look for signs of instability (refer to Chapter 10). Posteriorly the neck is tender to palpation throughout. Due to generalized pain and muscle spasm, it may take several days for symptoms to subside enough to pinpoint the exact area of the tear. The effort of straightening the neck from a flexed position or elevating the head when the trunk is flexed from the waist is extremely painful. Paresthesia or weakness in the upper extremities may develop at the outset or after several hours.

Radiographs

Cervical spine films in patients with cervical sprain are usually normal. In the lateral view, a hyperflexion injury with disruption of the ligamentum nuchae and the interspinous ligament might reveal a widening of spinous processes at the level of the injury or avulsion fractures at the tips of the spinous processes. In cases of severe hyperflexion sprain, anterior vertebral body compression may be noted.

Emergency Management and Referral

Cases of very severe sprain with evidence of instability should be referred immediately. Cervical sprain of lesser severity is treated conservatively. Bedrest (with a hand towel rolled and placed under the cervical spine for maximal relaxation), heat, soft collars, and antispasmodics, anti-inflammatories, and analgesics are the mainstay of therapy in the acute setting. All patients should be referred.

☐ CERVICAL DISC DISORDERS

Complaints of either sudden or persistent pain in the neck with radiating symptoms to an upper extremity are usually the result of proximal cervical root compression. The meninges and dentate ligaments serve to keep spinal cord and nerve roots relatively fixed at the level of the cervical spine. Unlike nerve roots in the lower spine, cervical nerve roots run a direct transverse course past the cervical discs and through the intervertebral foraminae. It is at this area, posterolaterally, that the cervical intervertebral disc ruptures. Although the extrusion of disc material is very small, even minor impingement on the relatively immobile nerve root is significant.[5] The disc ruptures posterolaterally where the annulus fibrosus is weakest and the posterior longitudinal ligament is quite thin. Hence, symptoms are most commonly unilateral.

Pathologically, two different lesions are responsible for the identical clinical symptoms of cervical nerve root compression:[9]

1. Acute cervical disc rupture—An acute posterolateral rupture of the disc, usually associated with a specific traumatic incident, associated with immediate symptoms of nerve root compression. There is no previous evidence of disc degeneration and generally no prior symptomatology. This "soft" disc is comprised only of extruded disc material.
2. Chronic disc degeneration—Developing over a period of months to years, chronic degeneration, or cervical spondylosis, starts at the level of the disc, which becomes dehydrated. As the disc space narrows, hypertrophic changes occur at the apophyseal

joints, resulting in osteophyte formation into the intervertebral foraminae. This "hard" disc usually occurs where the cervical spine is most mobile, at C-5 and C-6 vertebrae, symptoms developing insidiously (Fig 11–4).

Although rare, midline disc lesions do occur, generally of the "hard" variety. These develop gradually and will produce radicular symptoms in both upper extremities. Even more rare is the acute "soft" midline lesion, which presents with acute cord compression and quadriplegia. This is a true emergency.

Axiom: *Acute spinal cord compression due to midline cervical disc rupture is a true emergency. Immediate evaluation and decompression are mandatory to prevent permanent cord damage.*

As both of these entities are so similar in terms of clinical presentation and treatment, they will be discussed together.

Clinical Features

Clinical presentation of both acute cervical disc rupture and chronic disc degeneration are essentially identical except for onset and acuity of initial symptoms. A patient with acute cervical disc rupture rarely has preceding symptoms and can generally localize a specific point in time or traumatic event that suddenly resulted in severe symptoms. Chronic disc degeneration, on the other hand, develops insidiously, as a series of exacerbations that gradually subside, each slightly more intense than the previous episode.

Symptoms and signs are otherwise identical. The primary complaint is one of pain in the middle of the

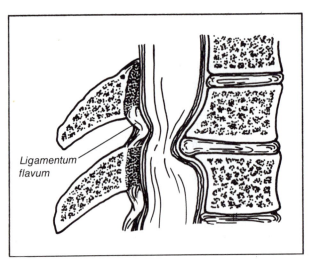

Ligamentum flavum

Figure 11–4. Cervical spondylosis.

neck that radiates to the occipital area and spreads downward across the shoulders. Pain is worse with motion, coughing, sneezing, and straining. Although it is relieved with rest, it is often worse at night if the head and the neck are improperly supported. Neck movement is limited due to the pain and muscle spasm. Forceful movement and pressure on the top of the head can increase symptoms.

Pain and numbness will radiate to the shoulder, chest, or arm and hand on one side. Table 11–1 lists the sensory findings consistent with nerve root compression at various levels of the cervical spine.[9] Sensory deficits are usually associated with motor deficits although not as readily perceived by the patient. Table 11–2 demonstrates motor weaknesses and reflex changes at various cervical levels.[9]

In the case of chronic degeneration, physical examination might also reveal muscular atrophy, particularly at the level of C-8, which supplies the small muscles of the hand. Chronic degeneration might also include significant myelopathy with a characteristic wide-based or jerky gait. Leg weakness develops gradually and is symmetric. Reflexes can be variable, with hyperreflexia seen commonly in the lower cervical segments. Abdominal reflexes are usually diminished but lower extremity reflexes are exaggerated. Sensory examination is extremely variable.

Although rare, marked osteophyte formation ante-

TABLE 11–1. SENSORY FINDINGS ASSOCIATED WITH NERVE ROOT COMPRESSION

Nerve Root	Disc Level	Symptoms
C-3	C2–3	Pain and numbness in back of neck, particularly around mastoid process and pinna of ear.
C-4	C3–4	Pain and numbness in back of neck, radiating along levator scapula muscle and occasionally down anterior chest.
C-5	C4–5	Pain radiating from side of neck to shoulder top; numbness over middle of body of deltoid muscle (axillary nerve distribution).
C-6	C5–6	Pain radiating down lateral side of arm and forearm, often into thumb and index fingers; numbness of tip of thumb or on dorsum of hand over first dorsal interosseous muscle.
C-7	C6–7	Pain radiating down middle of forearm, usually to middle finger, though index and ring finger may be involved.
C-8	C7–T-1	Pain down medial aspect of forearm to ring and small finger; numbness can involve small finger and medial portion of ring finger. Numbness rarely extends above wrist.

From Rothman RH, Simeone FA (eds): The Spine. Philadelphia, WB Saunders, 1982, p 387.

TABLE 11–2. MOTOR WEAKNESSES AND REFLEX CHANGES AT VARIOUS CERVICAL LEVELS

Nerve Root	Disc Level	Weakness: Reflex Change
C-3	C2–3	No readily detectable weakness or reflex change except by EMG.
C-4	C3–4	No readily detectable weakness or reflex change except by EMG.
C-5	C4–5	Weakness of extension of arm and shoulder, particularly above 90°; atrophy of deltoid muscle; no reflex change.
C-6	C5–6	Weakness of biceps muscle; depression of biceps reflex.
C-7	C6–7	Weakness of triceps muscle; depression of triceps reflex.
C-8	C7–T-1	Weakness of triceps and small muscles of the hand; no reflex change.

From Rothman RH, Simeone FA (eds): The Spine. Philadelphia, WB Saunders, 1982, p 387.

riorly in chronic disc degeneration can cause dysphagia (Fig 11–5).

Symptoms of headaches, dizziness, visual and auditory disturbance, and voice change have been described but their etiology is unclear.

Radiographs

Radiographic findings in patients with cervical disc disease can be quite different depending on etiology. X-ray evidence of acute disc rupture includes narrowing of the disc space, vacuum disc with the development of air in the disc space, or loss of the normal lordotic cervical curve. The latter is the least reliable finding; although previously attributed to muscle spasm, it can be shown that patient positioning can change the normal curve. Depending on the mechanism of injury, particularly in acute disc rupture, evidence of instability on flexion–extension views can be seen with coincident ligamentous damage.

Degenerative changes are a normal part of the aging process. X-ray findings, therefore, are significant only if they correlate clinically. Nevertheless, important x-ray findings include a narrowing of the anteroposterior diameter of the spinal canal due to bony intrusion (13 mm or less is suggestive of compression), narrowing of the intervertebral foraminae on the oblique views, narrowing of the disc space, irregularity of the apophyseal joints (particularly posterior slippage of the superior articular surface), and evidence of cervical instability. In chronic degeneration, the latter appears to occur due to a generalized laxity of supporting structures.

In patients with evidence of spinal cord or nerve root compression where surgery might be indicated, myelography, discography, and computed tomography are recommended.

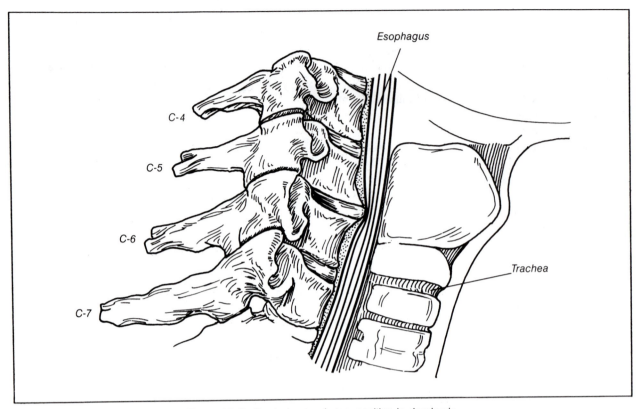

Figure 11–5. Cervical osteophytes resulting in dysphagia.

Complications

Significant bony spurs can cause compression of the vertebral artery. Turning the head to one side will cause compression of the contralateral vertebral artery, resulting in insufficient cerebral flow with dizziness and drop attacks.

Emergency Management and Referral

Patients with evidence of spinal cord compression due to cervical disc disease require immediate referral for decompression.

Patients with either acute disc rupture or chronic disc degeneration will respond favorably to conservative treatment. Cervical immobilization with complete bedrest and a properly fitted soft cervical collar promote healing of involved soft tissue damage in acute disc ruptures and reduce inflammation in both processes. Particularly in acute cervical injuries the collar is worn full time for 2 to 3 weeks. If not used at night, patients should be advised not to sleep in the prone position. Propping of the head with multiple pillows should be avoided. A small cylindrical pillow or rolled hand towel placed beneath the cervical spine while lying on the back will maintain the cervical spine in a neutral position.

Drug therapy should include anti-inflammatories, analgesics, and muscle relaxants. The latter two should only be used in the acute setting. Anti-inflammatory

agents are useful throughout the recuperation period, which generally lasts 6 weeks. Patient education regarding daily habits is also necessary, including reduction of automobile riding due to vibration and changes in work habits, so as to avoid prolonged periods in a single position. All patients should be referred for convalescent care. Conservative treatment is recommended for approximately 1 year before surgical intervention is considered.

□ REFERENCES

1. Hohl M: Soft tissue injuries of the neck. Clin Orthop 109:42, 1975
2. MacNab I: Acceleration extension injuries of the cervical spine. In Rothman MD, Simeone F (eds): The Spine. Philadelphia, WB Saunders, 1982, p 648.
3. MacNab I: Acceleration: Extension injuries of the cervical spine. In AAOS Symposium of the Spine. St. Louis, CB Mosby, 1969, pp 10–17
4. Ommayay AK, et al: Whiplash and brain damage. JAMA 204 (4):285, 1968
5. Turek SL: Cervical spine. In Orthopedics, Principles and their Application, 4th ed. Philadelphia, JB Lippincott, 1984, p 830
6. Hohl M: Soft tissue neck injuries. In The Cervical Spine,

The Cervical Spine Research Society. Philadelphia, JB Lippincott, 1983, p 283

7. Weir DC: Roentgenographic Signs of Cervical Injury. Clin Orthop 109:10, 1975

8. Greenfield J, Ilfeld F: Acute cervical strain. Clin Orthop 122:196, 1977

9. Simeone FA, Rothman RH (eds): Cervical disc disease. In The Spine, Philadelphia, WB Saunders, 1982, p 387

12

Specific Syndromes and Disorders

□ THORACIC OUTLET SYNDROMES

A number of physical abnormalities responsible for compression of the subclavian and axillary artery and vein and the trunks of the brachial plexus as they pass from the neck to the arm are described. Primary among these are cervical rib, costoclavicular syndrome, scalenus anticus syndrome, and hyperabduction syndrome. A number of mechanisms come into play: (1) constriction of the subclavian artery and brachial plexus at the insertions of the scalene muscles near the first thoracic rib; (2) compression between the first thoracic rib and the clavicle and subclavian muscle; (3) compression at a narrowing formed by the coracoid, the pectoralis minor tendon, and the costocoracoid membrane; and (4) compression of the axillary artery by the heads of the median nerve.[1] Numerous other factors come into play including increased muscle bulk or extreme lack of muscular tone, congenital anomalies including cervical ribs or bifid first ribs, previous local fractures particularly of the clavicle with malunion or excess callus, local tumors, and atherosclerosis.

Common to all is neurovascular compression between the clavicle and the first rib near the thoracic outlet. When these conditions present classically, a good history and physical examination suggest the specific location of the obstruction. Because of the number of intervening factors, however, specific localization of the actual lesion usually requires plain radiography, angiography, and electrodiagnostic studies.

Symptoms depend on whether nerves, blood vessels, or both are compressed, although usually one predominates, the most common being with neurologic symptoms. Pain and paresthesias referable to C-8 and T-1 along the medial aspect of the arm, the forearm, and the hand are noted.[2] Neurologic deficits are usually absent. Neurologic pain is distinguished from vascular pain in that the former is often burning and intermittent, the latter, constant and diffuse. Vascular compression results in pallor and a cyanosis of the fingers,

coolness of the extremities and, in 25% of the patients, Raynaud's phenomenon. Complete distal occlusion is generally due to embolic phenomena.

Decreased vascular flow can be quite subtle, but a number of physical maneuvers can aid in the diagnosis:

Intermittent claudication test—When both arms are elevated, abducted, and externally rotated, and the patient rapidly opens and closes the fist, pain will develop within seconds, in states of decreased vascular flow. The healthy person is able to continue the exercise for at least 1 minute.

Costoclavicular maneuver—In the seated position the patient draws the shoulders downward and backward as if standing at attention. Evidence of a bruit, heard inferior to the clavicle at the junction of the lateral and middle thirds, or decrease in palpation of the radial pulse constitutes a positive test.

Hyperabduction maneuver—Complete hyperabduction of an upper extremity will diminish distal pulses. This is generally indicative of hyperabduction syndrome.

Adson maneuver—The patient is instructed to turn the head to the side of the symptoms and take a deep breath with the neck fully extended. A decrease or obliteration of the radial pulse is considered a positive test, due to increased entrapment by the scalene muscles. This test is specific for the scalene anticus syndrome.

Allen test—With the hand tightly clenched in a fist, the examiner compresses both the radial and ulnar arteries. When the hand is opened, the examiner releases the ulnar artery; a patent ulnar artery permits flow to the entire hand. In the case of a distal ulnar artery obstruction the hand remains pale (Fig 12–1). This differentiates a distal from a more proximal etiology.

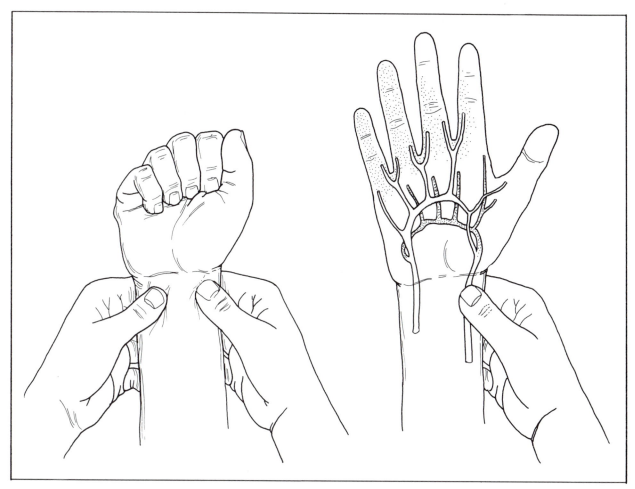

Figure 12–1. Allen test.

It is important to note that for the above maneuvers there is a high incidence of false-positive results, particularly for the costoclavicular compression and hyperabduction tests. Although suggestive, further evaluation is necessary. What follows is a brief description of each of the four syndromes. In particular, specific points are described to differentiate each entity.

Cervical Rib

Cervical rib is a supernumerary small rib fibrous band emanating from C-7, usually bilaterally (Fig 12–2). It is seen in about 0.5% of the healthy population, yet only about 10% produce symptoms.[2] The neurovascular bundle must pass over or beneath the cervical rib or fibrous band. Symptoms are enhanced particularly in the older patient with droopy shoulders or with downward traction on the arms.

Clinical Features

Neurologic symptoms of pain and paresthesias are attributed to the C-8 and T-1 roots with either sharp or dull pain along the ulnar aspect of the hand. Vascular compression usually results in a tingling sensation of "falling asleep" in the forearm and the hand. There are subjective complaints of weakness. Symptoms are generally increased with traction on the arm, particularly in lifting heavy objects. The Adson test is frequently positive, as use of the scalene muscles adds to the compression.

On physical examination, the cervical rib may be palpated, but might only consist of a fibrous band. There is tenderness to deep palpation behind the sternocleidomastoid muscle. Distally there may be atrophy of the interossei and lumbrical muscles, and weakness with flexion of the metacarpophalangeal joints, extension of the interphalangeal joints, abduction and adduction of the fingers, and adduction of the thumb.[1] Sensory deficits, if present, are in the ulnar distribution in the forearm and the hand. Vascular compression is manifested by a decreased radial pulse with coolness and pallor of the hand with thin shiny skin.

Radiographs

A cervical rib is present and generally emanates from C-7 bilaterally, although rarely from C-5 or C-6.

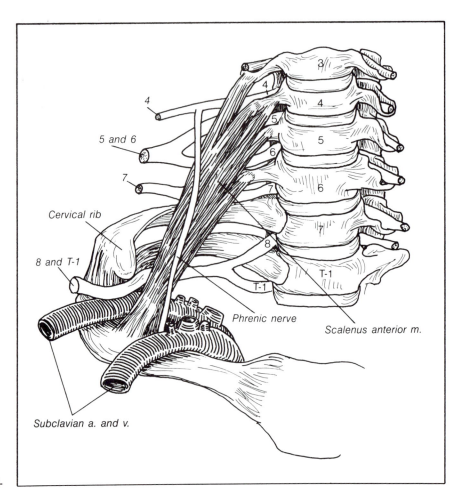

Figure 12–2. Cervical rib. The clavicle is omitted.

Complications

Poststenotic aneurysmal dilatation of the subclavian artery can be seen. It can occasionally be palpated in the supraclavicular fossa. This can result in thrombosis formation and distal embolization. Acute venous thrombosis is also seen.

Emergency Management and Referral

Conservative treatment consisting of exercises to improve tone in the trapezius and levator scapulae muscles reduces compression by elevating the shoulder girdle. The patient should avoid heavy lifting, and the arm on the involved side should be elevated when at rest. When symptoms are severe, surgical removal of the cervical rib is indicated.

Costoclavicular Syndrome

The costoclavicular syndrome is characterized by neurovascular compression at the level of the clavicle and the first rib, frequently associated with anomalies of the first rib, previous history of fractures, and significant callus formation of the clavicle, or an associated cervical rib.

Clinical Features

This syndrome is characterized by a relatively proximal vascular compression. Symptoms are similar to those of cervical rib, with pain and paresthesias along the ulnar aspect of the hand and the little fingers attributable to C-8 and T-1 with compression. Vascular symptoms include tingling or "falling asleep" noted in the forearm and the hand. Characteristically, these symptoms are significantly increased with the costoclavicular maneuver. Having the patient draw the shoulders back and downward increases the neurovascular symptoms particularly reducing the radial pulse. With partial compression bruits may be heard in the supraclavicular or infraclavicular areas, which will disappear if compression is significant enough to stop the flow entirely. Taking a deep breath will elevate the first rib and increase compression. The intermittent claudication test is also frequently positive.

Radiographs

Although frequently normal, abnormalities of the first rib or clavicle, evidence of previous fracture of the clavicle, or cervical rib may be evident.

Complications

Poststenotic aneurysmal dilatation of arteries with thrombus formation and embolization, and venous thrombosis are possible, but rare.

Emergency Management and Referral

Initial treatment is conservative therapy, including exercises to improve posture and elevate the shoulders, changing sleeping positions; work and recreational activities can frequently alleviate situations where compression may be increased. If symptoms become progressively severe, with signs of persistent neurologic deficit or increasing ischemia, surgical intervention may be necessary. Referral is recommended.

Scalenus Anticus Syndrome

Neurovascular compression can occur as the subclavian artery and the brachial plexus pass between the anterior scalene and middle scalene muscles, particularly where large tendons insert into the first thoracic rib creating a narrow interscalene triangle. Overlapping of the tendons, bony prominences of the first rib, or the addition of a cervical rib may significantly narrow this triangle. Physiologic use of the scalene muscles contributes to the compression (Fig 12–3).

Clinical Features

This is a proximal neurovascular compression. Signs and symptoms are similar to those of cervical rib. The picture is one of a mixed neurovascular compression; neurologic findings consistent with C-8 and T-1 compression, and vascular tingling along the medial forearm. The Adson maneuver, by increasing tension on the anterior and middle scalene muscles, increases compression and can significantly decrease the radial pulse or accentuate neurologic findings. A bruit may be audible in the supraclavicular fossa, which will completely disappear, as will the radial pulse, in complete compression.

Radiographs

As this syndrome is reproduced largely by compression between the scalene muscles, x-rays are frequently normal. It is possible to note abnormalities of the first thoracic rib, particularly of a large bony prominence, or cervical rib.

Complications

Poststenotic aneurysmal dilatation with thrombus formation and embolization, and venous thrombosis, can occur.

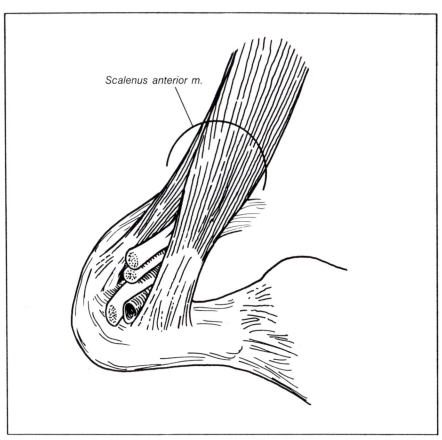

Scalenus anterior m.

Figure 12–3. Scalenus anticus syndrome.

Emergency Management and Referral

As this syndrome is usually produced by basic anatomic tightness of the interscalene triangle, conservative treatment of rest and avoidance of heavy lifting, as well as patient education regarding sleep position and severe craning of the neck, are frequently adequate. Surgical scalenotomy, however, is frequently indicated.

Hyperabduction Syndrome

Where the subclavian artery and brachial plexus pass the coracoid process and posterior to the pectoralis minor they are stretched across the coracoid process and compressed with hyperabduction of the arm, along with strong contraction of the pectoralis minor (Fig 12–4).

Clinical Features

Neurologic and vascular symptoms are referable first to the fingers, then progress proximally to involve the rest of the hands and the forearms. Compression can occur with occupational activity, but is most commonly noted due to hyperabduction when the patient is asleep. Swelling of the hands, distal weakness, occasional ulceration to the fingertips, and Raynaud's phenomenon can be seen. The hyperabduction maneuver has the patient seated and the examiner, while palpating the radial pulse, passively abducts the arm in an arch of 180 degrees. A positive test is noted with a decrease or disappearance of the pulse. Pulses generally return to normal when the arm is returned to the patient's side, but may remain decreased due to vascular spasm.

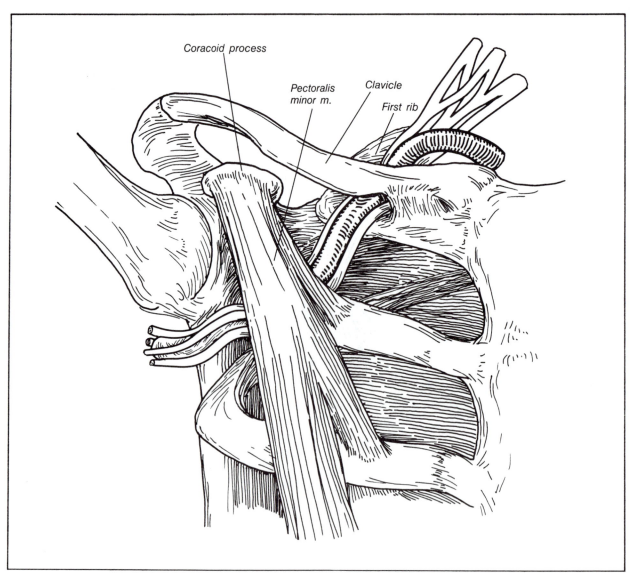

Figure 12–4. Hyperabduction syndrome.

Radiographs

Plain radiography is usually normal. Arteriography, done at intervals as the arm is abducted, will reveal the exact site of occlusion.

Complications

Poststenotic arterial dilatation, thrombus formation, and embolization, as well as venous thrombosis, can be seen.

Emergency Management and Referral

Conservative therapy including patient education to avoid hyperabduction during sleep and work, or recreational activities involving extreme hyperabduction, as in painting or ceiling repair, should be avoided. Sur-

gery is indicated if these measures are inadequate and symptoms persist. Referral for this and all thoracic outlet syndromes is recommended.

☐ BRACHIAL PLEXUS INJURIES

The brachial plexus is composed of the anterior rami of the fifth, sixth, seventh, and eighth cervical nerve roots and the first thoracic nerves. A "prefixed" plexus develops more cranially and includes the fourth cervical nerve; a "postfixed" plexus is more caudally developed and includes the second thoracic nerve. Figure 12–5

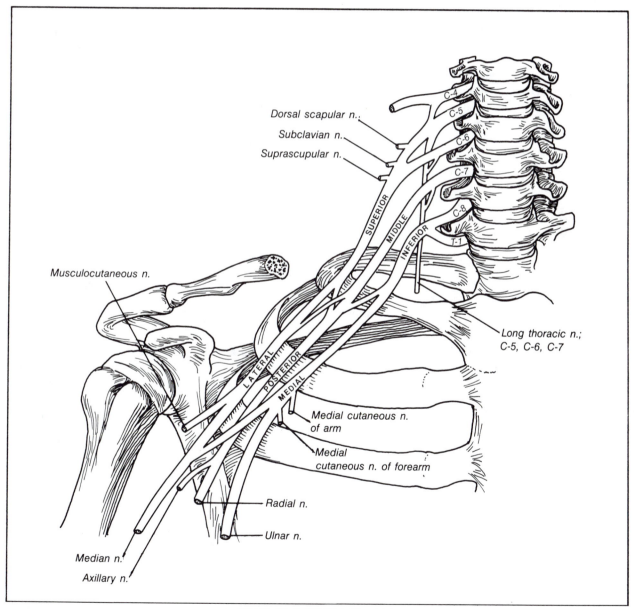

Figure 12–5. Brachial plexus injury.

traces the interconnections at the level of the roots, trunks, and cords. Specific innervations will be discussed later. Generally, the upper or lateral portion of the plexus innervates muscles of the scapula, shoulder, and flexor muscles of the arms. The medial portion innervates the intrinsic muscles of the hand and the cervical sympathetic. The posterior portion innervates the deltoids and extensor muscles of the arms and the forearms. The first thoracic ganglion is at this level and connects with the first thoracic ramus. Injuries at this level will produce a Horner's syndrome.[1]

Injury to the nerves of the brachial plexus can occur through multiple mechanisms. Traction on the brachial plexus occurs when the head is flexed laterally toward the opposite side. This is seen in birth trauma, shoulder dislocation, or automobile and athletic accidents with severe lateral forces applied to the cervical spine. Rupture of individual nerve fibers occurs most commonly, generally at the area where the plexus is most subject to stress at C-5 and C-6. Actual avulsion of nerve roots from the cord is rare.

A second mechanism of injury is compression due to clavicular fracture and callus formation, tumors, hemorrhage, or a direct blow to the side of the neck.

Penetrating wounds to the area occur from stabbings or gunshot wounds. Nerves in the plexus can be completely severed, but temporary dysfunction occurs from concussion and local edema.

Clinical Features

The mechanism of injury is usually obvious from the history. On presentation to the emergency department, the upper extremity is usually completely paralyzed. Due to concussion forces and local edema induced by all of the above mechanisms, the extent of the injury appears to be due to swelling. Many symptoms will rapidly resolve, revealing a truer picture of the actual damage.

Classical distinctions of upper (Erb) or lower (Klumpke) plexus injuries can be used to localize injuries, but frequently there is a mixed picture.

The mechanism of injury can help to localize the lesion. Stretching injuries usually are at the area of greatest stretch, the C-5 and C-6 roots in the upper trunk and lateral cord. Evidence of stretching from the lower brachial plexus is less common and is generally a milder injury, which spontaneously recovers. Penetrating injuries will damage the most exposed areas of the plexus, C-5, C-6, C-7, and the upper trunk. High velocity gunshot wounds will have significant concussion effects and will require a period of time for physiologic symptoms to subside. Axillary or infraclavicular wounds generally involve individual nerves or large blood vessels.

In the absence of significant concussion or local edema, localization of a specific injury can be made by close physical examination. Proximal injury to the nerve roots or trunk results in large areas of motor and sensory loss; C-5, C-6, and the upper trunk correspond to the shoulder girdle and the upper part of the extremity; C-7, C-8, T-1, and the middle and lower trunks refer to the forearm and the hands; T-1 or the spinal nerve result in Horner's syndrome. Table 12–1 delineates actual muscle innervation by each nerve root.

Several large nerves emanate from the plexus proximally. The long thoracic nerve innervates the serratus anterior muscle, injury resulting in winging of the scapula. The dorsal scapular nerve innervates the rhomboids and levator scapulae muscles, which rotate the scapula, but are difficult to test.

More distally, injury to the cords will result in smaller areas of specific peripheral involvement.

Lateral cord—Injury results in damage to the musculocutaneous nerve (biceps) and upper half of the median nerve (flexor carpi radialis and pronator teres)

Medial cord—Involves injury to the ulnar nerve, the medial cutaneous nerve to the arm and the forearm, and the lower half of the median nerve.

Posterior cord—Includes the radial nerve, the axillary nerve (deltoid, teres minor muscles), the subscapular nerve (subscapular and teres major muscles), and the thoracodorsal nerves (latissimus dorsi muscle).

Radiographs

Because these are soft tissue injuries, radiography is of little value. The mechanism of injury, however, might result in damage to the cervical spine, clavicle, or shoulder, and should be evaluated radiographically.

Emergency Management and Referral

The prognosis for recovery of brachial plexus injuries is extremely variable depending on the location of the injury. Regeneration of an avulsed nerve root is impossible. Neurorrhaphy at the level of the upper trunk or

TABLE 12–1. MUSCLE INNERVATION BY CERVICAL NERVE ROOT

Nerve Root	Muscles
C-5	Rhomboids, deltoid, supraspinatus, infraspinatus, biceps, brachialis, clavicular head of pectoralis major
C-6	Sternal head of pectoralis major and triceps
C-7	Extensors of wrist and fingers
C-8	Flexors of wrist and fingers
T-1	Intrinsic muscles of hand and cervical sympathetic

outer cord usually results in a good recovery; however, repair of the lower trunk and inner cord is poor. The extent of recovery of nerve function is dependent on the amount of time to surgery. As such, all brachial plexus injuries should be immediately referred.

□ "STINGERS"

The exact etiology of stingers ("burners" or "tinglers") is unknown. Seen commonly in football players as a result of forceful lateral impact to the head and the neck, it is believed to be a traction injury of the brachial plexus.

Clinical Features

After a severe block or tackle with lateral traction to the head and the neck, the patient describes a burning pain, numbness, or tingling extending from the shoulder down into the arm and the hand. Symptoms are referable to the C-5 and C-6 levels. There can be a momentary paralysis, but recovery is usually complete within a few minutes. Repeated insults can cause biceps and deltoid weakness or paresthesia.[3]

Three grades of the injury have been described.[4] Grade 1 injuries are minor, with full resolution of symptoms within minutes. Grade 2 injuries cause a decrease in muscle strength of the deltoid, infraspinatus, and biceps muscles for approximately 3 weeks with resolution usually within 6 months. Grade 3 injury motor and sensory deficits last longer than 1 year. Persistent symptoms should be evaluated by electromyography.

Associated Injuries

Severe lateral forces to the cervical spine can result in cervical spine fracture.

Radiographs

This is strictly a soft tissue injury; cervical spine films will be negative.

Emergency Management and Referral

Conservative therapy. Grade 1 injuries resolve spontaneously after a brief time. Grade 2 and 3 injuries should be referred. No further physical contact should be allowed until all neurologic symptoms resolve. Strengthening of the neck musculature is recommended. If the patient returns to playing football, correct head and neck techniques and blocking–tackling should be taught. Cervical rolls as part of the football equipment will limit extreme range of motion. Complaints of pain in the neck are generally not seen and

are suggestive of a more severe injury to the cervical spine.

□ GREATER OCCIPITAL NERVE SYNDROME (Occipital Neuritis)

Pain at the base of the neck associated with unilateral headache can be attributed to compression of the greater occipital nerve. Also called syndrome of the sensory root of the second cervical nerve, this nerve emanates from between the atlas and the axis. Its posterior primary ramus is subjected to compression with movements of extreme rotation and hyperextension of the neck. It is more common in patients with degenerative joint disease of the atlantoaxial region.

Clinical Features

Patients complain of pain in the suboccipital region usually with referred pain unilaterally over the parietotemporal area extending to the vertex and periorbital area. Pain is frequently constant with severe exacerbations. Numbness and tingling are described over the parietoccipital area. The patient may frequently complain of nausea, blurred vision, lacrimation, and dizziness, and is frequently labeled with a diagnosis of migraine headache.

Physical examination may reveal significant tenderness along the course of the second cervical nerve root and greater occipital nerve. It can be reproduced by rotating the head with hyperextension toward the side of symptoms. Decreased sensation may be noted. Injection of local anesthetic in the area of the second cervical nerve with resolution of symptoms is diagnostic. It is suggested that there may be significant psychologic overlay. A thorough history and mental status examination are necessary.

Radiographs

Cervical spine films are frequently normal. Degenerative changes may be seen at the atlantoaxial joint.

Emergency Management and Referral

Conservative therapy should be initiated, including the use of a cervical collar with the neck kept in mild flexion, nonsteriod anti-inflammatory agents, and, where indicated, relaxation exercises. Local injection of steriods may be helpful. All patients should be referred, as persistent symptoms may require surgical therapy by section of the greater occipital nerve or the sensory root of the second cervical root. Because there is significant overlap from the trigeminal nerve onto the scalp, little sensation is lost.

□ VERTEBAL ARTERY SYNDROME

Vertebral artery syndrome (vertebrobasilar artery insufficiency) is generally seen in the elderly and consists of episodes of dizziness and drop attacks due to compression of the vertebral artery. Partial occlusion of the vertebral artery due to cerebral vascular atherosclerosis, combined with significant degenerative joint disease of the spine, will result in decreased cerebral flow. More significant compression and relative ischemia are caused by rotation and hyperextension of the neck.

Clinical Features
Patients are usually elderly. At first, symptoms are relatively subtle, largely limited to dizziness, particularly when the patient hyperextends the head to look upward. With more significant compression, symptoms progress to episodes of unconsciousness. Examination should be cautious. By hyperextending and rotating the head, the patient will become dizzy and nystagmus can be observed.

Radiographs
Cervical spine x-rays can be completely normal or demonstrate evidence of degenerative joint disease. The definitive diagnosis is made by arteriography.

Complications
Chiropractic manipulation or aggressive examination can lead to permanent neurologic defects from prolonged ischemia due to compression or thrombosis.

Emergency Management and Referral
In patients with mild symptomatology, conservative therapy should be attempted. Hyperextension of the neck should be avoided by use of a soft cervical collar. Manipulation is contraindicated. Conservative measures are maintained while collateral circulation is established. If symptoms progress, carotid endarterectomy may be necessary to improve collateral circulation.

□ TORTICOLLIS

Also known as wryneck, torticollis is a contraction (often spasmodic) of the muscles of the neck, largely those supplied by the spinal accessory nerves, resulting in a rotational deformity with the chin pointing to the opposite side. The longer the deformity remains, the more resistant it is to therapy due to bony changes and contractions of the soft tissue. There are multiple etiologies.

Trauma
Usually due to sprain, dislocation, or fracture of the cervical spine. Most commonly this is seen in unilateral facet dislocation or subluxation. Patient describes turning the head and sensing a painful snap in the neck; the neck remains locked in this position and is associated with localized tenderness and muscle spasm.

A common variant of subluxation is seen in children, frequently after a respiratory tract infection. The child complains of a "crick in the neck" and torticollis is seen on examination. Of note is that the sternocleidomastoid muscle is not in spasm.

Congenital Torticollis
This is seen at birth and characteristically involves unilateral sternocleidomastoid muscle spasm of fibrous tumor.

Myositis
The exact etiology is unknown, but the condition of stiff neck after exposure to the cold is seen.

Spasmodic Torticollis
The etiology of spasmodic torticollis is unknown, involving spontaneous, painful, and persistent muscle contractions of the neck. Many muscles are involved including the sternocleidomastoid, trapezius, and splenius.

Neuritis of the Spinal Accessory Nerve
Neuritis of the spinal accessory nerve is a unilateral neuritis; it is temporary and involves local tenderness at the lateral border of the sternocleidomastoid in the area of the second cervical vertebra. The condition is temporary.

Infections
Infections include tuberculosis involving the spine and the discs. Poliomyelitis, although rare, will result in rotation of the head to the side of the paralyzed sternocleidomastoid muscle.

Clinical Features
A thorough history and physical examination are necessary to determine the cause of torticollis. A history of trauma, snapping of the neck, or recent upper respiratory infection in children with physical findings of local tenderness and muscle spasm are suggestive of subluxation. In these patients it is important to rule out a severe cervical spine injury. Localized spasm and tenderness of the cervical muscles are also seen in myositis and spasmodic torticollis. Tenderness of the spinal accessory nerve is suggestive of neuritis. Signs of acute or chronic illness will be suggestive of infectious etiology.

Radiographs

Unfortunately, cervical spine films are difficult to interpret due to the severe rotation of the cervical spine. They are, nevertheless, recommended in an effort to rule out severe fracture or dislocation in the event of trauma.

Emergency Management and Referral

Specific treatment will depend on etiology. Acute subluxation can be reduced with traction under anesthesia. Spontaneous luxation in children resolves gradually over several days and is assisted by the use of a soft cervical collar. Myositis and neuritis of the spinal accessory nerve are treated conservatively with heat, soft collar, and sedation. Spasmodic torticollis can be quite resistant to conservative measures, and might require intradural section of both spinal accessory nerves and the first three anterior cervical nerve roots. Resolution of infectious etiologies of torticollis involves treating the underlying illness.

The longer torticollis is allowed to continue, the more refractory it is to conservative measures. As such, all patients should be referred for follow-up care.

□ REFERENCES

1. Turek SL: Cervical brachial region. In Orthopedics, Principles and Their Application, 4th ed. Philadelphia, JB Lippincott, 1984, p 890
2. Imparato AM, Spencer FC: Peripheral arterial disease. In Schwartz (ed): Principals of Surgery, 5th ed. New York, McGraw-Hill, 1979, p 946
3. Jackson DW, Lohr FT: Cervical spine injuries. Clin Sports Med 5(2):373, 1986
4. Clancey W, et al: Upper trunk brachial plexus and injuries in contact sports. Am J Sports Med 5:209, 1977

□ BIBLIOGRAPHY

Turek SL: Cervical brachial region. In Orthopedics, Principles and Their Application, 4th ed. Philadelphia, JB Lippincott, 1984

PART IV

The Thoracolumbar Spine

13

Anatomy

□ INTRODUCTION

An understanding of the anatomy of the thoracic and lumbar spine, particularly as it relates to function, is essential to the proper diagnosis and treatment of disorders in this region. This is especially true in the setting of trauma as the bony and neurologic abnormalities found by physical examination often disclose the specific anatomic injury. This often can direct the patient's emergency management from very early on in the course, even before radiographic or laboratory data have been obtained.

□ FUNCTIONAL ANATOMY

There are 12 vertebrae in the thoracic region and 5 in the lumbar region. The first thoracic vertebra is the smallest, with each bony segment being slightly larger in a cranial to caudal progression. This pattern is also seen in the intervertebral discs (Fig 13–1). The thoracic spine is distinctive in two respects: (1) the normal curvature is kyphotic in contradistinction to the lordosis of the cervical and lumbar segments and (2) each vertebra articulates with a pair of ribs. The head of each rib articulates with the two adjacent vertebral bodies and the intervening intervertebral disc. This articulation is with the superior demifacet (costal facet) of one vertebral body and with the inferior demifacet of the vertebral body above (Fig 13–2). Each of the first ten ribs also articulates with the transverse process of its segment. The radiate and costotransverse ligaments lend stability to these articulations (Fig 13–3).

In both the thoracic and lumbar regions, the pedicles of each vertebra arise from the posterolateral aspect of the body and form the lateral part of the vertebral foramen with the laminae constituting the posterior aspect (Figs 13–2 and 13–4A). The articular processes are located at the junction of the pedicles and the laminae (Figs 13–2, 13–4A, and 13–4B). The neural foramina, through which the peripheral nerve roots exit, are bordered superiorly and inferiorly by the pedicles of the adjacent levels, anteriorly by the disc, and posteriorly by the articular processes (Figs 13–1 and 13–5). In the thoracic spine, the cartilaginous surface of the superior facet faces posteriorly and articulates with the anteriorly facing inferior facet from the vertebra above forming a true synovial joint (Figs 13–2 and 13–5). This vertical orientation combined with the articulation with the ribs adds greatly to the stability of the thoracic spine, but markedly reduces mobility.

The anatomy of the two most caudal thoracic vertebrae represents a transformation from the characteristics of T-1 through T-10 to those of the lumbar segments. The eleventh and twelfth ribs are much smaller and are independent from the rib cage. In addition, they do not articulate with the transverse processes of T-11 and T-12. In the thoracolumbar and lumbar region, the spinous processes are directed more horizontally. The vertebral bodies as well as the discs become progressively larger and more broad (Fig 13–1). The facet joints become more sagitally oriented (Figs 13–4A and 13–4B), thus leading to significant resistance to rotation while allowing more motion in flexion, extension, and lateral bending.

The major ligamentous structures from anterior to posterior are the anterior longitudinal ligament, the annulus fibrosus, the radiate ligaments (thoracic), the posterior longitudinal ligament, the costotransverse (thoracic) and intertransverse ligaments, the facet capsules, the ligamentum flavum, the interspinous ligaments, and the supraspinous ligaments (Figs 13–3 and 13–6).

□ STABILITY AND MOBILITY

Whereas the structure of the cervical and lumbar spine enhances mobility but reduces stability, that of the tho-

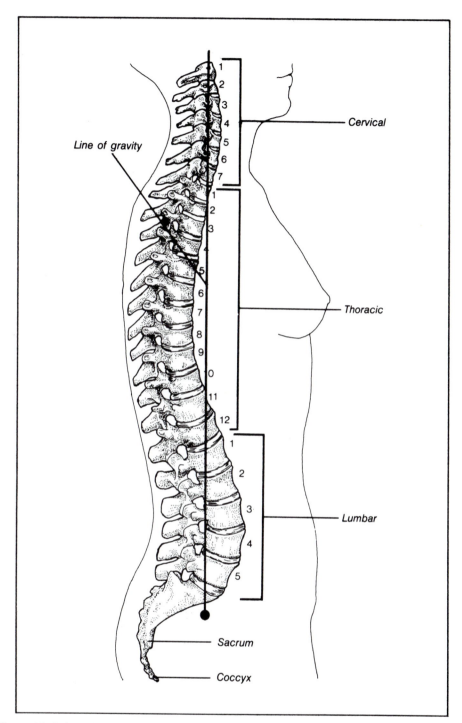

Figure 13–1. Lateral view of the spinal column. Note that the discs enlarge as one goes inferiorly.

racic spine leads to the reverse. The principle stabilizing elements include the rib cage, the intervertebral discs and the annulus fibrosus, the ligaments, and the facet joints. The ribs with their ligamentous attachments to the thoracic spine are a tremendous source of stability and lead to decreased mobility in flexion, extension, lateral bending, and rotation. Rotation is the motion that is least affected by these attachments. In addition to being an elastic shock absorber,[2] the intervertebral disc with its annulus fibrosus is an important stabilizing structure, particularly in the thoracic region. The discs in this region are thinner than in either the cervical or lumbar regions[3] and thus minimize the motion taking place between vertebral segments.

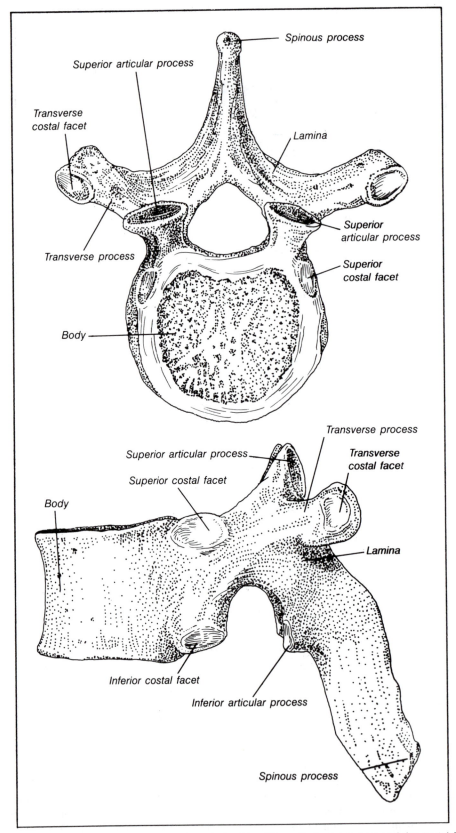

Figure 13–2. A typical thoracic vertebra. Note the relationship of the articular processes and the costal facet joints.

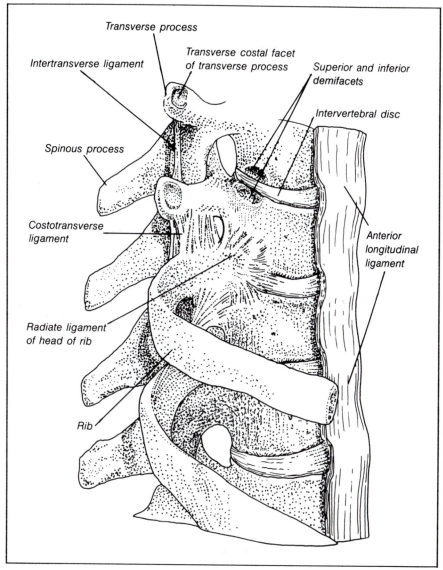

Figure 13–3. Lateral view of the thoracic spine with ligaments and rib attachments.

The ligamentous structures of the thoracic and lumbar spine are extremely important to their mechanical integrity. Holdsworth's pioneering work[4,5] on spinal stability in relation to trauma has added a great deal to our understanding of how the spine responds to injury. Holdsworth divided the ligamentous complexes of the spine into two columns. The anterior ligamentous complex (column) consists of the anterior and posterior longitudinal ligaments and the annulus fibrosus. The posterior complex consists of the ligamentum flavum, the facet joint capsules, the interspinous ligament, and the supraspinous ligament. The posterior complex was thought to play the key role; its integrity is necessary for stability and its disruption leads to clinical instability. More recent investigation has altered this concept[6] and views stability on the basis of a three-column theory.[7–9] The posterior column remains the same, whereas

the anterior portion is represented by two columns, the anterior and middle columns (Table 13–1, Fig 13–7). There is strong evidence to suggest that disruption of both the posterior and middle columns is required for acute instability of the spine (see Chapter 16).

As already described, the capsules of the facet joints are important stabilizing structures, but the anatomy of the joints themselves also lends to structural integrity. In the thoracic region, these joints are oriented in the frontal plane (Fig 13–2). Thus, motion is restricted in flexion, extension, and lateral bending. In addition, this anatomic feature makes facet dislocation extremely rare in the thoracic region.

Several anatomic differences make the lumbar region inherently more mobile than the thoracic spine. The stability provided by the rib cage is absent. The intervertebral discs are thicker and thus allow greater

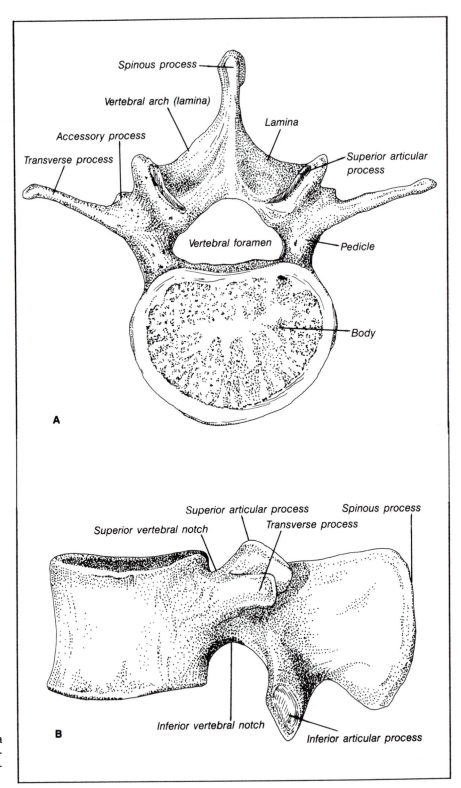

Figure 13–4. A. Superior view of a typical midlumbar vertebra. **B.** Lateral view of a typical midlumbar vertebra.

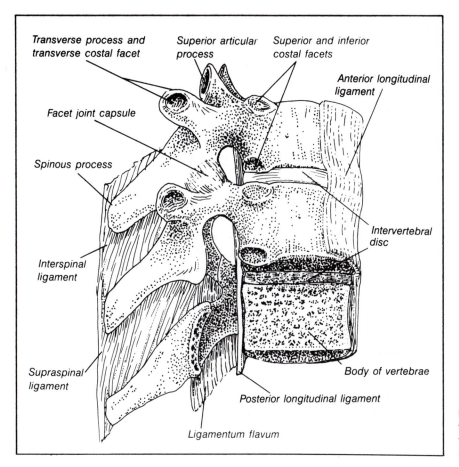

Figure 13–5. A schematic showing the capsule of the facet joints and the relationship of the various ligamentous attachments.

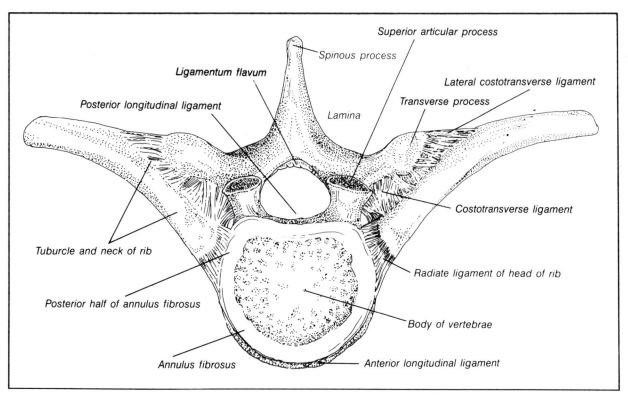

Figure 13–6. The important ligaments of the thoracic spine.

TABLE 13–1. ELEMENTS OF THE THREE-COLUMN SPINE

Anterior Column	Middle Column	Posterior Column
Anterior longitudi-nal ligament	Posterior longitudi-nal ligament	Supraspinous ligament
Anterior annulus fibrosus	Posterior annulus fibrosus	Interspinous ligament
Anterior half of vertebral body	Posterior half of vertebral body	Facet joint capsule Neural arch

movement between vertebral bodies. The sagittal orientation of the facet joints resists rotation but allows for significant flexion, extension, and lateral bending. The converse is true in the thoracic spine. It is this transition in anatomic and mechanical characteristics that makes the thoracolumbar region so vulnerable to unstable fractures and dislocations.[10]

Axiom: *Most unstable injuries of the thoracic and lumbar spine occur in the T-10 to L-1 region due to its vulnerable location between the relatively more stable thoracic and more mobile lumbar regions.*

□ SPINAL CORD AND NERVE ROOTS

There are several anatomic considerations that make the neurologic consequences of injuries in certain parts of the thoracic and lumbar spine unique. As already discussed, the thoracic spine has great stability and, therefore, requires tremendous forces to cause fracture–dislocations. If adequate force is achieved, however, significant displacement usually occurs. The spinal canal is very narrow between the levels of T-1

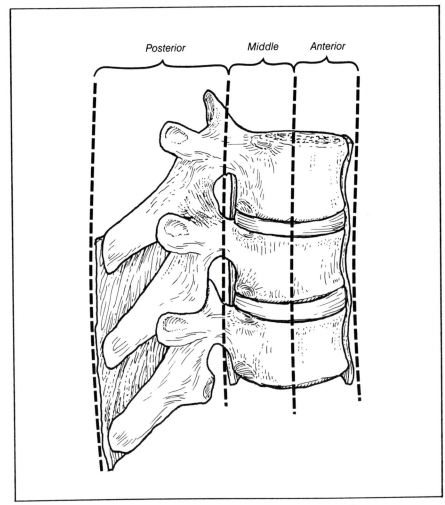

Figure 13–7. The three-column concept used to classify thoracic and lumbar spine fractures.

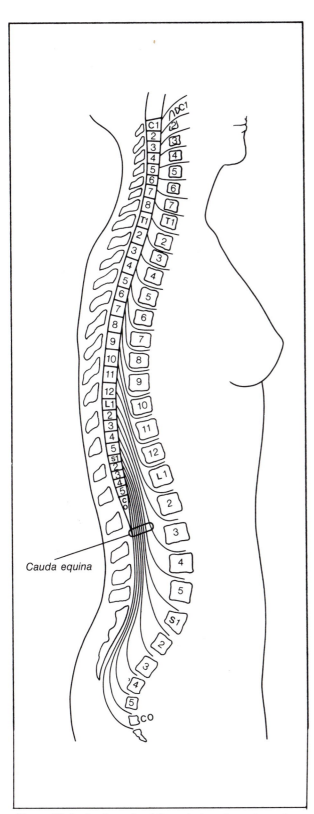

and T-10 and thus even a relatively small displacement can lead to catastrophic neurologic sequelae. For this reason, when fracture–dislocation occurs at these levels, complete transection of the cord usually results.

In the adult, the spinal cord terminates at the L1-2 interspace. Between the upper border of T-10 and this level, the lumbar enlargement contains the lumbar and sacral cord levels and gives rise to the concomitant nerve roots. The nerve roots course downward making up the cauda equina and exit the intervertebral foramina at their designated levels (Fig 13–8). Because the loss of several thoracic nerve roots has essentially no clinical consequence, significant neurologic damage is due only to cord damage from injuries above T-10. On the other hand, injuries below L-1 cause damage to the roots of the cauda equina, but not to the cord. Injuries between T-10 and L-1 produce combinations of cord and root damage and may lead to mixed patterns of injury (Fig 13–9). Injury to lumbar and sacral nerve roots has significant clinical consequences because of their motor innervations.

□ VASCULAR SUPPLY OF THE CORD

The anterior and paired posterior spinal arteries extend caudally down the entire length of the cord. The anterior spinal artery supplies the anterior and central portion of the cord, whereas the posterior spinal arteries supply the posterior and lateral substance. In the thoracic and lumbar region, small branches of the segmental arteries provide additional blood supply. Usually there are also several larger anastomosing vessels at the high thoracic and thoracolumbar levels.[11] Historically, the thoracic spinal cord has been thought to have a relatively poor blood supply between the T-4 and T-8 levels although this concept has been challenged.[12] In any case, neurologic impairment on the basis of vascular insufficiency is rare in thoracic and lumbar injuries.[13]

Figure 13–8. A schematic of the spinal cord, cauda equina, and the nerve roots exiting. See text for discussion.

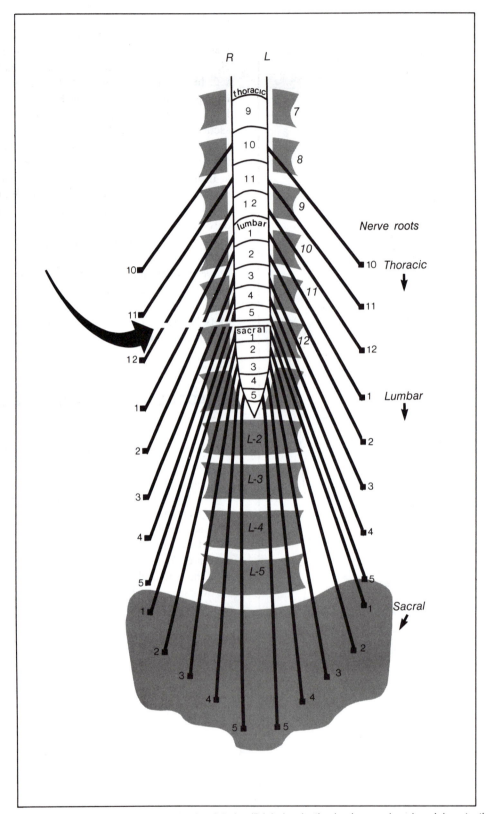

Figure 13–9. A schematic of the anatomic basis of "mixed" injuries in the lumbosacral region. Injury to the 12th thoracic vertebra has transected the cord between the lumbar and the sacral segments; the roots are lost on the right side, "spared" on the left side.

□ REFERENCES

1. Gregersen GG, Lucas DB: An in vivo study of the axial rotation of the human thoracolumbar spine. J Bone Joint Surg 49A:247,1967
2. Roaf R: A study of the mechanics of spinal injuries. J Bone Joint Surg 42B:810, 1960
3. Hollinshead WH: Anatomy for Surgeons: The Back and Limbs (Vol 3). New York, Paul Hoeber, 1958
4. Holdsworth FW: Fractures, dislocations, and fracture–dislocations of the spine. J Bone Joint Surg 45B:6, 1963
5. Holdsworth FW: Fractures, dislocations, and fracture–dislocations of the spine. J Bone Joint Surg 52A:1534, 1970
6. Bedbrook GM: Stability of spinal fractures and fracture–dislocations. Paraplegia 9:23, 1971
7. Denis F: The three-column spine and its significance in the classification of acute thoracolumbar spinal injuries. Spine 8:817, 1983
8. Denis F: Spinal stability as defined by three-column spine concept in acute spinal trauma. Clin Orthop 189:65, 1984
9. Ferguson RL, Allen BL: A mechanistic classification of thoracolumbar spine fractures. Clin Orthop 189:77, 1984
10. Scher AT: Radiological assessment of thoracolumbar spinal injuries. S Afr Med J 64:384, 1983
11. Keim HA, Hilal SK: Spinal angiography in scoliosis patients. J Bone Joint Surg 53A:904, 1971
12. Crock HV, Yoshizawa H: The Blood Supply of the Vertebral Column and Spinal Cord in Man. New York, Springer-Verlag, 1977
13. Schneider RC, Crosby EC, Russo RH, et al: Traumatic spinal cord syndromes and their management. Clin Neurosurg 20:424, 1973

14
Physical Examination

□ INTRODUCTION

Many physicians consider the back to be one of the most difficult regions of the body to examine; however, this need not be the case for several reasons. First, the anatomy is relatively simple, and proper examination is based on an understanding of the anatomy. Second, many of the important structures are relatively superficial and are, therefore, palpable. Third, the motion of the spine is much simpler than many other regions of the skeleton (i.e., the shoulder). And finally, other aspects of the physical examination can provide important hints regarding spinal pathology (i.e., neurologic examination). This final point also brings up the fact that a good back examination includes a good general physical examination as so many spinal disorders are associated with significant physical findings in other regions of the body.

The purpose of this chapter is to be comprehensive. This is contrary to the general approach in the practice of emergency medicine. In fact, it would be truly rare (and essentially impossible) to carry out all of the parts of the examination on a single patient in the emergency department. The emergency physician however, must know *all* of the parts of the examination to manage patients with the diverse clinical problems that present on essentially a daily basis. Only then can they know which parts of the examination may be reasonably and safely deleted without loss of important clinical information.

A final point of introduction is to reiterate the importance of the back examination in victims of multiple trauma. Amazingly enough, evaluation of this region may be postponed or entirely forgotten. This occurs despite the fact that so many significant injuries may be easily picked up by a "brief look" at the back. More importantly, the patient's most serious injury may remain unnoticed until this simple maneuver is carried out. Unfortunately, in some cases this may not occur until hours after arrival at the hospital.

□ INSPECTION

Examination of the back must occur with the patient undressed. Small undergarments may be worn if they do not make the examination more cumbersome.

Inspection begins from the front. The shoulders and the pelvis should be level and leg length equal. The general proportion of the torso to the legs is noted as it may be abnormal in patients with spinal curves or Marfan's syndrome. Note is made of obesity, malformations, general posture, and facial expression.

Next the patient is viewed from behind. Abnormal skin findings may be important and provide useful diagnostic information. Bruising or other signs of trauma are noted as are unusual skin markings. Cafe-au-lait spots, lipomata, birthmarks, neurofibromata, patches of hair, or areas of bulging may indicate underlying spinal or neurologic anomalies. Herpes zoster is a cause of back pain that may be totally missed unless the physician examines the skin carefully.

Once again, the shoulders should be level as should the scapulae, elbows, hands, pelvis, gluteal folds, and popliteal fossae. Asymmetry in any region should be further investigated as it may be associated with or even cause the "back problem." Pelvic obliquity is most easily noted by placing the hands on the iliac crests. Normally these heights are equal. If they are unequal, a shortened extremity is a likely cause of back pain.

Normally, the head and the spine are directly above the pelvis with the spine being perfectly straight when viewed from behind. Any lateral curve or prominence of one side of the chest should be noted as these suggest scoliosis (Fig 14–1). If this is a possibility, a "plumb line" is helpful in the evaluation. This test is accomplished by placing a string on the spinous process of T-1 with a "bob" at the end. Normally, the plumb line will rest in the gluteal cleft. It will be lateral to this, however, if a significant curve is present (Fig 14–2). A shortened leg may result in nonstructural

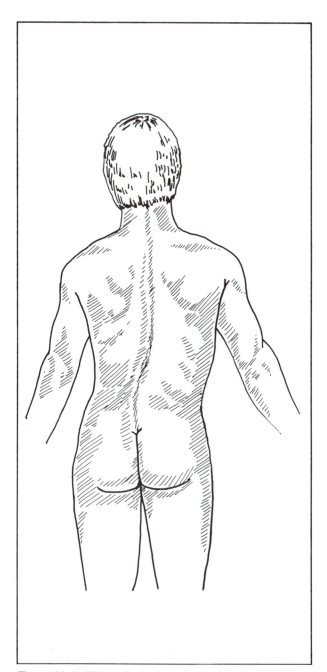

Figure 14–1. With scoliosis, the spine is shortened and the chest is asymmetrical.

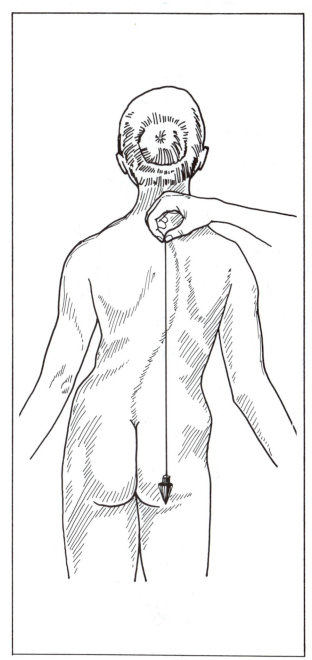

Figure 14–2. A plumb line dropped from the occiput is not on the midline in a patient with scoliosis.

scoliosis, but this should resolve when the patient is examined in a sitting position (Figs 14–3A and 14–3B.). The leg length is measured from the anterior superior iliac spine to the ipsilateral medial malleous and should be performed in anyone in whom unequal leg length is suspected as a cause of back pain.

Finally, the patient is observed from the side. This gives the best view of general posture as well as the "normal" spinal curvature. Normally, there is a lordosis of the cervical and lumbar regions of the spine with a kyphotic curve of the thoracic spine and sacrum. Alterations in the normal curvature are best seen when viewing the patient from the side. These include increased thoracic kyphosis (Scheuermann's disease, osteoporotic wedge fractures), gibbus deformity (tuberculous spondylitis, tumor), increased lumbar lordosis (obesity, pregnancy, poor abdominal muscle tone), and loss of the normal lumbar lordosis (ankylosing spondylitis, paravertebral muscle spasm) (Figs 14–4 through 14–7).

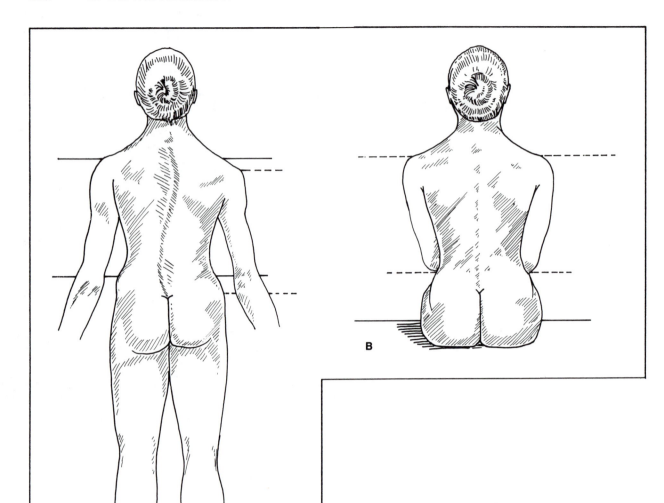

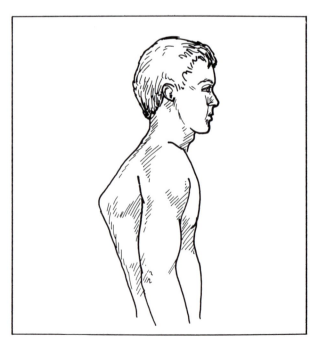

Figure 14–3. The nonstructural scoliosis secondary to a shortened leg **(A)** disappears when the patient is examined in the sitting position **(B)**.

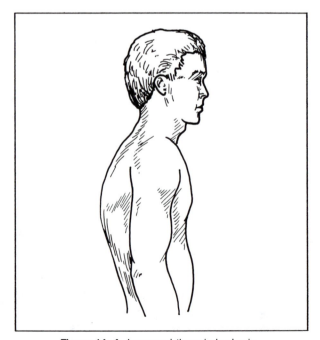

Figure 14–4. Increased thoracic kyphosis.

Figure 14–5. Gibbus deformity.

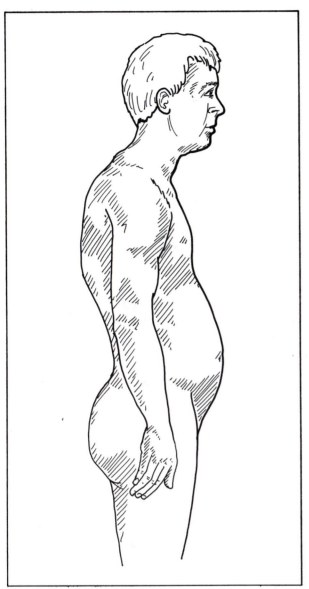

Figure 14–6. Increased lumbar lordosis in a patient with a protuberant abdomen causing postural abnormality and back pain.

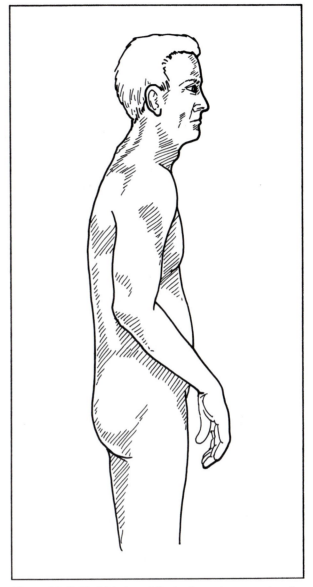

Figure 14–7. Straightening of the lumbar spine secondary to paravertebral muscle spasm.

☐ RANGE OF MOTION

There is significant variation in the range of motion of the thoracic and lumbar spine in the general population.[1,2] In addition, subtle changes in spinal mobility are often difficult to notice by physical examination alone. These two facts may make the diagnosis of impaired mobility difficult in a given patient. With experience, however, range-of-motion testing can become a powerful adjunct to the other aspects of the back examination.

Although a patient's complaint may refer only to one region of the back, it is still imperative to test the mobility of the entire thoracic and lumbar region on *all* patients with back symptoms. The reason for this is twofold: first, specific pathologic problems may present with reduced range of motion in a specific direction and region (extension is reduced with facet pathology). Second, *symptoms* in one region of the back may be due to *pathology* in another. For example, thoracic kyphosis tends to increase the lumbar lordosis. Thus a patient with a primary thoracic disorder may present with symptoms in the lumbar region. For this reason, we present the testing of range of motion of the back as a single set of maneuvers rather than as two individual regional examinations. The movements of the thoracic and lumbar spine are flexion, extension, lateral bending, and rotation. The examination for each begins with the patient standing erect.

Flexion

Testing begins by having the patient bend forward, attempting to touch the toes. From the lateral view, the back should appear as a single, gentle, smooth curve without areas of acute angulation. The lumbar region normally will either flatten out or go into a slight flexion curve. If a lordosis remains, it is abnormal. A kyphotic deformity may be accentuated by this maneuver, thus increasing the likelihood of making an early diagnosis (Fig 14–8). The distance from the fingertips to the floor should be measured. It should be noted that the vast majority of flexion occurs at the hip during this maneuver. In fact, some patients with completely immobile backs can touch their toes. Thus this measurement is most useful for following changes in the finger–floor distance with progressive spinal or hip disease. The most accurate indicator of spinal flexion is obtained by measuring the distance between the spinous processes of T-1 and S-1 in the standing position and then after forward bending (Figs 14–9A and 14–9B). Normally, the measured increase is approximately 10 cm. If the increase is less than normal, the T-1 to T-12 and T-12 to S-1 measurements should be obtained to determine whether the abnormal mobility resides in the thoracic or the lumbar region, or both. Normally, the difference is 2.5 cm for the thoracic region and 7.5 cm for the lumbar region. Limitation of flexion is seen in thoracic vertebral body fractures, injuries of the posterior longitudinal ligament in the lumbar region, interspinous ligament strain, and myofascial syndromes. Finally, while the patient is bending over, the back should be observed from the "skyline" view (Fig 14–10). Both sides of the chest should be equal in height and size. If the patient has a structural scoliosis, one side of the chest will be prominent and will appear as a humpback deformity (Fig 14–11).

Extension

To test extension, instruct the patient to bend backward as far as possible. Observe the patient from the side using the spinous processes of T-1 and S-1 as landmarks. Extension is usually about 30 degrees from this vertical line. Disorders that decrease a patient's ability to extend the back include a dorsal kyphosis and ankylosing spondylitis. This maneuver will often exacerbate pain caused by a herniated disc, facet joint problems, or spondylolisthesis; therefore, these problems may also decrease mobility in extension.

Lateral Bending

Lateral bending is tested by asking the patient to lean to the side while running the hand down the side of the leg (Fig 14–12). Make sure that no flexion or rotation of the torso occurs during this maneuver, as this will falsely increase the amount of "lateral" bending that the patient can accomplish. Now have the patient bend toward the opposite side and grossly compare mobility in the two directions. Any difference indicates pathology (i.e., scoliosis, paraspinous muscle spasm, herniated disc) (Fig 14–13). At the extreme of lateral bending, a finger–floor measurement should be made and both sides compared. This is also useful for comparing with future measurements that may indicate decreasing mobility over time. An additional measurement is obtained by viewing the patient from behind. An imaginary line between T-1 and S-1 will be 30 to 35 degrees from the vertical if lateral bending is normal (Fig 14–14).

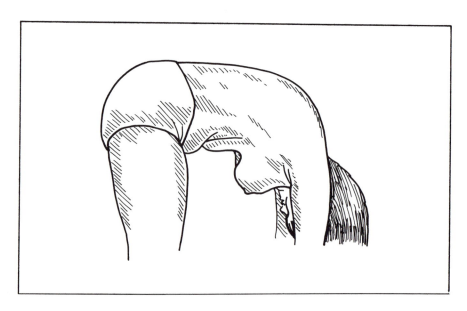

Figure 14–8. In a patient with thoracic kyphosis, the abnormal curve is accentuated on flexion.

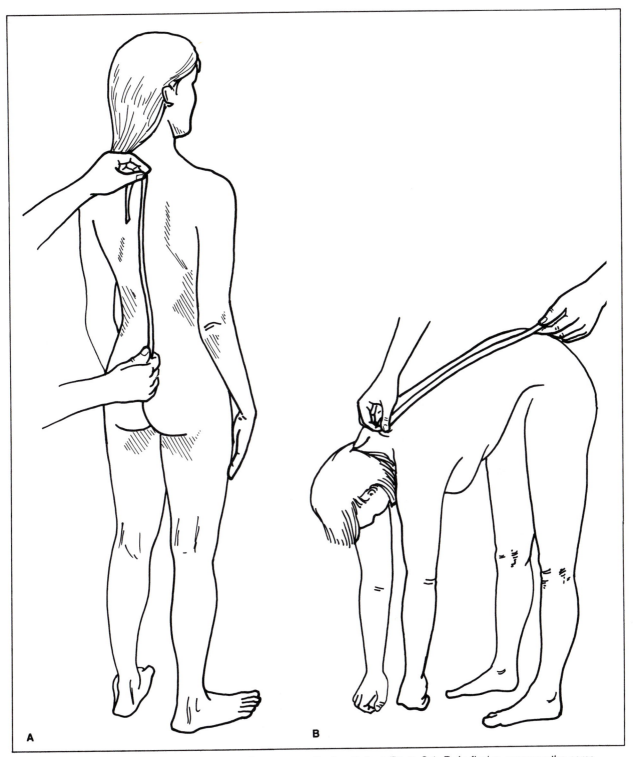

Figure 14–9. A. While the patient is standing measure the length from T-1 to S-1. **B.** In flexion, measure the same distance. In patients with ankylosing spondylitis or other disorders affecting the spine, the change in distance will be much less than 10 cm.

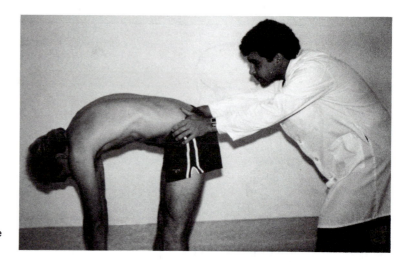

Figure 14–10. Performing a skyline view of the spine.

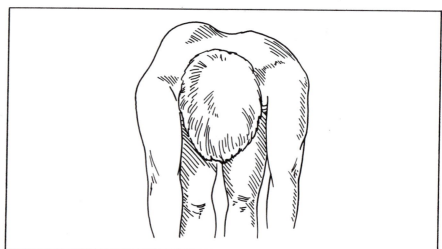

Figure 14–11. The typical hump-back seen on skyline view in a patient with scoliosis.

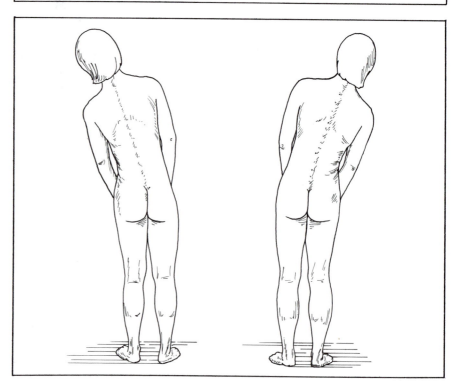

Figure 14–12. Normal right and left lateral bend of the spine.

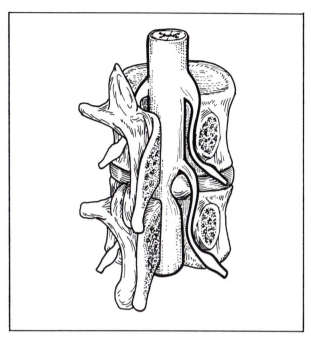

Figure 14–13. Herniated disc causing irritation of the nerve root and radicular pain.

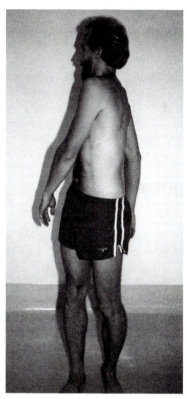

Figure 14–15. Testing for rotation in a standing patient.

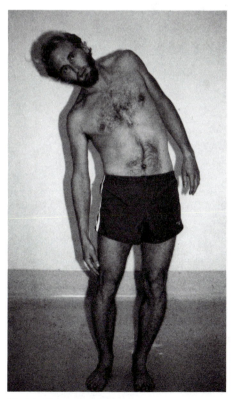

Figure 14–14. Examining "line" between T-1 and S-1 in lateral bending to see if less than 30 degrees from vertical.

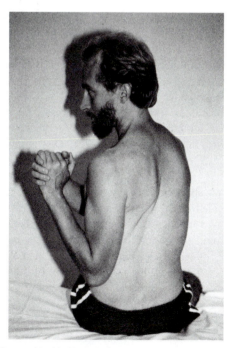

Figure 14–16. Testing for rotation in a sitting patient.

Rotation

Rotation is tested by asking the patients to turn the shoulders and torso as far as possible to either side without rotating the pelvis (Fig 14–15). To prevent pelvic rotation from occurring it may be helpful to have the patients sit down (Fig 14–16) or to aid them with the maneuver by holding the pelvis steady. Normal rotation is 40 to 45 degrees and any asymmetry should be considered abnormal.

☐ PALPATION

As with the examination of any region of the body, palpation of the back is often directed by abnormalities detected by inspection. The examiner is seeking areas of tenderness, warmth, swelling, induration, tumor, and alterations in structure or symmetry.

Bony Palpation

The bony landmarks of the thoracic, lumbar, and sacral regions are shown in Figures 14–17 and 14–18. The scapulae and the rib cage should be palpated in search of asymmetry, tenderness, or other abnormalities. Lack of symmetry may represent scoliosis.

Except in extremely obese individuals, the spinous processes are quite easy to palpate and identify individually. Each should be in the midline, whereas deviation laterally represents a rotational abnormality (i.e., scoliosis, fracture). The distance between adjacent spinous processes (interspinous distance) is nearly identical from one segment to the next and should be palpated at each level (Fig 14–19). In the setting of trauma, an increase in this distance may indicate an unstable injury with ligamentous rupture (Fig 14–20). A decreased interspinous distance is often present in the setting of burst fractures (see Chapter 16). Defects, such as spina bifida or secondary to previous spinal surgery, are also easily palpable. If a step-off is palpated in the low lumbar or lumbosacral region it may represent spondylolisthesis (Figs 14–21 and 14–22). This is most common at L-5 to S-1, but can occur at L-4 to L-5 and L-3 to L-4.

If an abnormality is found by palpation, the level can be identified by counting spinous processes from one of two landmarks. T-1 is easily identifiable as the most prominent spinous process at the upper end of the thoracic spine. In the lumbar region, the L-4 to L-5 interspace is reliably located at the level of the superior aspect of the iliac crests (Fig 14–22).

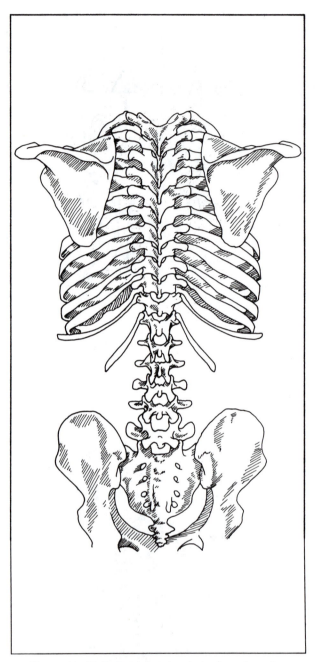

Figure 14–17. Bony landmarks of the thoracic region.

After examining the spinous processes, each of the facet joints should be palpated. These are located approximately 2.5 cm lateral to and between the spinous processes bilaterally. Although the joints themselves are

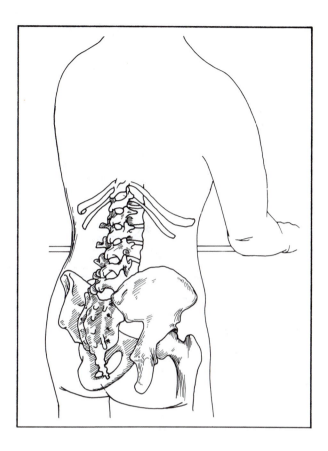

Figure 14–18. Bony landmarks in the lumbar region.

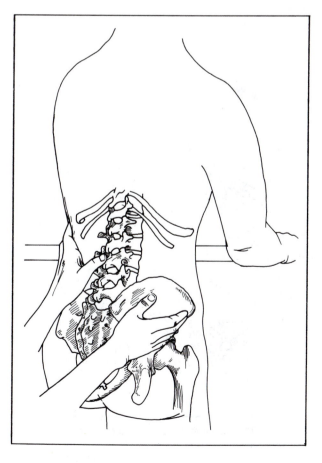

Figure 14–19. Palpating the spinous processes.

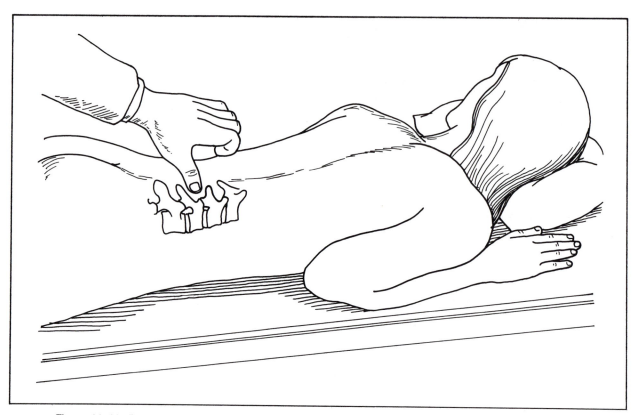

Figure 14–20. Palpating the interspinous and supraspinous ligaments. An increased interspinous distance may represent an unstable injury.

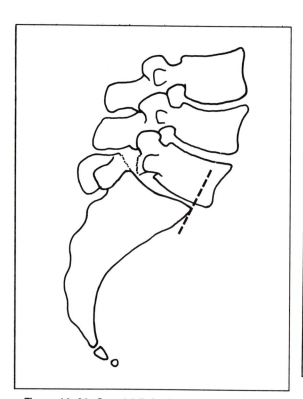

Figure 14–21. Spondylolisthesis at the L-5 to S-1 level.

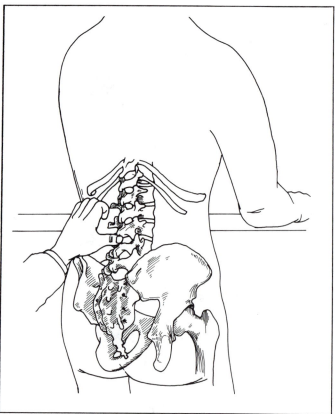

Figure 14–22. A step-off is demonstrated in a patient with spondylolisthesis.

deep to the paraspinous muscles and cannot be felt directly, tenderness and overlying muscle spasm may result from pathology in these structures. Next the sacrum should be palpated for tenderness or deformity. The S-2 spinous process is located at the level of the posterior superior iliac spines (Fig 14–23). The sacroiliac (SI) joints are then palpated and may suggest disorders, such as SI strain or ankylosing spondylitis, if tenderness is present. Several other tests have been described that may help detect SI joint disease.[3] First, with the patient lying supine, press downward on the iliac wings (attempting to spread them apart). Next, turn the patient on the side and press downward on the iliac wing (attempting to push the iliac wings toward each other). Finally, with the patient prone, press firmly over the body of the sacrum. Each of these maneuvers applies a unique stress to the SI joints and if pain is elicited, it implies an inflammatory process.

The coccyx is palpated last and may be very tender after direct blows or a fall even if no fracture is present (Fig 14–24).

Complete examination of the coccyx requires a rectal examination. This allows the coccyx to be grasped between the thumb and the index finger.

In thin patients, the lumbosacral region of the spine can be palpated anteriorly "through" the abdomen. The patient should lie supine with the hips slightly flexed and is instructed to relax the abdominal muscles. The umbilicus is located at the L-3–L-4 interspace and also at the level of the aortic bifurcation.[4] Below the umbilicus, in thin patients, the anterior aspect of L-4, L-5, and S-1 (the sacral promontory) can be palpated as well as the overlying anterior longitudinal ligament. In some patients with spinal pathology, this will cause or exacerbate pain in the lumbosacral region of the back. Abdominal tenderness may be due

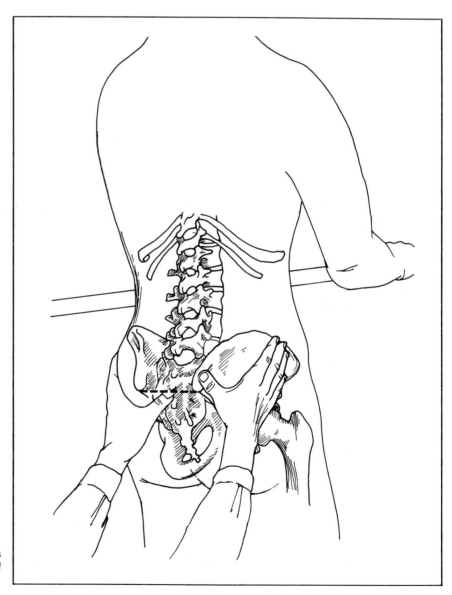

Figure 14–23. The S-2 spinous process is palpated at the level of the posterior superior iliac spine.

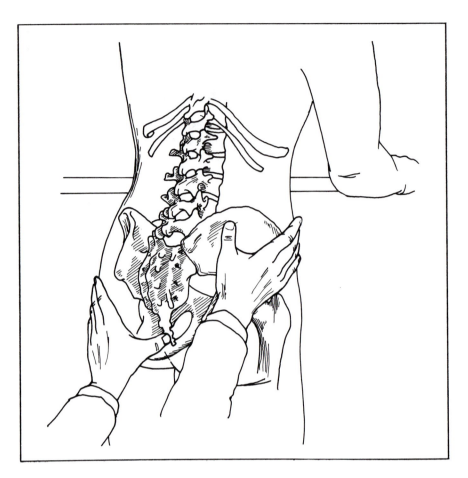

Figure 14–24. Palpating the coccyx.

to pathology anywhere between the anterior abdominal wall and the spine. The finding of abdominal tenderness should be viewed with this fact in mind and thus may direct further work-up.

Axiom: *When examining the abdomen in patients who present with low back pain check for an aortic aneurysm. In addition, retrocecal appendix and pelvic pathology can present with low back pain.*

Soft Tissue Palpation

All of the regions of the back should be briefly "scanned" with the palpating hands in search of abnormalities. Tense, bulging, tender muscle masses indicate spasm. A search is made for soft tissue masses, hematomas, and any asymmetry. Midline masses or cystic structures may indicate underlying spinal and neurologic anomalies such as spina bifida or myelocele. Fluctuant masses in the paraspinous or flank region may represent an abscess extending from spinal tuberculosis or bacterial osteomyelitis.

Supraspinous Ligament

The supraspinous ligament is attached to and connects each of the vertebral spinous processes and is felt as a firm, fibrous structure when palpating the recesses between adjacent vertebrae (Fig 14–25). Each level should be palpated in search of tenderness. In major trauma, a disrupted posterior ligamentous complex will be palpable as a widened interspinous distance. When the supraspinous (and interspinous) ligaments are disrupted, the palpating finger advances deeper into the interspinous space than at the adjacent normal segments.

Paraspinous Muscles

The paraspinous musculature is made up of three layers. Table 14–1 gives a summary of these layers (Fig 14–26). The erector spinae muscles are the most superficial and thus are most amenable to palpation. Exami-

TABLE 14–1. PARASPINOUS MUSCULATURE

Layer	Musculature
Superficial (erector spinae)	Iliocostalis
	Longissimus
	Spinalis
	Sacrospinalis
Middle	Semispinalis
Deep	Multifidus

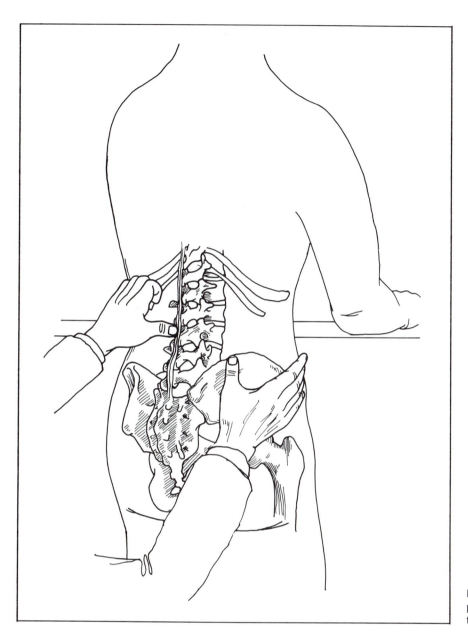

Figure 14–25. Palpation of the supraspinous ligament while the patient is standing.

nation should include palpation of the entire thoracic, lumbar, and sacral region as spasm may be noted in areas distant from the primary pathology. When spasm occurs, it may be unilateral or bilateral and may lead to nonstructural spinal deformities (scoliosis, loss of lumbar lordosis). Areas of tenderness should also be noted. Muscular asymmetry is of importance as it may represent atrophy and an underlying neurologic lesion.

Gluteal Region

The gluteal muscles are palpated in search of tenderness, spasm, atrophy, or other abnormalities. Palpation of the sciatic nerve is a very important part of the examination in this region. Have the patient flex the hip to 90 degrees by placing the foot on a chair while standing erect. In this position, the ischial tuberosity

and greater trochanter can easily be palpated. The sciatic nerve trunk passes into the lower extremity midway between these two structures and can be palpated there (Fig 14–27). If palpation of the nerve elicits pain, a lesion compressing a nerve root (i.e., herniated disc, narrowed intervertebral foramen, tumor) may be present and requires further investigation.

□ PERCUSSION

At times, percussion is useful to differentiate spinal tenderness from a deeper source of pain (i.e., kidney). Beginning from T-1 and progressing downward, each spinous process is percussed firmly with a reflex ham-

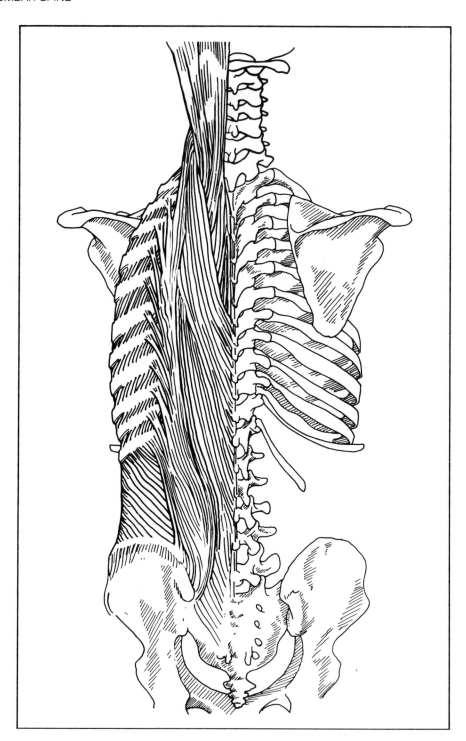

Figure 14–26. The paraspinal muscles and their relation to the spine and thorax.

mer or clasped hand. Continue down to the sacrum and then percuss the SI joints. Generally, pain caused by percussion results from a spinal pathology (i.e., infection, fracture) rather than retroperitoneal organ disease.

ated with or that cause back pain that may be picked up by the listening ear (aortic insufficiency in Marfan's syndrome, spinal malformation with congenital heart defects, abdominal aortic aneurysm).

☐ AUSCULTATION

Although not classically described as an aspect of the back examination, there are certainly diseases associ-

☐ NEUROLOGIC EXAMINATION

Although there is no true neurologic examination of the spine itself, an intimate relationship exists between tho-

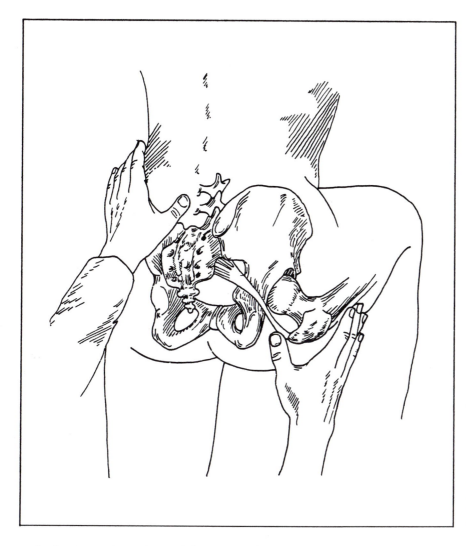

Figure 14–27. Palpation of the sciatic nerve, which is located between the greater trochanter and the ischial tuberosity, is most easily done with the leg flexed 90 degrees at the hip.

racic, lumbar, and sacral spinal disorders and the neurologic examination of the torso and lower extremities. Thus, the combination of motor, sensory, and reflex tests often provides specific information on the segment(s) involved and can be powerful clinical tools if carried out in a careful manner. This interaction is discussed at length in the chapter on neurologic and cord syndromes (Chapter 2). Some of that material is repeated here but this section will primarily deal with the neurologic examination of the lower extremities as it relates to spinal pathology.

Motor Testing

The motor examination of the thoracic region should have already been accomplished during inspection and palpation. Because the innervation of the paraspinous musculature is segmental, atrophy may occur at specific levels and can often be correlated with sensory findings, especially if a lesion involves several segments. The motor examination of the lower extremities begins with observation of the patient while standing and walking. Any abnormalities in gait suggest pathology either in the spine or extremities and should be

investigated further. Three quick, simple tests are then performed that "scan" for pathology in the lumbosacral cord and roots:

Squat test—The patient is asked to slowly drop to a squatting position and then return to standing (Fig 14–28). Weakness implies pathology at L-3 and L-4 (quadriceps femoris).

Heel walk—The patient is asked to walk on the heels (dorsiflexing the ankle). This tests L-4 and L-5 (tibialis anterior, extensor digitorum longus) (Fig 14–29).

Toe walk—The patient is asked to walk on tip-toes. This tests S-1 and S-2 (gastrocnemius, soleus) (Fig 14–30).

Any abnormalities that are found should be investigated by more formal motor testing (Table 14–2).

The circumference of several points on the thighs and the calves should be measured and compared on the two extremities. The patellae are used as references to insure measurement of corresponding regions of the legs. A difference of more than 1 cm is abnormal and

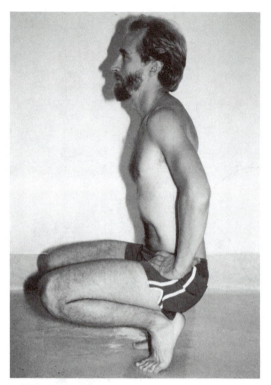

Figure 14–28. The squat test. (See text for discussion.)

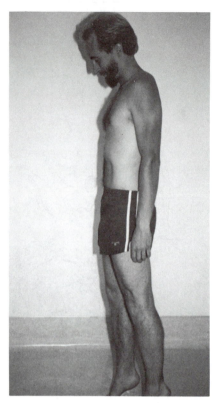

Figure 14–30. Plantar flexors are tested by walking on the toes.

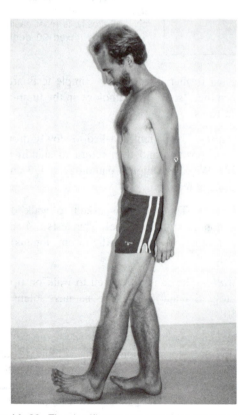

Figure 14–29. The dorsiflexors are tested by the heel walk.

implies atrophy of the musculature on the leg with the smaller circumference.

S-2 to S-4 innervate the anal sphincter, bladder, and intrinsics of the foot. Thus, a history of urinary retention or incontinence, or the findings of decreased rectal tone or atrophy of the intrinsics of the foot, should lead one to suspect pathology in the S-2 to S-4 region.

Sensory Testing

The segmental dermatomal distribution of the body is very specific with surprisingly little variation from one person to the next. This generally allows exact localization of a root or cord lesion when a sensory deficit is present (see Fig 2–1). It should be noted that there is a significant amount of dermatomal overlap in the thoracic, abdominal, and groin region (Fig 14–31), and thus a lesion at a single level may not result in any sensory deficit at all.

Generally, the testing of light touch and pinprick are adequate in the vast majority of patients. Certain cord lesions, however, lead to specific deficits of temperature sensation or proprioception, and these modalities should be tested in appropriate settings (see Chapter 2).

TABLE 14–2. MOTOR INNERVATION

Body Area	Muscles	Motion	Nerve Roots
Hip	Quadriceps femoris, sartorius, iliopsoas	Flexion	L-2 to L-4
	Gluteus medius and minimus, tensor fasciae latae	Abduction	L-4, L-5
	Gluteus maximus, biceps femoris	Extension	L-5 to S-2
Knee	Quadriceps femoris	Extension	L-3, L-4
	Semimembrano-sus, Semitendinosus, biceps femoris	Flexion	L-4 to S-1
Ankle	Tibialis anterior, extensor digitorum longus	Dorsiflexion	L-4, L-5
	Gastrocnemius, soleus	Plantar flexion	S-1, S-2
Foot	Peroneus longus and brevis	Eversion	L-5, S-1
Toes and great toe	Extensor digitorum and hallucis longus	Extension	L-5
	Flexor digitorum and hallucis brevis and longus	Flexion	S-1, S-2

Reflex Testing

Deep Tendon Reflexes

There are only two deep tendon reflexes (DTRs) of significance in the entire region below the cervical spinal cord: the knee jerk (L-2 to L-4) and the ankle jerk (S-1) (Table 14–3). They are of great importance for two reasons. First, a tremendous amount of pathology occurs in the lumbosacral region and thus these reflexes are "well placed" for localizing segmental lesions. Second, cord lesions anywhere above the lumbosacral region will often manifest themselves in the abnormalities of knee and ankle jerks by the findings typical of an upper motor neuron lesion.

The knee jerk is tested by briskly striking the patellar tendon just below the patella while the patient sits relaxed with the legs dangling at the bedside. This

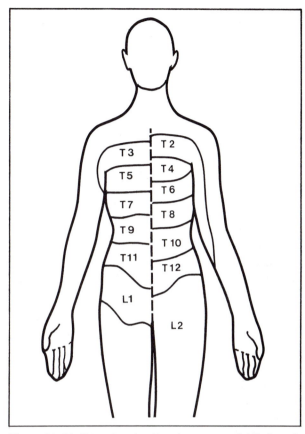

Figure 14–31. Dermatomal pattern for sensory distribution of the thoracic and upper lumbar nerve roots.

causes contraction of the quadriceps and extension of the knee. The ankle jerk is best tested by having the patient kneel on a chair with the feet extending beyond the seat. The Achilles tendon is struck with a reflex hammer, and the foot plantar flexes in response. Both DTRs should have a brisk and brief contraction and relaxation phase and should be bilaterally symmetrical.

Because so much pathology occurs at the lumbosacral junction (i.e., degenerative joint disease with root impingement, disc herniation), the specific motor, sensory, and reflex findings resulting from lesions in this region should be memorized (Figs 14–32 to 14–34).

TABLE 14–3. REFLEXES

Reflex	Spinal Segment
Knee jerk	L-2 to L-4
Ankle jerk	S-1
Cremasteric	T-12 to L-2
Epigastric	T-7 to T-10
Abdominal	T-7 to L-1
Hypogastric	T-12 to L-1
Bulbocavernosus	S-2 to S-4
Anal wink	S-2 to S-4

Cutaneous Reflexes

The cutaneous reflexes are mediated by the cerebral cortex (upper motor neurons) as opposed to DTRs, which are spinal reflexes dependent on lower motor neuron function. An upper motor neuron lesion will decrease or obliterate a cutaneous reflex, whereas it will exaggerate the DTRs (due to loss of inhibition).

Epigastric Reflex. Gentle cutaneous stimulation beginning in the midline of the epigastrium stroking inferiorly leads to contraction of the upper abdominal muscles and subtle movement of the umbilicus superiorly. The muscles of the upper quadrants are innervated by the T-7 to T-10 spinal levels.

Abdominal Reflex. With the patient lying supine each quadrant of the abdomen is gently stroked. The umbilicus should move toward the quadrant that is stimulated. This test is most easily interpreted in thin patients and is generally not useful in the obese patient.

Cremasteric and Hypogastric Reflexes. Stroking the inner aspect of the upper thigh causes contraction of the ipsilateral cremasteric (T-12 to L-2) and lower abdominal musculature (T-10 to L-1). Thus the scrotal sac is pulled superiorly (Fig 14–35) and the umbilicus makes a subtle inferior movement toward the side of stimulation. Generally the hypogastric reflex can only be observed in thin patients.

Anal Wink. Gently stroke the perianal skin. Normally this causes contraction of the external sphincter and results in the anal wink. This reflex is mediated by S-2 to S-4.

Pathologic Reflexes

Pathologic reflexes occur in the setting of an upper motor neuron lesion that results in the loss of normal inhibition on the lower motor neurons. It should be noted that during acute spinal cord injuries, a state of "spinal shock" exists that results in no reflex activity at all for 12 to 72 hours. As this resolves, the pathologic reflexes appear.

Babinski Sign. Run a pointed instrument along the plantar aspect of the foot (Fig 14–36). A positive test entails dorsiflexion of the great toe and splaying of the others and indicates an upper motor neuron lesion. The test is negative if the toes flex or do not move at all.

Oppenheim Test. The examiner runs a fingernail or knuckles down the crest of the shin toward the foot. A positive test is identical to a Babinski sign.

Chaddock Test. The examiner's fingernail is scraped firmly along the lateral aspect of the calcaneous and fifth metatarsal. A positive test is identical to a Babinski sign.

Bulbocavernosus Reflex. While performing a rectal examination, the glans penis is squeezed with firm pressure. Contraction of the anal sphincter around the examining finger is a positive test. In cord-injured patients the appearance of this reflex heralds resolution of spinal shock and indicates an extremely poor prognosis for recovery of neurologic function.

Special Maneuvers

Outline of Special Maneuvers
Tests for sciatic nerve and root pathology
   Straight leg raising (SLR)
   Contralateral SLR
   Lasegue sign
   Popliteal pressure test
Tests for meningeal, dural, or root pathology
   Kernig's sign
   Brudzinski's sign
   Naffziger test
   Milgram test
   Valsalva maneuver
Tests for sacroiliac joint pathology
   Pelvic splay test
   Pelvic compression test
   Sacral pressure test
   Pelvic rock test
   Gaenslen's sign
   FABERE (Patrick) test
Tests for femoral nerve and root pathology
   Femoral stretch test
   Knee hyperflexion test
Tests for innervation of the abdominal musculature
   Beevor's sign
   Epigastric reflex ⎫
   Abdominal reflex ⎬ See cutaneous reflexes
   Hypogastric reflex ⎭
Miscellaneous tests
   Soto-Hall test
   Gluteal skyline test
   Trendelenburg test
   T-1 root stretch test
   Scapular approximation test
Tests for determining functional pain
   "Sitting" straight leg raising test
   Hoover test
   Axial "compression" test
   Superficial "pinch" test
   Pelvic rotation test
   Toe walk/heel walk

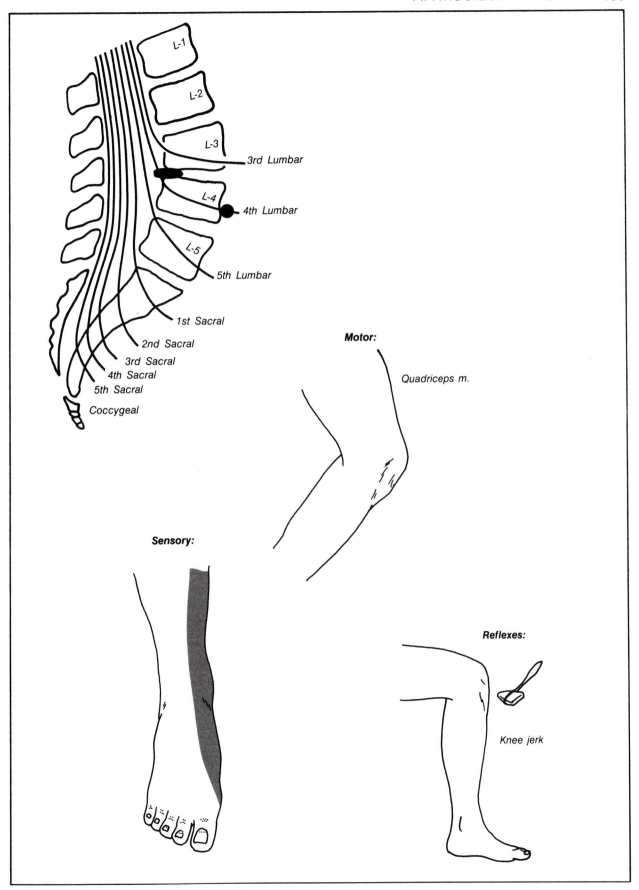

Figure 14–32. The L-4 nerve root innervations.

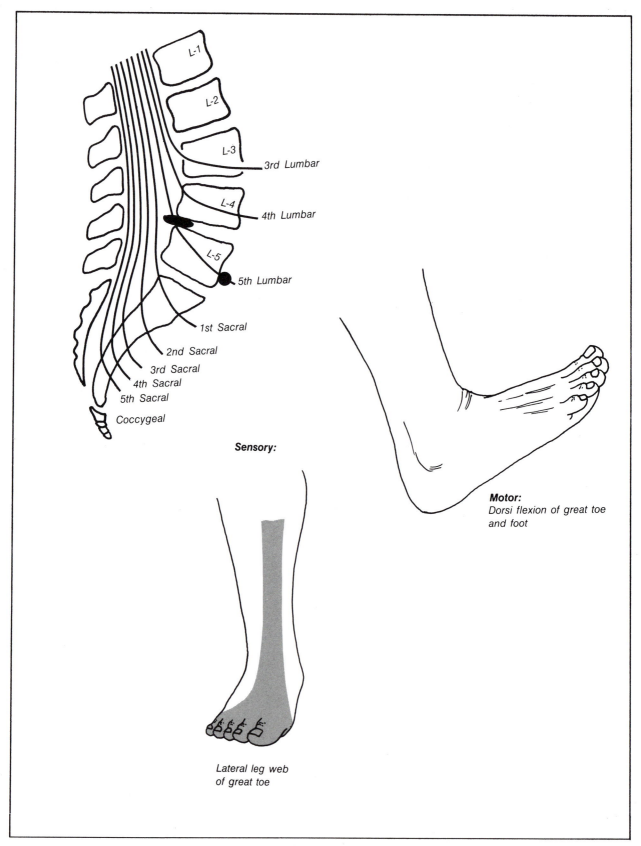

L-1

L-2

L-3

3rd Lumbar

L-4

4th Lumbar

L-5

5th Lumbar

1st Sacral

2nd Sacral

3rd Sacral

4th Sacral

5th Sacral

Coccygeal

Sensory:

Motor:
Dorsi flexion of great toe and foot

Lateral leg web of great toe

Figure 14–33. The L-5 nerve root innervations.

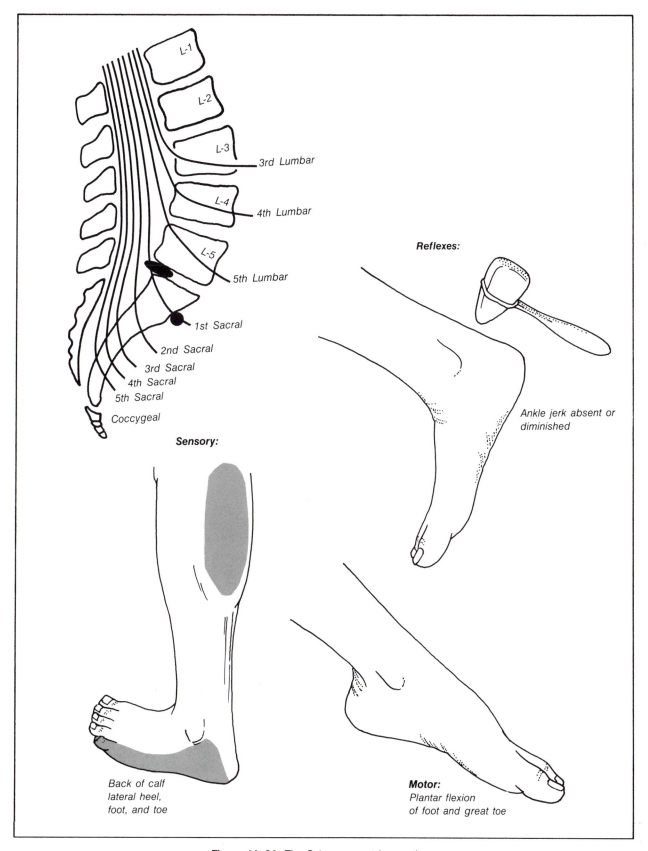

Figure 14–34. The S-1 nerve root innervations.

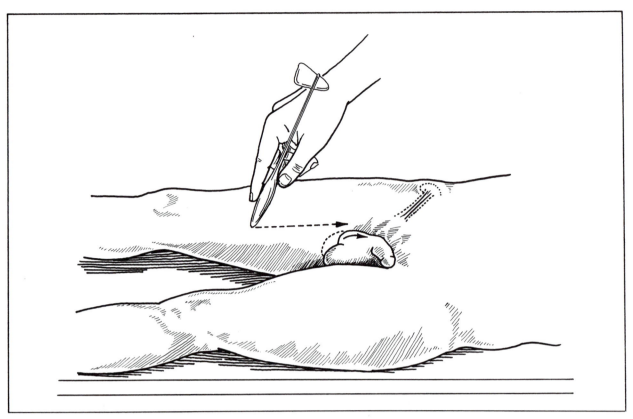

Figure 14–35. Testing for the cremasteric reflex.

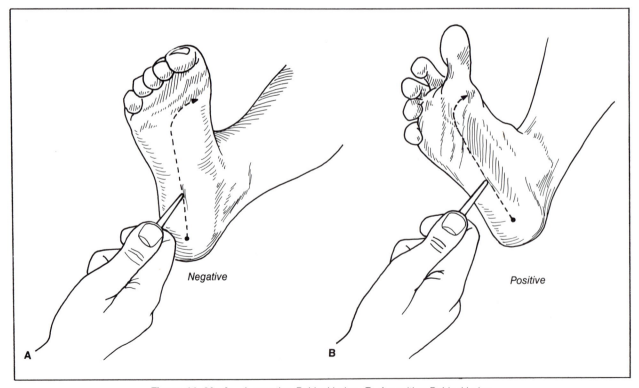

Figure 14–36. A. A negative Babinski sign. **B.** A positive Babinski sign.

Tests for Sciatic Nerve and Root Pathology

Straight Leg Raising (SLR). This maneuver is intended to stretch the sciatic nerve and thus indicates pathology in the nerve or its roots (primarily L-5 to S-2). With the patient supine, the leg is kept straight and the examiner lifts the leg (Fig 14–37). If no pain is elicited during the complete arc from 0 to 90 degrees, the test is negative. The presence of pain, however, does not necessarily imply a positive test. Several points must be made to understand a true positive test. Between 0 and 35 degrees, the sciatic nerve is not yet taut, and thus pain indicates hip, leg, or SI joint pathology or malingering. From 35 to 70 degrees, the sciatic nerve and lumbosacral nerve roots are stretched.[5–7] Precipitation or worsening of low back pain (with or without radiation) during this part of the test implies sciatic nerve or root irritation (i.e., herniated disc, narrowed intervertebral foramen). Beyond 70 degrees, the lumbar spine begins to flex, and pain implies pathology in the joints of this region.[5] Pain or tightness occurring only in the leg during the SLR test is generally due to muscle stretching and should not be interpreted as a positive test. One means of improving the specificity of the test is as follows: If back pain is elicited during the arc from 35 to 70 degrees, the examiner should drop the leg back slightly until the pain is relieved. The foot is then dorsiflexed by the examiner (stretching the sciatic nerve). If the back pain returns, the test is positive (Fig 14–38).

Contralateral (Well-Leg) Straight Leg Raising. This maneuver (first described by Fajersztajn[8]) is accomplished in the same manner as the SLR test but on the side opposite to the predominant symptoms. A positive test is highly significant and encountering a false-positive test is much less likely than with SLR.[9,10]

Lasegue Sign. Several maneuvers have been given this name; however, the original test consists of flexing the hip to 90 degrees on the side of the symptoms. The knee is initially kept flexed as well.[11] This does not stretch the sciatic nerve or roots, and thus pain at this point in the maneuver is due to hip, leg, or lumbar disease or malingering. When knee extension produces pain in the back (often with radiation into the sciatic distribution), the test is positive and has the same implications as a positive SLR test.

Popliteal Pressure Test. A SLR test is carried out until it is positive. Then the foot is placed on the examiner's shoulder and the knee is slightly flexed to relieve the pain. The examiner's thumbs are placed in the popliteal fossa and pressure is exerted. This stretches the sciatic nerve and the pain symptoms return (Fig 14–39).[12]

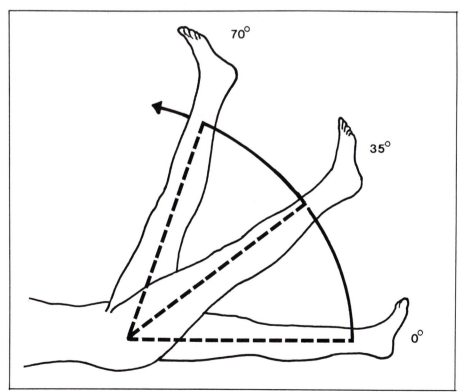

Figure 14–37. Performing a straight leg raising test. (See text for discussion.)

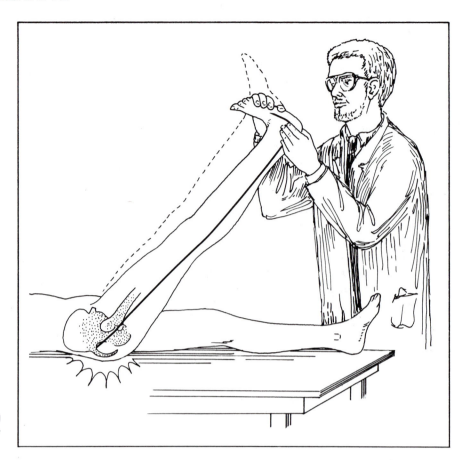

Figure 14–38. Straight leg raising test with pain accentuated by dorsiflexion of the foot.

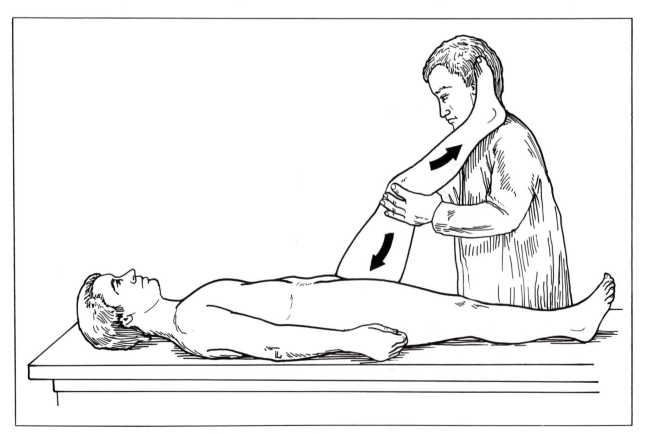

Figure 14–39. Popliteal pressure test.

Tests for Meningeal, Dural, or Root Pathology

Kernig's Sign. With the patient supine, one hip is flexed bringing the thigh onto the abdomen with the knee remaining flexed. The knee is then extended and a positive test is indicated by resistance to extension of the knee or pain in the spine (Fig 14–40). A positive test implies irritation of the meninges, dura, or nerve roots.

Brudzinski's Sign. With the patient supine and the legs straight, the neck is passively flexed by the examiner. A positive test is indicated by back pain and spontaneous flexion of the hips and knees to relieve the tension on the dura and nerve roots (Fig 14–41). The sensitivity and specificity of the Kernig's and Brudzinski's signs are not known but they have been advocated as confirmatory tests when the SLR test is positive.[13]

Naffziger Test. With the patient supine, gently compress the jugular veins for approximately 10 seconds. This increases the pressure in the cerebrospinal fluid and may cause pain if a space-occupying lesion is present (i.e., tumor, herniated disc, etc.) (Fig 14–42). If pain is not elicited by compression alone, the patient should be instructed to cough. If pain occurs, the test is positive. Radiation in the sciatic distribution is not uncommon.

Milgram Test. With the patient supine, he or she is instructed to raise both legs several inches off the table while keeping the legs straight. This increases cerebrospinal fluid pressure. If the patient experiences back pain within 30 seconds, the test is positive and implies the same possible pathologic processes as a positive Naffziger test. The pain may be so great that the patient drops one or both legs (Fig 14–43).

Valsalva Maneuver. With the patient sitting in a chair, ask him or her to bear down as if trying to have a bowel movement. As with the Naffziger and Milgram test this increases cerebrospinal fluid pressure, and back pain implies an irritating lesion involving the dura or the nerve roots.

Tests for Sacroiliac Joint Pathology

Pelvic Splay Test. With the patient supine, downward pressure is applied to the pelvic wings in an attempt to "splay open" the pelvis (Fig 14–44).[3] This is thought

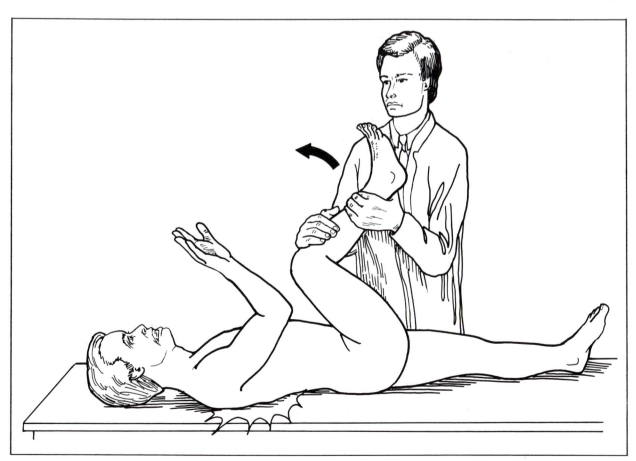

Figure 14–40. Kernig's sign.

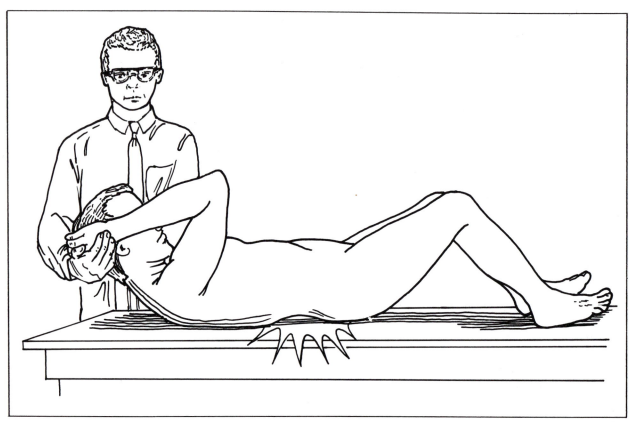

Figure 14–41. Brudzinski test.

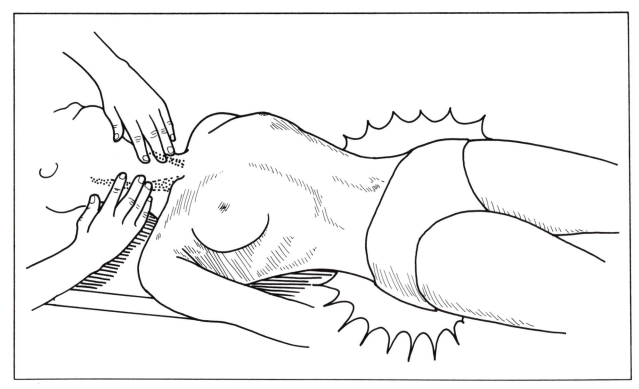

Figure 14–42. Naffziger test.

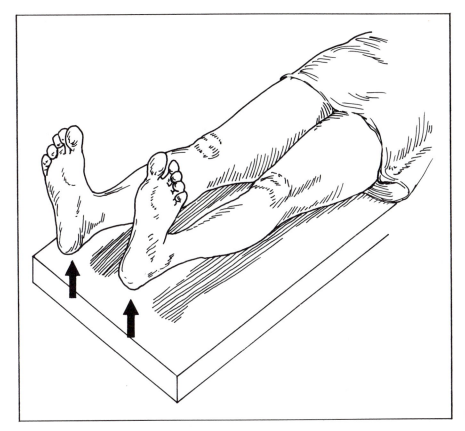

Figure 14–43. Milgram test.

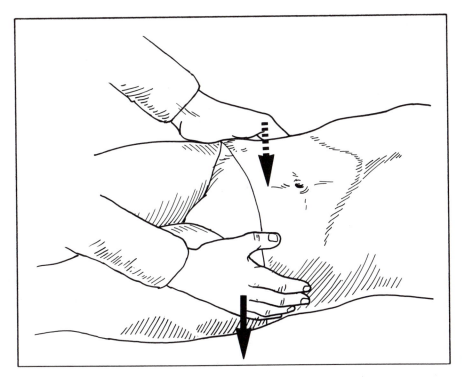

Figure 14–44. Pelvic splay test.

to stress the anterior part of the SI joints and thus causes pain if these joints are inflamed.

Pelvic Compression Test. Now instruct the patient to lie on the side. Downward pressure is applied to the iliac wing (as if attempting to push the iliac crests together). This is thought to stress the posterior part of the SI joints.[3]

Sacral Pressure Test. The patient now turns to the prone position and firm downward pressure is applied to the body of the sacrum. This places a rotational stress on the SI joints.[3] Pain implies pathology of the joints.

Pelvic Rock Test. With the patient supine, the examiner places the hands on the iliac wings and the thumbs on the anterior superior iliac spine. Pressure is then exerted toward the midline (Fig 14–45). This places the

same stress on the SI joints as the pelvic compression test.

Gaenslen's Sign. With the patient supine instruct him or her to flex both knees and hips and hold the knees in the knee–chest position (Fig 14–46A). The examiner then helps move the patient to the edge of the table with one buttock over the edge. The "suspended" leg is then allowed to drop (Fig 14–46B) placing stress on the SI joint. The test is generally negative (painless) unless SI joint pathology exists.

FABERE (Patrick) Test. The term FABERE is a mnemonic for flexion/abduction/external rotation/extension. With the patient supine, the hips and the knees are flexed and then the hip is abducted and externally rotated to bring the foot to rest on the opposite knee (Fig 14–47). When this has been accomplished, the examiner places one hand on the knee and the other on the

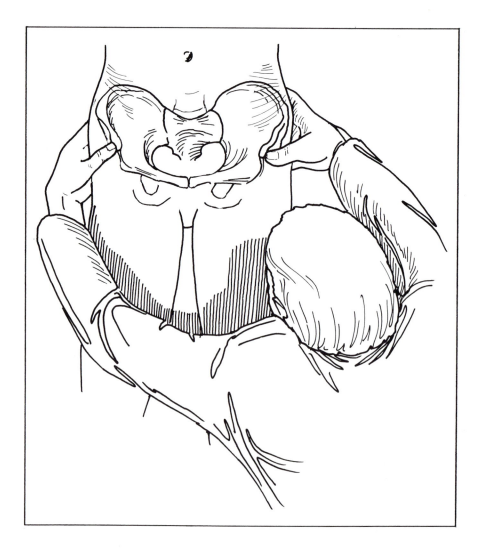

Figure 14–45. Pelvic rock test.

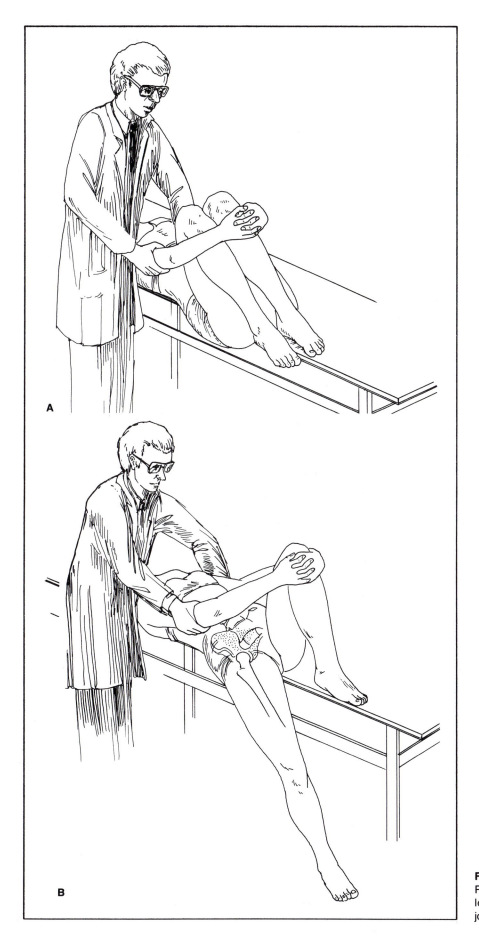

Figure 14–46. Gaenslen's test. **A.** Patient on edge of bed. **B.** Leg allowed to drop causing sacroiliac joint pain. (See text for discussion.)

195

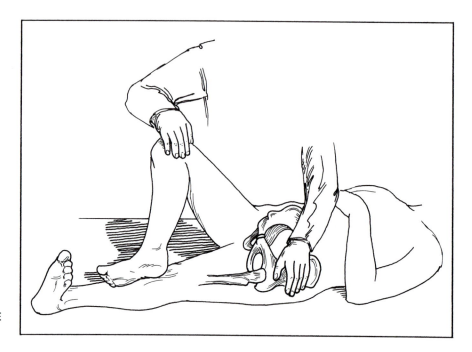

Figure 14–47. The FABERE (Patrick) test.

contralateral iliac wing and gently but firmly extends the hip by pushing downward on the knee. Pathology in the hip or ipsilateral SI joint will cause pain and indicates a positive test.

Tests for Femoral Nerve and Root Pathology

Femoral Stretch Test. With the patient prone, the examiner stabilizes the pelvis with one hand and extends the hip 10 to 20 degrees with the other by grasping the ankle and pulling upward (Fig 14–48). This stretches the femoral nerve.[14] Pain represents a lesion in the L-2 to L-4 region and may radiate in a dermatomal pattern.

Knee Hyperflexion Test. With the patient prone, the knee is fully flexed onto the ipsilateral buttock. Pain in the thigh is thought to represent an L-3 lesion, although the data to support this test are minimal (Fig 14–49).[15]

Tests for Innervation of the Abdominal Musculature

Beevor's Sign. The supine patient is instructed to lift the head and upper back off the table as if starting a sit-up. This requires contraction of the abdominal muscles. Because these muscles are segmentally innervated (T-7 to L-1), cord or root lesions will lead to weakness in specific areas. If the muscles are weakened or atrophic on one side, this maneuver causes the umbilicus to move toward the normal side, as this contraction is unopposed (Fig 14–50).

Miscellaneous Tests

Soto-Hall Test. With the patient supine, the examiner places one hand on the clavicles and the other behind the head. While stabilizing the chest by pressing firmly on the clavicles, the neck is passively flexed (Fig 14–

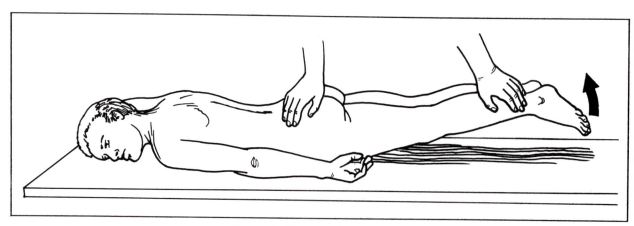

Figure 14–48. Femoral stretch test.

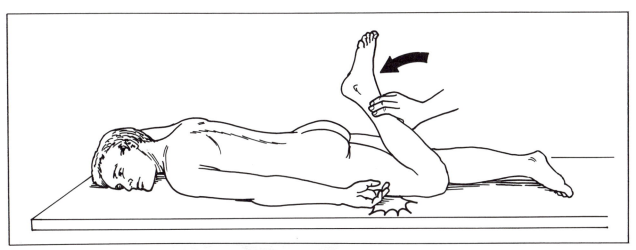

Figure 14–49. The knee hyperflexion test.

51). This stresses the supraspinous and interspinous ligaments in the cervical and thoracic region and results in localized pain if any of these are sprained. Obviously, this test should be done gently and only in patients who have had unstable injuries ruled out.

Gluteal Skyline Test. The patient lies prone with the arms at the sides and the head straight, resting the forehead on a pillow. The buttocks are then exposed and are observed from the skyline views both from the head and the foot of the bed. Atrophy of the gluteus maximus will cause flattening of one buttock. The patient is then instructed to contract the gluteal muscles. Flattening or failure to contract one side implies a lesion in the L-5 to S-2 region or in the inferior gluteal nerve.[16]

Trendelenburg Test. The patient is observed in the standing position and is instructed to stand on one foot. If the abductors of the hip (gluteus minimus and medius, tensor fasciae latae muscles) are weak, the opposite side of the pelvis will sag (Fig 14–52). If this occurs, the test is positive and a lesion in the L-4 to S-1 region or the superior gluteal nerve should be suspected.

T-1 Root Stretch Test. The patient abducts the arm to 90 degrees, then flexes the elbow and pronates the hand to bring the hand to rest behind the neck.[17] This stretches the nerve root of T-1 and causes pain in the lower neck, the upper back, or the scapular region if there is root irritation at this level.

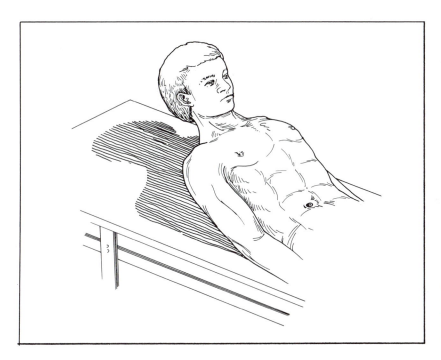

Figure 14–50. With paralysis of one side of the abdominal muscles, the umbilicus moves toward the opposite side when a partial sit-up is performed.

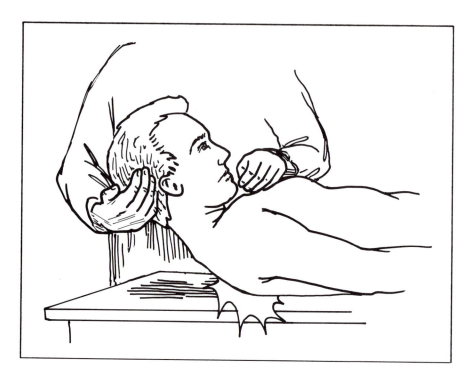

Figure 14–51. The Soto-Hall test.

Scapular Approximation Test. With the examiner standing behind the patient, the shoulders are lifted upward and rotated posteriorly, bringing the scapulae together.[17] A root lesion of T-1 or T-2 will cause pain on the ipsilateral side in the paraspinous or scapular region.

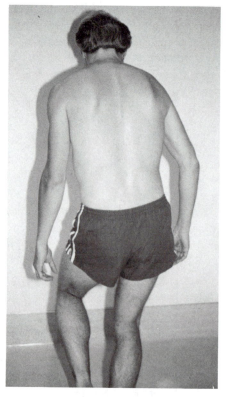

Figure 14–52. The Trendelburg test.

Related Examination

As discussed previously, back complaints may be caused by pathology in many organ systems. In most cases in which a back examination is indicated, an examination of the skin, lungs, chest, cardiovascular system, and abdomen is also necessary. In addition, rectal and pelvic examinations, as well as a thorough hip examination, should be considered in all but the most simple or obvious diagnostic situations.

Patients with back complaints should also be tested for abnormal chest expansion. This is accomplished by placing a tape measure around the chest at the level of the T-4 spinous process. Measurements are taken at maximum expiration and inspiration. The difference in these measurements should be at least 3 cm in adults.[18] Common causes of limited chest expansion include chronic obstructive pulmonary disease, ankylosing spondylitis, scoliosis, and kyphosis. It should be noted, however, that this is a late finding in these illnesses and is associated with advanced disease.

Determining Functional (Nonorganic) Pain

Patients frequently present to the emergency department with back pain that seems to have no organic basis. They may appear to be magnifying their symptoms if not frankly malingering (or drug-seeking). Although it can be very difficult to determine which patients have "true" pathology, a thorough examination coupled with a knowledge of several special maneuvers can be very helpful.

Many aspects of the history and physical examination that have been discussed in this chapter may lead the physician to suspect a functional component to a patient's complaint. A reaction may seem greatly exaggerated, manifesting as loud crying during only minimal bodily manipulation or the patient may collapse to the floor after walking into the emergency department under his or her own power. The physician may notice that the patient rests comfortably while left alone, only to complain bitterly of pain and writhe about the bed any time the physician passes by the patient's door or enters the room. Nonanatomic complaints such as glove or stocking distribution of paresthesias may also raise one's suspicion of functional pain.

Special Tests

The tests described here are often helpful in guiding one's suspicions that a back complaint is functional. If all of them are negative, an organic problem is probably the cause of the patient's symptoms. On the other hand, if several or most of the tests are positive, the probability that the complaint is functional is markedly increased.[19]

"Sitting" Straight Leg Raising Test. If the SLR test was positive, the patient is instructed to sit on the table "so that the back can be examined." This produces the same tension on the sciatic nerve as the SLR test does unless the patient flexes the knees. If the knees are flexed, the examiner should then "examine the knees" by extending them until the legs are straight. In this case, if the patient has sciatic pathology, he or she will complain of pain and lean backward to relieve the sciatic nerve stretch (Fig 14–53). If the patient is comfortable sitting up with the legs straight, the SLR test should be considered a false-positive test.

Hoover Test. With the patient supine, the examiner places the hands under the patient's heels and asks to lift the "weak" leg by flexing the hip. Normally, this will result in a downward pressure on the hand holding the contralateral heel. If this does not occur, either there is significant bilateral leg weakness or the patient is not really trying to lift the leg (Fig 14–54).[20]

Axial "Compression" Test. With the patient standing, the examiner applies gentle downward pressure to the head simulating pressure on the entire spine. This does not create any axial force on the lumbosacral spine and thus if it precipitates low back pain, the pain is functional (Fig 14–55).

Superficial "Pinch" Test. The examiner lightly pinches the subcutaneous tissue in the area of the back where

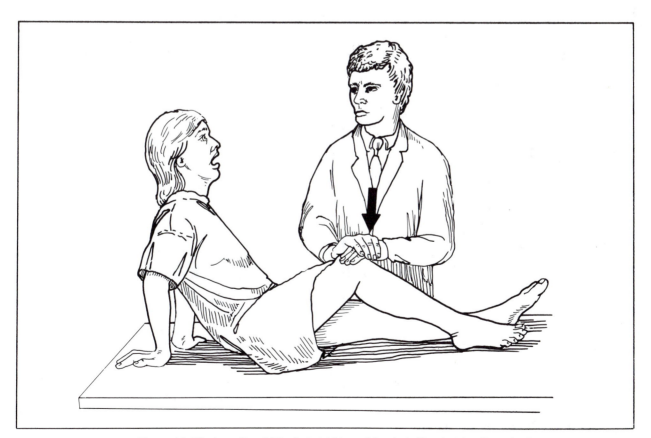

Figure 14–53. A positive "sitting" straight leg raising test. (See text for discussion.)

the patient complains of pain. If this reproduces or exacerbates the patient's pain, it is functional because the spine, the ligaments, and the paraspinous musculature are not perturbed in any way by this test.

Pelvic Rotation Test. With the patient standing, the examiner places the hands on the patient's iliac crests and rotates the pelvis back and forth to either side. This maneuver simulates rotation of the spine while in reality all of the rotation occurs at the hip joints. If severe pain in the thoracic or lumbar spine occurs, it is functional in origin as no significant stress has been placed on the spine or its supporting structures (Fig 14–56).

Toe Walk/Heel Walk. If weakness is found by testing plantar flexion, and/or dorsiflexion of the ankles is suspected to be secondary to lack of effort, gait testing is very useful. If the patient can walk normally on heels and toes, the "weakness" found by formal motor testing is feigned.

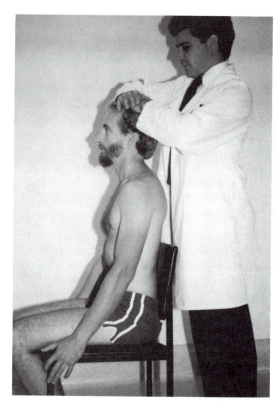

Figure 14–55. The axial "compression" test.

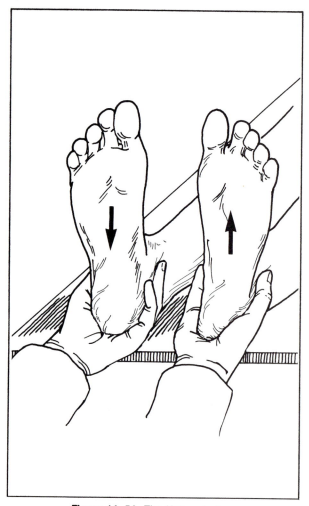

Figure 14–54. The Hoover test.

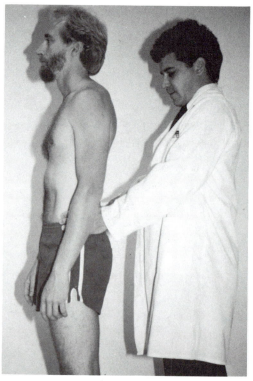

Figure 14–56. Rotation of the entire body through the hip joints should not elicit severe back pain in patients with root irritation as the spine itself is not moved with this maneuver.

□ REFERENCES

1. Moll JMH, Wright V: Normal range of spinal mobility: An objective clinical study. Ann Rheum Dis 30:381, 1971

2. Pennal GF, Conn GS, McDonald G, et al: Motion studies of the lumbar spine. J Bone Joint Surg 54B:442, 1972

3. Newton DRL: Discussion of the clinical and radiological aspects of sacroiliac disease. Proc R Soc Med 50:850, 1957

4. Hoppenfeld S: Physical examination of the spine and extremities. New York, Appleton, Century, Crofts, 1976

5. Fahrni WH: Observations on straight-leg-raising with special reference to nerve root adhesions. Can J Surg 9:44, 1966

6. Scham SM, Taylor TKF: Tension signs in lumbar disc prolapse. Clin Orthop Relat Res 75:195, 1971

7. Cyriax J: Dural pain. Lancet 1:919, 1978

8. Fajersztajn J: Ueber das gekreuzte ischiasphanomenon. Wien Klin Wochenschr 14:41, 1901

9. Hudgins WR: The cross straight leg raising test. N Engl J Med 297:1127, 1977

10. Woodhall B, Hayes GJ: The well-straight-leg-raising test of Fajersztajn in the diagnosis of ruptured intervertebral disc. J Bone Surg 32A:786, 1950

11. Frost JJ: Contributions to the clinical study of sciatica. Neurologic classics. Arch Neurol 21:220, 1969

12. Cram RH: A sign of sciatic nerve root pressure. J Bone Joint Surg 35B:192, 1953

13. Beals RK, Hickman NW: Industrial injuries of the back and extremities. J Bone Joint Surg 54A:1593, 1972

14. Dyck P: The femoral nerve traction test with lumbar disc protrusion. Surg Neurol 6:163, 1976

15. Quinet RJ, Hadler NM: Diagnosis and treatment of backache. Semin Arthritis Rheum 8:261, 1979.

16. Katznelson A, Nerubay J, Level A: Gluteal skyline (G.S. L.): A search for an objective sign in the diagnosis of disc lesions of the lower lumbar spine. Spine 7:74, 1982

17. Cyriax J: Textbook of Orthopaedic Medicine: 1; Diagnosis of soft tissue lesions. London, Bailliere Tindall, 1982

18. Moll JMH, Wright V: An objective clinical study of chest expansion. Ann Rheum Dis 31:1, 1972

19. Waddell G, McCulloch JA, Kummel E, et al: Nonorganic physical signs in low back pain. Spine 5:117, 1980

20. Hoover CF: A new sign for the detection of malingering and functional paralysis of the lower extremities. JAMA 51:746, 1908

15

Radiology

□ INTRODUCTION

The cornerstone of the diagnostic armamentarium available for evaluation of traumatic and nontraumatic disorders of the spine is radiography. Thus, an understanding of the indications for the use of the various radiographic modalities as well as the shortcomings and risks involved in each is essential to their appropriate use as tools to aid in rapid, specific diagnoses.

In the setting of multiple major trauma, spinal injury must be ruled out in all cases. In the vast majority of these situations, radiographs are necessary to accomplish this with a high degree of confidence. In the authors' experience, the thoracic and lumbar regions of the spine are often overlooked in the evaluation of patients with major trauma, and significant delays in the diagnosis of injuries to this region are a frequent occurrence (Fig 15–1). There are three contributing factors that lead to this problem: first, because very large forces are required to cause unstable fractures in this region, these injuries are relatively uncommon. This leads to a low index of suspicion for the injury. Second, physical examination of the back is frequently deferred or overlooked altogether in the setting of major trauma. Finally, although an anteroposterior (AP) supine chest radiograph is essentially always obtained in this setting, the film is often too underpenetrated to evaluate the thoracic spine or, if it is visible, it is ignored.

Axiom: *In the setting of multiple trauma, evaluation of the chest film should always include a careful look at the thoracic spine. If the patient has back pain, always obtain an AP and lateral thoracolumbar spine view before movement.*

□ PLAIN RADIOGRAPHY

Standard radiography is always the first line diagnostic study in the evaluation of spinal trauma (Figs 15–2 and 15–3). In the thoracic and lumbar regions, AP and lateral views can be obtained with relative ease and without risk of spinal displacement if the proper log roll technique is used in obtaining the films. In fact, in many trauma suites, these views can be obtained without any patient manipulation at all.

In the AP view, alignment of the vertebral bodies is carefully assessed as displacement may be subtle even in the setting of very unstable fractures. The height of each vertebral body should be noted. This may be decreased in wedge and burst fractures, although these fractures are usually more obvious in the lateral view. Lateral wedge fractures are easily seen in the AP view. The distance between spinous processes is examined. Widening of this distance implies posterior ligamentous complex rupture, a very unstable situation. In normal conditions, an imaginary line can be drawn through all of the spinous processes. In displaced fractures and dislocations, this line will be disrupted. In addition, injuries with rotational displacement will result in the spinous processes being malaligned in the vertical plane. In the AP view, the pedicles are seen nearly end-on and appear as ovals at the lateral aspects of each vertebral body. Disruption of this normal oval appearance or widening of the distance between the pedicles at a given level implies posterior arch injury (Fig 15–4). The transverse processes should also be evaluated in the AP view. In the thoracic region the

---

Axiom: *On the AP view, widening of the distance between the pedicles at one level implies posterior arch fracture until proven otherwise.*

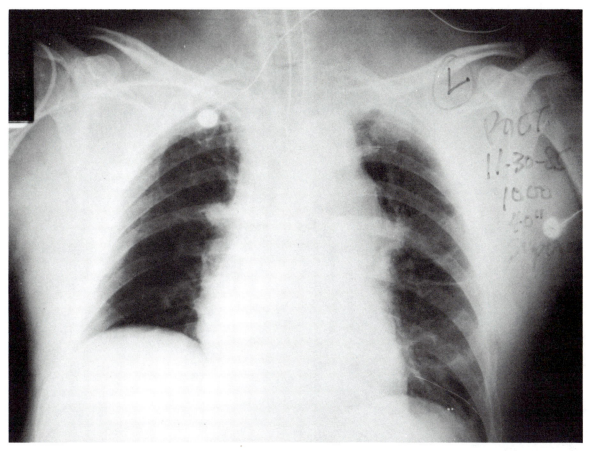

A

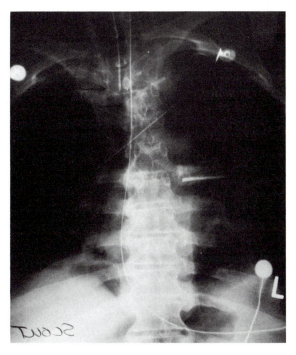

B

Figure 15–1. Thoracic spine fracture with delayed diagnosis. The fracture was not picked up until several hours after the accident. Even then, the diagnosis was made serendipitously during angiographic aortography. Note that the fracture was not evident in the initial chest film.

paraspinous soft tissues and ribs should be noted. Significant injuries may cause bleeding and formation of a hematoma leading to widening or bulging of the paraspinal line (Fig 15–5).

In the lateral view, alignment of the vertebral bodies is examined as well as the spinal curves (kyphosis in the thoracic region, lordosis in the lumbar). The height of the vertebral bodies is once again evaluated in search of wedge or burst fractures. The pedicles, facets, and laminae of each level are examined for injury. Finally, the spinous processes are evaluated for fractures and the interspinous distances are noted once again.

Standard radiographs should never be deleted from the evaluation of thoracic or lumbar spinal injuries as they are by far the best means of identifying the level(s) of damage[1] and thus accurately guide further workup such as tomography or computed tomography (CT).

Only a careful, methodical approach to reading films such as that described above will prevent the misdiagnosis of significant injuries and pathology.

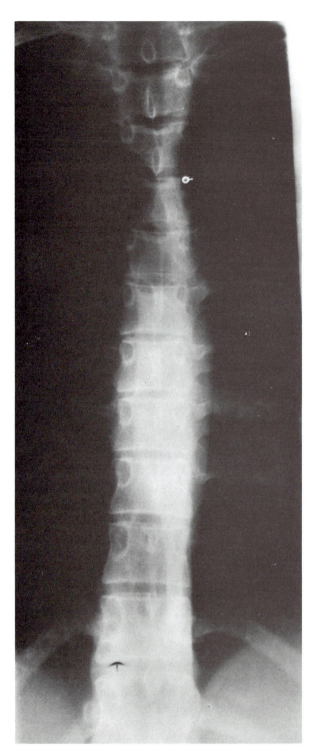

A

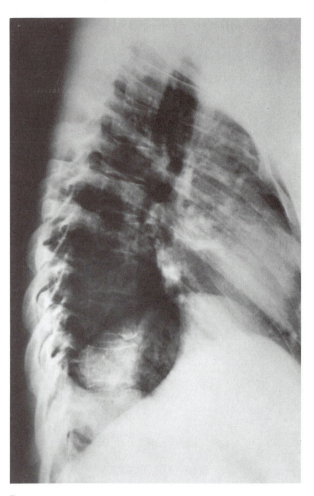

B

Figure 15–2. Normal anteroposterior and lateral thoracic spine x-rays.

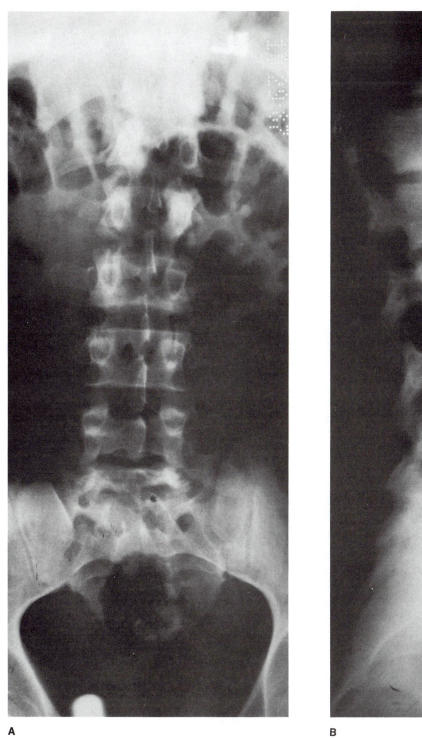
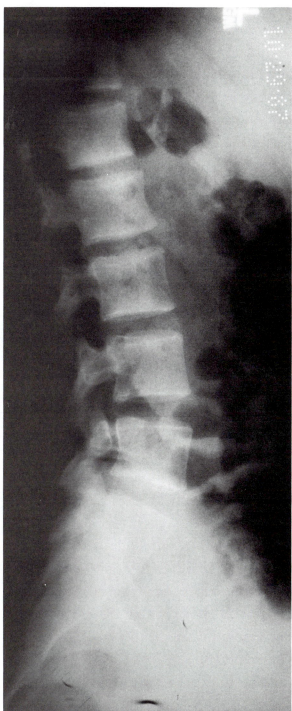

A

B

Figure 15–3. (A) Normal anteroposterior and **(B)** lateral lumbosacral spine x-rays.

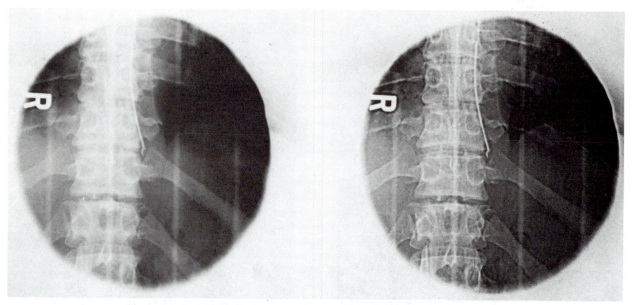

Figure 15–4. Anteroposterior x-ray showing widened interpedicular distance at L-1.

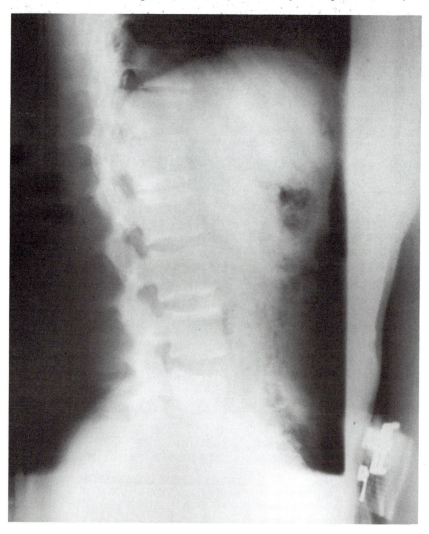

Figure 15–5. Thoracic spine fracture x-ray showing paraspinal hematoma.

□ COMPUTED TOMOGRAPHY

The advent of CT scanning in the evaluation of spinal injuries is unquestionably a major one.[1-6] It is ideal in this setting as it is widely available, can be accomplished without patient manipulation or risk of spinal displacement, and can give valuable information about other potentially injured organ systems. On the other hand, it should by no means be considered a replacement for standard radiography.[1,3] Its use generally requires a significant amount of time and usually necessitates moving the patient out of the emergency department into an environment less conducive to close monitoring and observation. In addition, in the setting of trauma, patients often require sedation or even pharmacologic paralysis to obtain an adequate study. This can lead to significant complications. Despite these disadvantages, CT of the spine can be exceptionally helpful in the diagnosis and the management of spinal injuries.

In recent years it has become apparent that CT is ideal for evaluating injuries to the posterior elements and the integrity of the neural canal. This is an important advance as these same areas have proven difficult to evaluate by standard radiography alone. Fractures of the pedicles, lateral masses, laminae, and facets as well as facet dislocations are seen with excellent detail (Figs 15–6 to 15–8).[1-3] A study by Keene[1] showed standard radiography to be an inadequate assessment in 19% of 27 patients with these injuries. This same investigation found that standard radiography and tomograms underestimated the degree of neural canal impingement by 20% or more in 12 of 22 in which CT was also obtained. CT is particularly helpful in distinguishing between wedge and burst fractures. In burst injuries, retropulsion of bone fragments from the posterior vertebral body tends to occur at the upper aspect of the body, and thus the pedicles may obscure this finding on the lateral radiograph (Fig 15–9).[3] CT nicely details this region and can show loss of integrity of the posterior vertebral body[7] that may otherwise remain undetected (Fig 15–10).[8] Very small bony fragments can be detected in the neural canal.[9] In the setting of penetrating trauma, CT is superior to standard radiographs and tomography for evaluating fractures and metallic fragments in the spinal canal.[5]

As previously noted, CT is inadequate for assessing the level of spinal injury. It also is inadequate for evaluating the amount of anterior compression in wedge fractures. Horizontal fractures and spinal displacement

TABLE 15–1. INJURIES IN WHICH CT PROVIDES IMPORTANT DIAGNOSTIC INFORMATION

Posterior element fractures
Facet dislocations
Bony fragments in neural canal
Penetrating injuries (metallic fragments)
Burst fractures
Concomitant organ damage

may also be missed by this modality, particularly if sagittal and coronal reconstruction are not available.

In summary, CT is a powerful tool when used as an adjunct to standard radiography in spinal trauma. It is the modality of choice for evaluating injuries to the posterior elements, burst fractures, penetrating injuries, and whenever the integrity of the spinal canal is in question.[4-7] It is safe, widely available, and useful for evaluating concomitant injuries to other organ systems (Table 15–1).

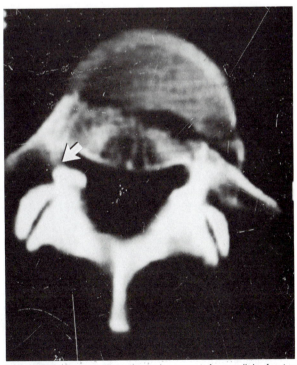

Figure 15–6. Computed tomography scan of a pedicle fracture. The scan shows a disruption in the area where the pedicle attaches to the vertebral body.

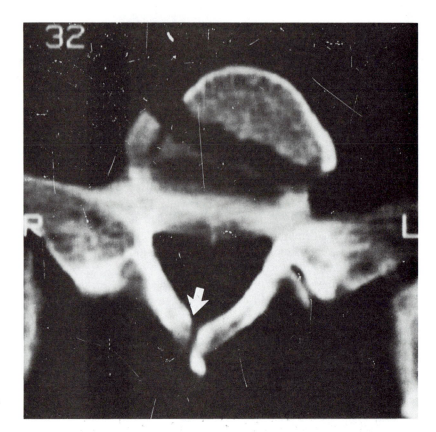

Figure 15–7. Computed tomography scan of a lamina fracture.

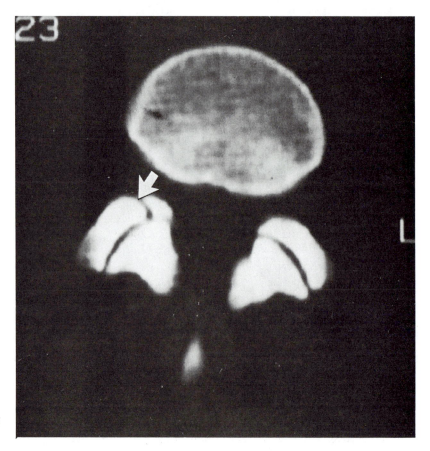

Figure 15–8. Computed tomography scan of a facet fracture.

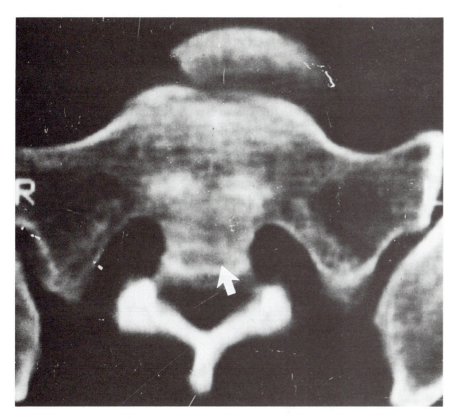

Figure 15–9. Computed tomography scan of a burst fracture showing a retropulsed bone fragment.

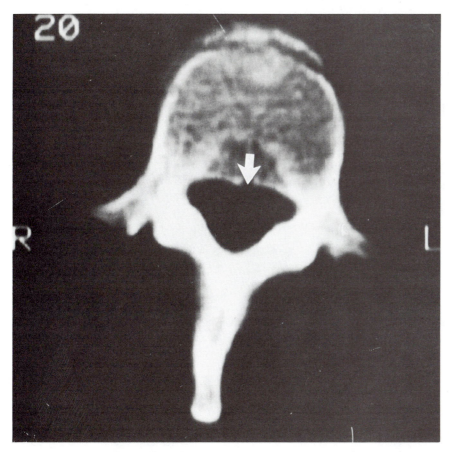

Figure 15–10. Computed tomography scan showing a disruption of the posterior cortex of the vertebral body (middle column) that was not detected on plain radiographs.

□ TOMOGRAPHY

For many years, tomography has been a powerful adjunct to standard radiography for the evaluation of spinal injuries. The neural arch, facets, vertebral bodies, and small fracture fragments are all seen well. CT has several advantages over tomography, however, and when available is considered the modality of choice.[8] Tomography is generally more time-consuming and leads to significantly greater radiation exposure. It is inferior to CT for evaluating the integrity of the neural canal. Most importantly, obtaining lateral tomograms requires the patient to be placed in the lateral decubitus position, thus leading to unnecessary risk for spinal displacement.[1]

Axiom: *In the setting of acute thoracic and lumbar spinal trauma, CT is more accurate at determining neural canal impingement and is faster and safer than conventional tomography.*

□ MYELOGRAPHY

For decades, the use of myelography in the setting of acute spinal trauma has been controversial primarily because the results generally do not significantly affect therapeutic decisions. There are several situations, however, in which intrathecal contrast studies may reveal important information: (1) when the level of neurologic damage is not consistent with the level of skeletal injury; (2) when neurologic abnormalities are present despite normal radiographs and CT; (3) when there is increasing neurologic deficit, and (4) when disruption of the dura is suspected. CT myelography is superior to conventional myelography and is the procedure of choice when it is available.[2,7]

□ PITFALLS

Under the best of circumstances, the radiographic evaluation of the thoracic spine is difficult. Interpretation of the lateral view is particularly difficult due to the overlying rib cage and shoulders. As discussed earlier, failure to diagnose significant spinal injuries in both the thoracic and lumbar regions is often the result of failure to examine the back and having a low index of suspicion for the injury. The diagnosis of a spinal fracture at one level may create "tunnel vision" and precipitate the failure to diagnose fractures at other levels.[10] The difficulty in evaluating neural arch injuries and protrusion of fracture fragments into the neural canal has already been stressed. Particularly in the setting of major trauma, a cursory analysis of the films for gross

spinal alignment without a careful, methodical reading is fraught with danger. This point is punctuated by the paradoxical fact that the most unstable injuries are also the most likely to be spontaneously reduced when the patient is placed in a supine position.[2,11-15] Finally, it should be reemphasized that CT must never be used alone to evaluate spinal fractures as it is inadequate to determine the level(s) of injury and may altogether miss fractures that are oriented in the horizontal plane.

Axiom: *Very unstable thoracic and lumbar spine injuries may be spontaneously reduced simply by placing the patient in a supine position. This fact mandates a careful evaluation of all films when spinal injury is a possibility.*

□ REFERENCES

1. Keene JS: Radiographic evaluation of thoracolumbar fractures. Clin Orthop 189:58, 1984
2. Angtuaco EJC, Binet EF: Radiology of thoracic and lumbar fractures. Clin Orthop 189:43, 1984
3. Trafton PG, Boyd CA: Computed tomography of thoracic and lumbar spine injuries. J Trauma 24:506, 1984
4. Suomalainen O, Kettunen K, Saari T: Computed tomography of spinal and pelvic fractures. Ann Chir Gynaecol 72:337, 1983
5. Plumley TF, Kilcoyne RF, Mack LA: Computed tomography in evaluation of gunshot wounds of the spine. J Comp Assist Tomo 7:310, 1983
6. Keene GCR, Hone MR, Sage MR: Atlas fracture: Demonstration using computerized tomography. A case report. J Bone Joint Surg 60A:1106, 1978
7. McAfee PC, Yuan HA, Fredrickson BE, et al: The value of computed tomography in thoracolumbar fractures: The analysis of 100 consecutive cases and a new classification. J Bone Joint Surg 65A:461, 1983
8. Post MJ, Green BA, Quencer RM, et al: The value of computed tomography in spinal trauma. Spine 7:417, 1982
9. Lindahl S, Willen J, Irstam L: Computed tomography of bone fragments in the spinal canal. Spine 8:181, 1983
10. Calenoff L, Chessare JW, Rogers LF, et al: Multiple level spinal injuries: Importance of early recognition. AJR 130:665, 1978
11. Kaufer H, Kling TF: The thoracolumbar spine. In Rockwood CA, Green DP (eds): Fractures in Adults. Philadelphia, JB Lippincott, 1984
12. Kaufer H, Hayes JT: Lumbar fracture–dislocation. A study of 21 cases. J Bone Joint Surg 48A:712, 1966
13. Scher AT: Radiological assessment of thoracolumbar spinal injuries. S Afr Med J 64:384, 1983
14. Holdsworth FW: Fractures, dislocations and fracture–dislocations of the spine. J Bone Joint Surg 45B:6, 1963
15. Holdsworth FW: Fractures, dislocations, and fracture–dislocations of the spine. J Bone Joint Surg 52A:1534, 1970

16

Fractures, Dislocations, and Major Ligamentous Injuries

□ INTRODUCTION AND GENERAL CONCEPTS

Injuries to the back are extremely common and result in a vast number of emergency department visits. Fortunately, only a small percentage of these injuries lead to unstable fractures and neurologic sequelae. Nevertheless, the major thoracolumbar injuries are often devastating and occur most frequently during the prime of life. The economic impact on society and these injured individuals is very high in terms of medical care, lost wages and productivity, and quality of life.

A significant percentage of the serious thoracolumbar injuries occur in the setting of major, multisystem trauma. As discussed in Chapter 15, it is in this particular setting that the diagnosis is often delayed, if not missed altogether, in the emergency department. There are several reasons for this problem. First, more obvious or more immediately life-threatening injuries may result in tunnel vision. Second, the signs and symptoms of spinal injury may be subtle or nonexistent due to unconsciousness, altered mental status, or other sources of pain that distract the patient. Third, although anteroposterior (AP) chest and pelvis x-rays are always obtained in this setting, the spine is often overlooked when these films are read. Fourth, and most important, examination of the back is frequently deferred during trauma evaluation and resuscitation. When these pitfalls are kept in mind, missed fractures are very rare.

□ NEUROLOGIC INJURY

The anatomy of the thoracolumbar spine and spinal cord results in patterns of neurologic damage that vary depending on the level of injury (see Chapter 13 for detailed discussion). In the thoracic region from T-1 to T-10 the stability of the spine is such that great forces are required to cause fracture–dislocations. Thus, when this does occur, it usually results in significant displacement of the adjacent segments. In addition, the spinal canal is very narrow in the T-1 to T-10 region. These two factors explain the high proportion of significant neurologic damage that results from injuries at these levels. One study of 152 patients with upper thoracic spine fractures (T-1 to T-10) and cord damage revealed 82% to have sustained complete cord lesions.[1]

In adults, the spinal cord terminates at the L1-2 interspace. The lumbar and sacral cord segments are located in the conus medullaris between the upper aspect of T-10 and the lower portion of L-1. Below L-1, the lumbar and sacral nerve roots course downward as the cauda equina to exit at their respective intervertebral foramina. Because the loss of several nerve roots in the thoracic region is of little clinical consequence, significant neurologic sequelae that result from injuries above T-10 are due solely to cord damage. On the other hand, injuries below L-1 result in damage to the cauda equina with no cord involvement. Unlike nerve root injuries above T-10, damage to lumbosacral roots may

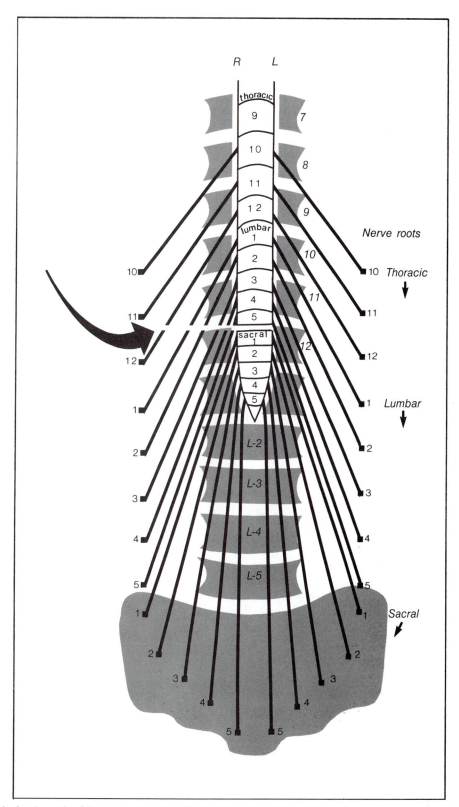

Figure 16–1. A schematic of the anatomic basis of "mixed" injuries in the lumbosacral region. Injury to the 12th thoracic vertebra has transected the cord between the lumbar and the sacral segments; the roots are lost on the right side, "spared" on the left side. Variations of these patterns occur in different patients even with identical bony injuries.

be very deleterious because of their motor innervation. Injuries between T-10 and L-1 may damage the conus, the cauda equina, or both in varying combinations. A given fracture in this region may present with varied neurologic pictures in different patients (Fig 16–1). The difference between cord and root damage is not trivial. The motor roots contain axons of lower motor neurons (i.e., peripheral motor fibers). Thus, motor deficits that result from damage to the cauda equina may improve even if the axons are severed as long as the epineurium remains intact.[2] This explains why injuries to the cauda equina generally have a better prognosis than injuries to the conus or the cord.

☐ STABILITY

The anatomic factors that affect the stability and mobility of the thoracic and lumbar spine are discussed at length in Chapters 13 and 19. In brief, the anatomy of the thoracic spine enhances stability at the expense of mobility, whereas the converse is true in the lumbar spine. The thoracolumbar region represents an area of transition between the two and by virtue of this location is rendered most vulnerable to unstable fractures and fracture–dislocations. This accounts for the disproportionately large number of major injuries that occur in the T-10 to L-1 region.

Our understanding of spinal instability in the setting of traumatic injury was greatly advanced by the work of Holdsworth.[3,4] Since that time the thoracolumbar spine has been conceptually separated into two columns or complexes (Compare Tables 16–1 and 16–2.) for the purpose of predicting the stability or instability of spinal fractures. This theory held that disruption of the posterior column was both necessary and sufficient to render a fracture unstable. Additional evidence has made it clear, however, that posterior column disruption alone is not sufficient to create instability.[5–8] The disruption of the posterior part of the annulus fibrosus is also required to render the spine

TABLE 16–1. ANATOMIC STRUCTURES IN TWO-COLUMN CONCEPT OF SPINAL STABILITY

Anterior Column	Posterior Column
Anterior longitudinal ligament	Supraspinous ligament
Anterior annulus fibrosus	Interspinous ligament
Anterior vertebral body	Facet joint capsule
Posterior longitudinal ligament	Ligamentum flavum
Posterior annulus fibrosus	Neural arch
Posterior vertebral body	

TABLE 16–2. ANATOMIC STRUCTURES IN THREE-COLUMN CONCEPT OF SPINAL STABILITY

Anterior Column	Middle Column	Posterior Column
Anterior longitudinal ligament	Posterior longitudinal ligament	Supraspinous ligament
Anterior annulus fibrosus	Posterior annulus fibrosus	Interspinous ligament
Anterior vertebral body	Posterior vertebral body	Facet joint capsule
		Ligamentum flavum
		Neural arch

acutely unstable. With this information and data from a large series of patients, Denis[9–11] introduced a three-column concept of spinal stability. According to this theory, disruption of both the posterior and middle columns is required to create an unstable spine (Figs 16–2A and 16–2B, Table 16–2).

Instability can be defined in several ways depending on the time frame over which a given injury is to be managed. For example, although several adjacent thoracic wedge fractures create almost no risk for acute cord damage, they may result in a progressive kyphotic deformity that may lead to cord impingement and neurologic sequelae if not properly corrected. For the purpose of this text, however, only injuries that are acutely at risk for greater displacement and/or neurologic injury will be considered unstable.

Axiom: *Both posterior and middle column disruption are required to render a thoracic or lumbar spinal injury acutely unstable.*

☐ CLASSIFICATION AND MECHANISM OF INJURY

Although Holdsworth's classification was a monumental advancement in the understanding of thoracolumbar fractures,[3,4] he did not perceive the importance of the middle column. In addition, the potential for instability of burst fractures was not appreciated, and flexion–distraction injuries were not included. The classification by Denis, based on 412 thoracolumbar injuries, has markedly improved on Holdsworth's. It is descriptive rather than mechanistic and is also quite cumbersome detailing five types of compression fractures and five types of burst fractures. Since the introduction of the

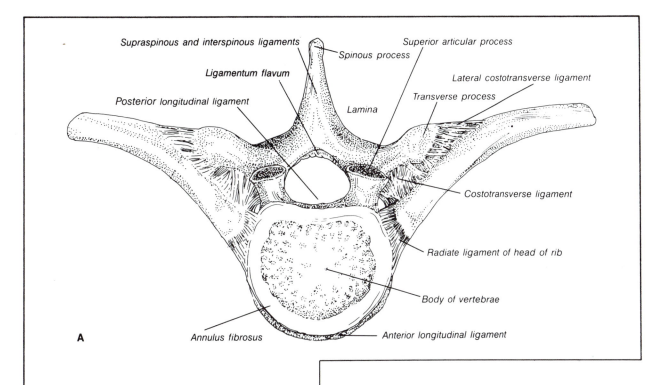

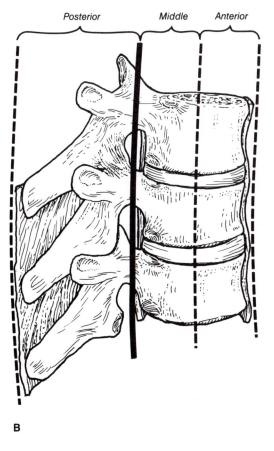

Figure 16–2. A. The important ligaments of the thoracic spine. **B.** The three-column concept used to classify thoracic and lumbar spine fractures.

three-column concept by Denis, several other investigators have also introduced fracture classifications based on this new information.[12,13] McAfee and colleagues[12] created a classification system based on the computed tomographic results of 100 patients with thoracolumbar fractures. They have emphasized the importance of the middle column. They describe each injury only in relation to three forces (axial distraction, axial compression, and translation), however, and only as these forces pertain to the middle column. Although this mechanistic classification is internally consistent, it is rather nonintuitive when related to the forces acting on the injured person as a whole. Ferguson and Allen[13] developed a mechanistic classification with considerable merit. We feel, however, that several fractures are misclassified with respect to injury mechanism. In emergency medicine, the knowledge of *how* a person was injured is an extremely important aid in rapid patient assessment and helps lead one to a timely diagnosis of specific injuries. In fact, in certain circumstances this single piece of information is the only initial clue as to what is going on with a traumatized patient. Because of this fact and because specific fracture patterns follow intuitively from the mechanisms that produce them, the following classification is based on the various forces that act on the spine to produce osseous and ligamentous injury. Injuries with similar mechanisms and identical implications for stability, management, and referral have been grouped together for simplicity. Injuries with significant differences in stability or management have been separated, however, even if the mechanisms producing them are identical, to punctuate these management differences.

An important distinction of our classification as compared with those mentioned above is that the labels of *stable* or *unstable* in this case hold implications primarily for emergency management. By design we have kept away from issues of surgical management. Consequently, several injury types considered stable from the perspective of the spinal surgeon should be viewed and managed as unstable by the emergency physician. To prevent confusion, these differences will be discussed where they occur.

□ FLEXION

PURE FLEXION

■ Anterior Wedge Fracture   (Fig 16–3)

Pure Flexion

Stable Injury

Mechanism. Some authors maintain that severe flexion injuries may result in disruption of the posterior ligamentous complex,[10,13] but anterior flexion alone cannot accomplish this.[14–16] Rotational forces must be added to disrupt the posterior ligaments.[3,4,17,18] Because only the anterior column has failed, the injury is stable.

Clinical Features. This is the most common fracture in the thoracic and lumbar spine. Pain and tenderness at the site are nearly universally present in conscious patients. It generally results from falls, jumps, or motor vehicle accidents, but also may be caused by grand mal seizures. This fracture is extremely common in osteoporotic patients and may result from such trivial trauma as coughing or sneezing. It occurs most commonly in the midthoracic or upper lumbar region.[10] The anterior column is compressed but the middle column remains intact. Because of this, acute neurologic damage does not occur.[11]

Associated Injuries. Because this injury occurs most frequently in the setting of falls or motor vehicle accidents, it may present as an insignificant finding in the setting of major trauma. On the other hand, in the more typical presentation the fracture is the only injury. Coexistent fractures at other spinal levels are not infrequent.[10] Calcaneal fractures are associated with these injuries when they occur in the setting of vertical plunges.

Radiographs. This fracture is best seen in the lateral view. The vertebral body is compressed anteriorly with the posterior aspect remaining normal. The body thus takes on the form of a wedge (Fig 16–3). A kyphotic deformity may be present especially in the setting of multiple adjacent fractures. The entire posterior cortex of the vertebral body remains intact. This is the key feature that differentiates the injury from a burst fracture. Care must be taken to insure that disruption of the posterior cortex is not missed since significant neurologic sequelae may result in this setting. The posterior elements remain intact. In the AP view this fracture may be difficult to appreciate although an increased interspinous distance will be noted if a kyphotic deformity is present. No subluxation is seen in any view.

The sole use for computed tomography (CT) in this setting is to evaluate the posterior cortex of the vertebral body if standard radiographs do not document that this area is intact.

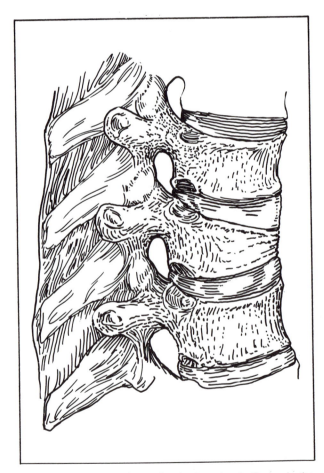

Figure 16–3. An anterior wedge fracture due to flexion in the thoracic region (ribs removed for visualization).

Complications. As previously discussed, acute neurologic injury almost never occurs. In rare instances with multiple wedge fractures at adjacent levels and a resultant severe kyphotic deformity there can be some cord damage.[12,18] Although some authors feel that an increasing kyphotic deformity may present as a delayed complication,[19] it occurs rarely, if at all.[4,12,13]

Ileus is a relatively frequent early complication and may develop up to 24 hours after the injury. As with any disorder requiring lengthy bedrest, pulmonary embolism and other thromboembolic problems may occur.

Emergency Management and Referral. The treatment for this injury is pain relief and bedrest. Because this fracture is stable and without risk for neurologic sequelae, these patients may be discharged unless an ileus is present. If this is the case, they should be admitted. Early mobilization is advisable with ambulation at 2 to 3 weeks and increasing activity as the pain subsides.[3,4,10]

Referral to an orthopedist for follow-up is often appropriate as some professionals feel that increasing deformity may occur in some cases. This also allows for an exercise program to be established and physical therapy as deemed necessary by the follow-up physician. These patients generally do very well with restrictions in physical activity being unusual after 3 to 4 months.

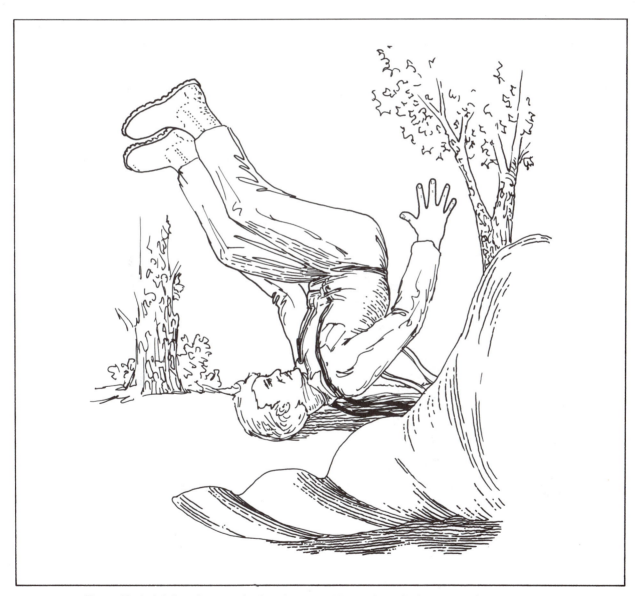

Figure 16–4. A fall on the upper back and one shoulder produces flexion–rotation forces on the spine.

FLEXION WITH ROTATION

- "Slice" Fracture   (Figs 16–5 and 16–6)
- Fracture–Dislocation Through
  Disc   (Fig 16–7)
- Posterior Ligamentous Disruption
  Without Wedge Fracture   (Fig 16–8)
- Posterior Ligamentous Disruption
  With Wedge Fracture   (Fig 16–9)

Flexion With Rotation

Unstable Injury

Mechanism. All of these injuries are very unstable. There is failure of all three complexes rendering the spine extremely vulnerable to further displacement. The slice and disc fractures occur in the setting of relatively more rotation than flexion, whereas the converse is true for the posterior ligamentous disruptions.[3,4] This explains the lack of facet fractures in the latter case.[4,18] Although pure dislocations are not uncommon in the cervical spine, due to the orientation of the facet joints these injuries are quite uncommon in the lumbar region and indeed rare in the thoracic spine.[3,4,21] The slice fracture thus accounts for the vast majority of flexion–rotation injuries in the thoracic and lumbar spine. Ferguson and Allen[13] classified the posterior ligamentous disruption with anterior wedging as being caused by compressive flexion. As previously discussed, this cannot be the case because flexion alone is not adequate to result in posterior ligamentous failure. Rotational forces must also be present.[3,4,14–18]

Clinical Features. These fractures account for only about 10% of all thoracic and lumbar fractures.[10,14,22] They are most frequently seen in the setting of major falls or motor vehicle accidents. A fall ending with a "tuck-and-roll" landing is a classic mechanism that creates flexion–rotation forces on the thoracolumbar spine (Fig 16–4). The majority of these injuries occur at the level of the thoracolumbar junction (T-10 to L-2),[10,14,19] but a significant percentage are also found in

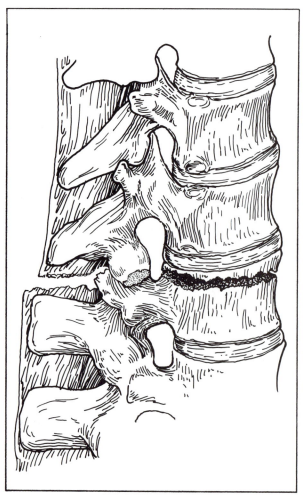

Figure 16–5. A "slice" fracture shown from the lateral view.

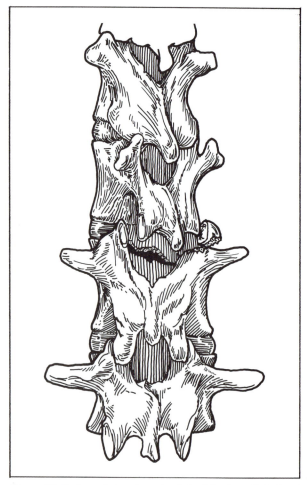

Figure 16–6. A posterior view of a "slice" fracture. Note facet dislocation on the left and facet fracture on the right.

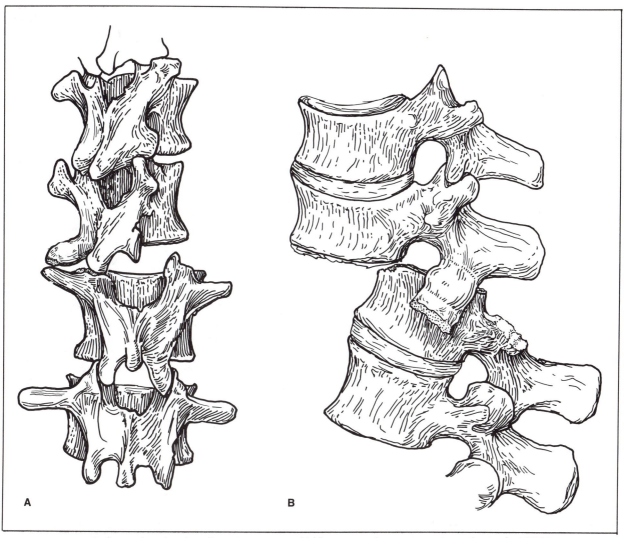

Figure 16–7. A fracture–dislocation through the disc. Note that the only bony disruption is a facet and a small chipped area on the anterosuperior aspect of the lower vertebral body. **A.** Posterior view. **B.** Lateral view.

the midthoracic region.[10,14] Examination reveals tenderness at the fracture site with the spinous process at the lower aspect of the dislocation being prominent. A gibbus will result if a significant kyphotic deformity is present. The distance between the spinous processes at the level of the dislocation will be widened and the spinous processes above the injury level will often be rotated off of the midline.

The majority of patients rendered paraplegic from thoracolumbar spinal trauma have this injury.[3] Sixty to 80% of these injuries result in permanent, major neurologic damage.[10,14,22,23] To make things worse, these patients often have serious trauma to other organ systems as well, further complicating their management and recovery.

Associated Injuries. In patients suffering a tuck-and-roll mechanism there may be a shoulder fracture or

dislocation but otherwise there are no specifically associated injuries. Often, however, the patient will have suffered multisystem trauma and thus can present with a myriad of problems.

Radiographs. The "slice" fracture is the classic thoracolumbar fracture–dislocation described by Holdsworth.[3,4] Generally, it is seen best in the lateral view with the superior segment being anteriorly subluxed on the inferior segment and a bony slice through the upper portion of the vertebral body below (Figs 16–5 and 16–6). Evidence of the posterior ligamentous rupture is seen as a widening between the spinous processes. Fracture of one or both of the superior articular processes of the lower vertebrae is noted. Care must be taken to prevent confusing this fracture with a simple wedge fracture in cases where displacement is minimal. The abnormalities on the AP view may be subtle. Displacement of the fracture is usually noted but may be minimal. The rotational component causes the spinous processes above and below the fracture to be malaligned (Figs 16–5 and 16–6). An increased interspinous space at the level of the injury may again be noted. The articular facet fracture may be appreciated but is often difficult to see in this view. It may be noted on the oblique films but great care must be taken to prevent movement of the spine when obtaining these views. The intervertebral disc is nearly always intact but on rare occasions the slice occurs through the disc rather than the body (Fig 16–7).[10,18] Slight wedging of the anterior aspect of the vertebral body may occur in this case.

This mechanism may also produce a pure dislocation. In this case the posterior ligamentous complex is completely disrupted with an increased interspinous distance and complete dislocation of the facet joints (Fig 16–8A) Radiographic evidence of rotation above the injury is similar to that seen with the slice fracture. Anterior subluxation may also occur with the articular processes of the superior vertebra being located anterior to the facets from the vertebra below (Fig 16–8B). Varying amounts of anterior wedging of the vertebral body below the dislocation may also be noted (Fig 16–9).

CT may be very helpful in evaluating these inju-ries (see Chapter 15). The decrease in the cross-sectional size of the spinal canal as well as cord impingement or disruption may be noted. Rotational malalignment is obvious as are articular process fractures. The vertebral body fracture may be missed as its orientation is very close to the horizontal plane. Myelography or CT myelography may be useful in certain settings (see Chapter 15).[12,20]

Complications. The high percentage of patients with serious neurologic damage has already been discussed and remains the most serious complication in most cases. For those with serious neural damage the long-term outcome is generally quite poor although a few patients with cauda equina injuries may show improvement. Even if no neurologic damage is sustained (20 to 40%), these patients must have surgical stabilization of their spine and subsequent prolonged bedrest. Thus the usual complications found in this setting are apt to occur. If not properly managed, increasing spinal deformity can present as a long-term complication.[24]

Emergency Management and Referral. Patients with these injuries generally have suffered a very significant force of injury. They must be managed from the outset as having sustained multisystem trauma even when this is not apparent. Hypotension may be secondary to spi-

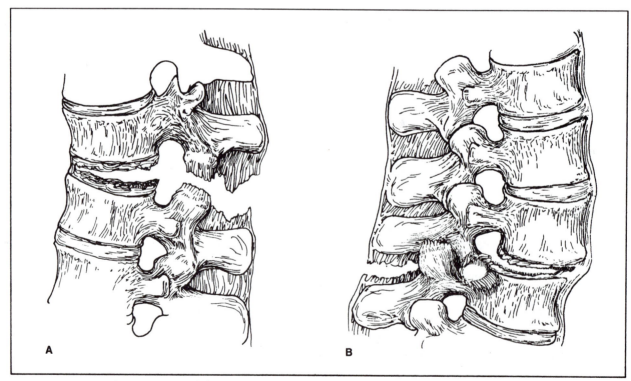

Figure 16–8. A. Ligamentous disruption without a wedge fracture caused by a flexion–rotation mechanism. **B.** Anterior subluxation. Note that the facets have been dislocated with the inferior facet from the upper vertebra lying anterior to the facet from the lower vertebra.

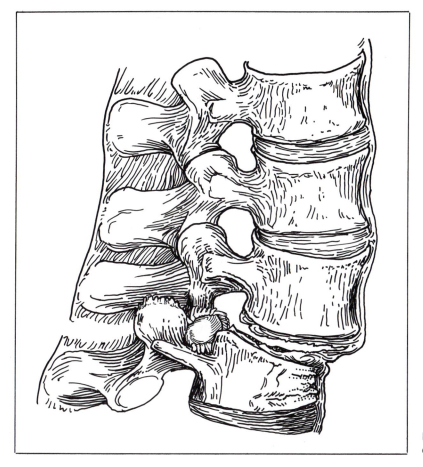

Figure 16–9. Posterior ligamentous disruption with a wedge fracture.

nal shock or hemorrhage, necessitating a careful search for abdominal, chest, and pelvic injuries. With cord damage in the thoracic region, the abdominal examination may be very misleading. Thus abdominal CT or peritoneal lavage must be undertaken to rule out intra-abdominal hemorrhage. Extreme care must be taken when moving these patients due to the inherent instability of the injuries. It must also be remembered that the x-ray findings may be very subtle because virtual re-alignment of the spine may occur when the patient is immobilized in the supine position.[3,4,18]

All of these patients require admission and those with neurologic deficits should have emergent neuro-surgical consultation. If the patient is neurologically intact, consultation with either an orthopedist or a neurosurgeon experienced in the care of spinal trauma is acceptable.

DISTRACTION (TENSION)

■ "Chance" Fracture   (Fig 16–10)
■ Ligamentous Disruption   (Fig 16–11)
■ Ligamentous Disruption With
   Posterior and/or Middle Element
   Fracture   (Fig 16–12)

☐ DISTRACTION (TENSION)

Unstable Injury

Mechanism. Some authors have considered the chance fracture to be stable because the bony parts reapproximate and often heal without surgical stabilization.[2,10,11,17] From the perspective of emergency management, however, in no way should any of the distraction injuries be considered stable. The posterior and middle columns are disrupted and, as such, prevention of displacement and neurologic damage is only insured as long as appropriate spinal immobilization is maintained. These injuries are acutely unstable in flexion.[11]

The pure bony injury was first described by Chance[25] and thus bears his name. All of the distraction injuries occur primarily in the setting of a lap seat belt mechanism.[10,11,12,17,26–28] Some have described it as a flexion–distraction injury.[10,11,26] Although there may be a minor component of flexion, clearly the primary mechanism is distraction.[12,15,17,29] The axis of flexion in this setting is in front of the spine at the point where the belt contacts the anterior aspect of the iliac wings. This point is significantly anterior to the nucleus pulposus, which is the axis in flexion injuries.[12,17,18] Thus, the entire spine is subjected to distraction forces which, if great enough, lead to disruption of the posterior and middle columns. This explains why compression of the anterior column (wedging) is unusual in these injuries.[17] Because there is no significant rotational or translational component to the force, displacement is very unusual.[17] Denis[10,11] attributed four fracture–dislocations with displacement (three with complete cord lesions) to a flexion–distraction mechanism. McAfee and colleagues[12] reported 11 such cases, four of which had suffered serious neurologic damage and also implicated a flexion–distraction mechanism. It is likely, however, that a significant rotational component was present in these cases rather than a pure distraction or flexion–distraction mechanism.[17]

Clinical Features. As discussed, almost all of these injuries occur in victims of automobile or airplane accidents who are wearing lap seat belts at the time of impact. The distraction injuries occur infrequently, accounting for only about 5% of thoracolumbar fractures and ligamentous disruptions.[10,14] The chance fractures and mixed injuries occur with similar frequencies and account for 75 to 90% of distraction injuries. Pure ligamentous disruptions account for the additional 10 to 25%.[10,17] Distraction injuries nearly always occur in the T-11 to L-4 region of the spine.[10,11,14,17,26]

As with most of the other major spinal injuries, multisystem trauma must be assumed during the evaluation. Tenderness at the fracture site is present and an increased interspinous distance may be noted. The majority of patients (80 to 90%) will ultimately develop ecchymosis on the lower abdomen in the area of contact with the belt.[17] Its absence in the emergency department by no means rules out a distraction injury as this sign may require several days to develop.[22] Neurologic damage is very unusual with these injuries, probably occurring in less than 5%.[10-12,17] In fact, all 19 patients with seat belt-type injuries in the series by Denis and all four patients with chance fractures in the report by McAfee and co-workers were neurologically intact.

Associated Injuries. Intra-abdominal injuries are common in this setting.[17,26,30] Intestinal contusions and tears occur most frequently,[26,30] but injuries to the spleen, liver, pancreas, diaphragm, gastrointestinal tract, and vascular structures also occur. Fractures of the iliac wing have also been reported.[30]

Radiographs. The "chance" fracture[25] is an entirely bony injury (Fig 16–10). A horizontal disruption occurs through the spinous process, the laminae, the transverse processes, the pedicles, and the vertebral body. This is seen best in the lateral view. Because the spinous process is split, the distance between the spi-

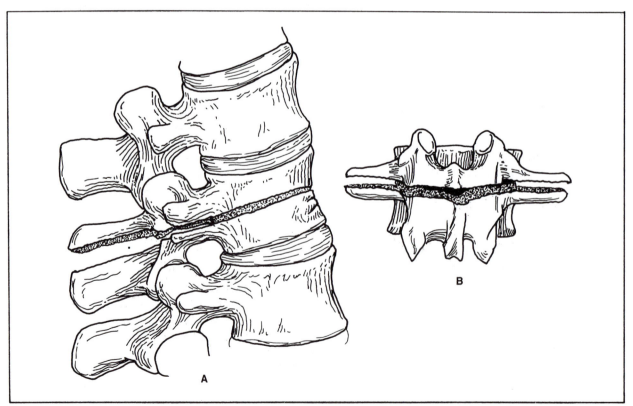

Figure 16–10. A "chance" fracture created by a distraction mechanism. **A.** Lateral view. **B.** Posterior view.

nous processes above and below the injury is widened. The height of the posterior aspect of the vertebral body is increased. Translational displacement in the horizontal plane is very rare[17] and the articular processes and facet joints remain intact. The findings in the AP view may be subtle but often show the split spinous process and pedicles, and again the increased interspinous distance is noted. The transverse process fractures are seen best in this view. In contrast to the chance fracture, there is no bony abnormality involved with the ligamentous disruption injury (Fig 16–11). In this case there is disruption of the posterior ligamentous complex, the facet joints and capsules, the posterior longitudinal ligament, the annulus fibrosis, and the intervertebral disc. An increased interspinous distance is revealed in both the AP and lateral views, and the oblique films often reveal the facet dislocations. In addition, a widening of the posterior aspect of the disc space is usually seen in the lateral projection. Radiographically this injury is similar to the "pure dislocation" of the flexion–rotation type except that no rotational or translational abnormalities are present (see previous section). Various combinations of lamina, pedicle, transverse process, posterior vertebral body, and disc disruptions also occur (Figs 16–12A through 16–12C) and are generally seen best in the lateral and oblique projections.

Computed tomography adds little information in these types of injuries as the disruption is oriented in the horizontal plane. Of all the thoracolumbar fractures, CT is probably the least helpful for these injuries.[10,12] Standard tomograms may yield useful information.[10]

Complications. As discussed, neurologic damage is very unusual. Often the more significant problem is associated abdominal injury. Although most of these patients do not require surgical stabilization of their spinal injury, prolonged bedrest leaves them at risk for a myriad of problems.

Emergency Management and Referral. Management is similar to that for the flexion–rotation injuries, although the problems of cord damage and spinal shock are rare in this instance. Again, one must have a high index of suspicion for the presence of serious intra-abdominal injury. Strict spinal immobilization must be

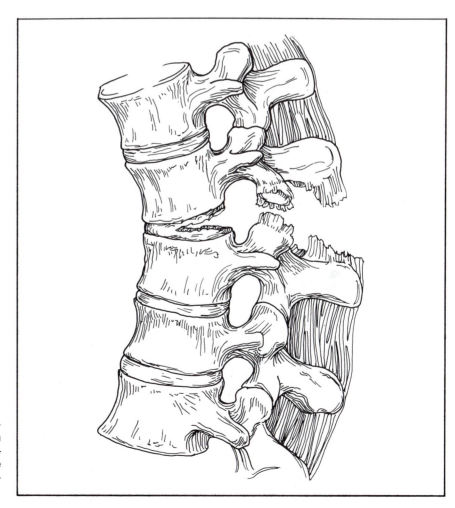

Figure 16–11. Ligamentous disruption. Radiographically this injury can be differentiated from the flexion–rotation dislocation by the absence of rotational and translational malalignment (see Fig 16–8).

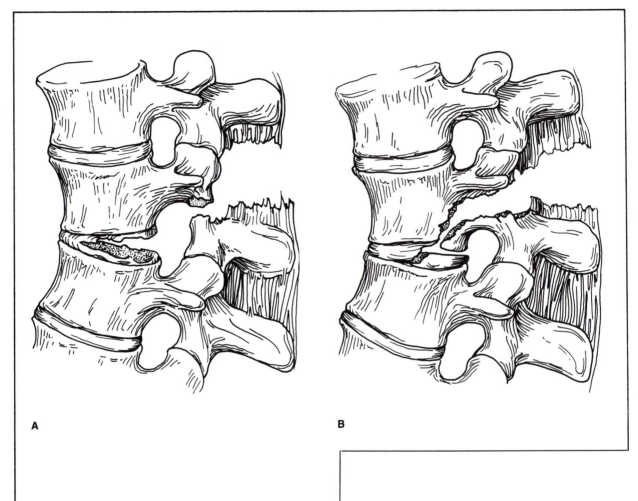

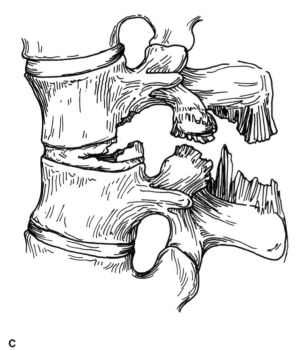

Figure 16–12. A. Ligamentous disruption with a posterior element fracture. **B.** Ligamentous disruption with a posterior and middle element fracture. **C.** Ligamentous disruption with a middle element fracture.

maintained even in patients with chance fractures to ensure alignment. Remember, they may be unstable in flexion.

CT scanning rarely adds significant information.[10,12] If the routine radiographs are not adequate or if further detail of the injury is necessary, standard tomography is probably the procedure of choice.

□ AXIAL LOAD

PURE AXIAL LOAD

■ Burst Fracture Without Posterior
  Element Fracture   (Fig 16–13A,B)
■ Burst Fracture With Posterior
  Element Fracture   (Fig 16–14)

Pure Axial Load

Unstable Injury

Mechanism. Historically, because the posterior ligamentous complex remains intact, these injuries have

been considered stable.[3,4,15] More recently, however, the high incidence of associated neurologic sequelae, posterior element fractures, and propensity for increasing deformity have altered this concept.[12–14,31–33]

At present, some authors feel that burst fractures may be either stable or unstable depending on the extent of bony injury.[12,13,32] McAfee and colleagues[12,32] consider posterior element fractures necessary to render a burst fracture unstable. These injuries are undoubtedly unstable since all three columns have failed. Others, however, consider all burst fractures to be potentially unstable even if the posterior elements remain intact.[14,16,31,38] When the posterior column is intact, there is no risk of displacement as is seen with the fracture–dislocations. There are several reasons, however, why all burst fractures should be considered acutely unstable in the emergency department setting. First, the early management of other significant injuries may preclude a careful evaluation of thoracolumbar fractures beyond insuring gross alignment. Second, as previously discussed, it has become clear that a significant number of posterior element fractures are missed by standard radiography. Thus, until CT is performed it should be assumed that all three columns have been

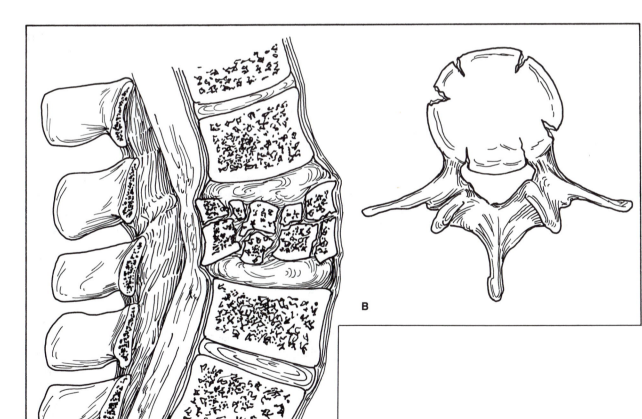

Figure 16–13. Burst fracture without posterior element disruption. Note retropulsion of bone fragments posteriorly into the spinal canal with cord injury. **A.** Lateral view. **B.** Superior view.

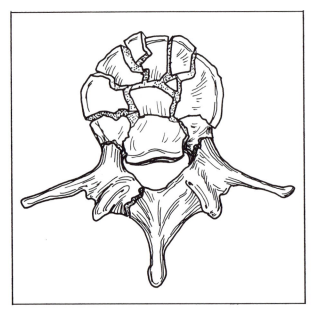

Figure 16–14. Burst fracture with posterior element fracture. Note disruption of both pedicles and one lamina as well as retropulsion of the bony fragment from the posterior aspect of the vertebral body.

disrupted. Third, even those burst fractures considered stable by some authors have a high incidence of neurologic damage. And finally, because the ability of the middle column to bear weight has been disrupted, any axial compressive load may cause the retropulsed bone fragment to move posteriorly toward the cord.[13] Thus, the risk of causing or increasing neurologic injury is significant.[10]

Some authors have considered axial compression and flexion as important forces in producing the majority of burst fractures.[10,11,13] Axial load, however, is the essential component required to disrupt the middle or the middle and posterior columns, whereas flexion plays little or no role in these injuries.[3,4,12,15,31,32]

Clinical Features. As suggested by the injury mechanism, these fractures are most often associated with falls,[14,33] although motor vehicle accidents also account for a significant number.[32] In several series of thoracolumbar fractures the percentage of burst injuries varied widely, representing anywhere from 1.5 to 66%.[12,14,39] Each of these studies, however, reported injuries occurring in selected populations. The 14% reported by Denis[10] is probably an accurate estimate. As discussed previously, burst injuries with and without posterior element fractures occur in similar proportions.[12,14,33] The vast majority of burst fractures occur in the T-12 to L-3 region.[10,14]

As with the other major thoracolumbar injuries, the evaluation and management of these patients must

be guided by the assumption that multiple system injuries are present. Physical examination of the spine reveals tenderness at the fracture level but unlike the fracture–dislocations, signs of rotation, displacement, and increased interspinous distance are not present. Neurologic sequelae are a frequent concomitant of burst injuries. Between 42 and 58% of patients with these fractures sustain some degree of neurologic injury.[10,12,14] The loss of all useful motor function may occur in as many as 36% of patients with these fractures.[10] Not surprisingly, patients with associated posterior element fractures are at higher risk for neurologic damage than those in whom these structures are intact.[12,33]

Associated Injuries. Due to the large forces required to produce these injuries, multiple organ systems may be injured. Pelvic and sacral fractures occur frequently[33] as do head injuries and multiple level spinal fractures.[32] Lower extremity fractures are very common, especially ankle and calcaneal fractures.[33] Retroperitoneal hemorrhage has also been reported in association with these injuries.[32]

Radiographs. With this injury, the entire vertebral body fails in compression resulting in a comminuted fracture. There is loss of height of the body both anteriorly and posteriorly. This results in protrusion of the posterior cortex of the body into the neural canal (Figs 16–13 through 16–15). These abnormalities are best seen in the lateral view, although the decreased vertebral body height is often visible in the AP view as well. The spine remains well aligned in the vertical planes and no increase in interspinous distance occurs.

Only recently has the high incidence of posterior element fractures associated with burst injuries been noted.[10–14,31–34] In fact, this probably occurs in one-half to two-thirds of these injuries.[12,14,33] Essentially any of the posterior elements can be fractured in association with burst fractures (Figs 16–14 and 16–16). Typically, the distance between the pedicles at the fracture level is increased when compared with the levels above and below in the AP view (Fig 16–17).

An important point is that the integrity of the posterior cortex of the vertebral body may be difficult to insure with standard radiographs. This is due in part to the fact that the retropulsed bone often occurs at the level of the pedicles, thus obscuring the abnormality.[14,31] In addition, bony fragments in the neural canal and posterior element fractures may be very difficult to see. For this reason, burst fractures (unstable) may be misdiagnosed as anterior wedge fractures (stable). Thus, great care must be taken to evaluate the posterior aspect of the vertebral body when viewing the lateral radiograph. If reasonable doubt remains after standard films are read, CT should be obtained.

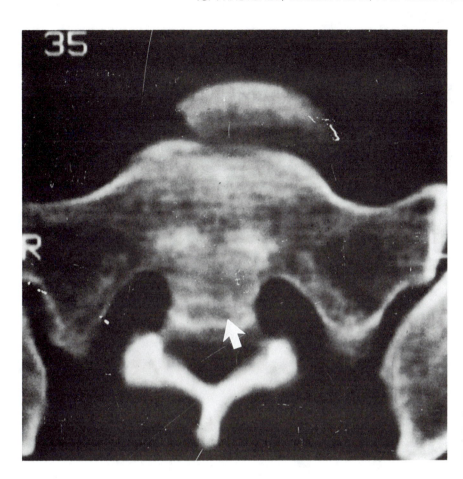

Figure 16–15. Computed tomography scan of a burst fracture with protrusion of the posterior cortex of the body into the neural canal.

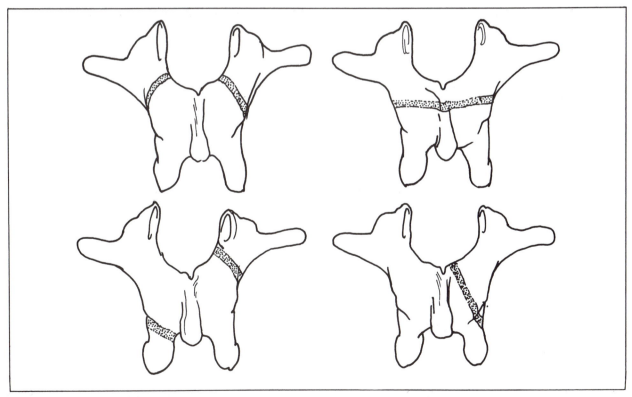

Figure 16–16. Various posterior element fractures associated with burst fractures. Definition and evaluation of these types of injuries are much improved by computed tomography. *From Smith GR, Northrop CH, Loop JW: Radiology 122:657, 1977.* [33]

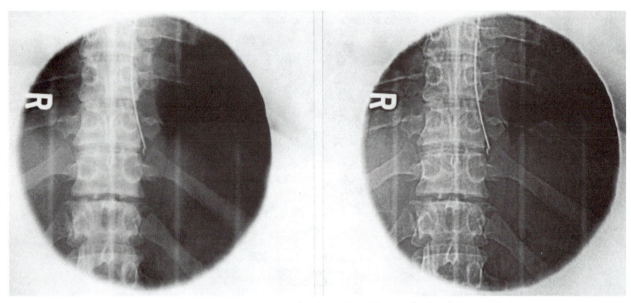

Figure 16–17. Anteroposterior x-ray showing widened interpedicular distance at L-1.

A large number of studies have documented the superb detail obtained by CT in the evaluation of these injuries.[10–12,14,20,31,32,34–37] Disruption and retropulsion of the posterior vertebral body are well seen (Fig 16–15). The degree of neural canal compromise can be assessed by measurement of the midsagittal diameter of the canal. Normally, this measurement should be no less than 14 mm at L-1.[12] A slightly smaller lower limit is seen above this level, and the canal is somewhat larger below. CT nicely details the elements of the neural ring and the facet articulations. Very small bony fragments in the neural canal can also be visualized.[12,37]

Axiom: *The posterior cortex of the vertebral body must always be carefully assessed when evaluating compression injuries. Failure to do so may lead to the misdiagnosis of an unstable burst fracture as a stable wedge fracture.*

Complications. As discussed, neurologic injury occurs frequently although complete paraplegia is significantly less frequent than with the fracture–dislocations.[10,12,14] Of note is that some patients who initially are neurologically intact develop signs of neurologic compromise in the first few days after the injury even with bedrest and appropriate spinal precautions. Trafton and Boyd[14] showed that this occurs primarily in patients in whom the neural canal is seriously compromised by a retropulsed bone fragment. The average decrease in midsagittal diameter of the canal in these patients was 66%, significantly greater than in those who remained neurologically normal.

The long-term neurologic outcome of these pa-

tients is better than for patients with fracture–dislocations. McAfee and colleagues[32] reported 12 patients with burst fractures and neurologic injury who improved after operative management. Interestingly, five patients with conus medullaris lesions recovered fully. Other complications suffered by these patients are similar to those seen with fracture–dislocations including increasing spinal deformity.[31,32,38] Chronic back pain may be severe enough to cause long-term disability and prevents some patients from returning to their previous vocation.[32]

Emergency Management and Referral. The emergency management and referral of these patients is essentially the same as described for those with flexion–rotation injuries. Several specific management issues, however, must be noted: First, as previously discussed, all burst fractures should be considered unstable and managed with strict spinal immobilization. Second, neurologic status should be reevaluated frequently as deterioration often occurs with these injuries. Patients in whom CT shows the midsagittal diameter of the neural canal to be 50% of normal or less appear to have an increased risk for progressive neurologic damage.[14] Third, posterior element fractures occur approximately half of the time with burst injuries and these may be missed by standard radiography. Finally, when evaluating compression injuries, great care must be taken to insure that the posterior aspect of the vertebral body is intact. If good quality radiographs do not accomplish this, a CT should be obtained. If CT is not available, standard tomography is appropriate. When suspicion remains after tomography, the patient may need to be transferred to another facility where CT is available if his or her clinical status does not preclude this.

AXIAL LOAD WITH ROTATION

■ Sagittal Slice Fracture   (Fig 16–18)

Axial Load With Rotation

Unstable Injury

Mechanism. These fractures are extremely unstable injuries because all three columns are disrupted and there is significant translational displacement.

This fracture results from a combination of axial load and rotational forces.[40] Although there are some differences in this fracture and the type D burst fracture described by Denis,[10,11] the mechanism is the same and they may represent the same injury. We have chosen not to categorize this fracture as a burst injury for three reasons: (1) a significant rotational component is required to produce this injury, whereas burst fractures are produced by pure axial load; (2) this injury is a true fracture–dislocation, unlike burst fractures that maintain spinal alignment; and (3) this injury is essentially always associated with a complete cord injury.[40] With burst fractures, on the other hand, about half of the patients are completely intact neurologically.[10,12,14]

Clinical Features. The setting in which this injury occurs is similar to that of burst fractures (falls and motor vehicle accidents). The incidence of this injury is unknown but it is probably rare. The clinical features are essentially the same as with the flexion–rotation slice fracture.

Associated Injuries. Because this injury occurs in the same setting as burst fractures, the associated injuries are similar.

Radiographs. The sagittal slice fracture was first described by Bohlman.[1,40] The vertebral body above the fracture "slices" down and laterally on the body below, resulting in a comminuted fracture and significant lateral displacement. This displacement is obvious in the AP view and without close inspection may be diagnosed as a flexion–rotation slice fracture (Fig 16–18). The transverse process on the side of the displacement may be fractured. Articular process fractures may also be noted. In the lateral view, the vertebral bodies overlap and the comminuted vertebral body fracture is noted. Retropulsion of the posterior aspect of the body is also apparent.[10,11] Various posterior element fractures may also occur.

As expected, CT is very useful in delineating the extent of bony damage as well as impingement on the cord.

Complications, Emergency Management, and Referral. Essentially the same as for flexion–rotation slice fractures.

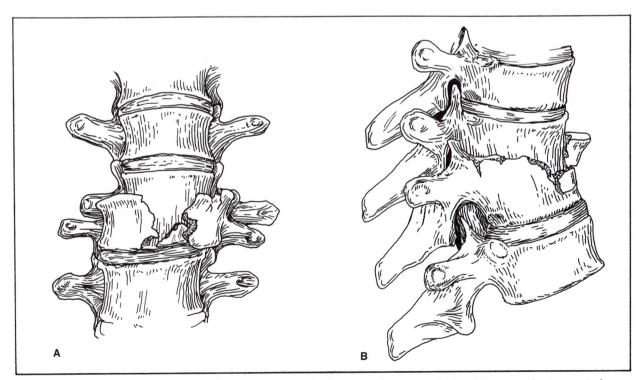

Figure 16–18. Sagittal slice fracture created by an axial load with rotation mechanism. Note the tremendous amount of bony damage in addition to the significant malalignment. This explains the very high incidence of neurologic involvement with these injuries. **A.** Anterior view. **B.** Lateral view.

□ EXTENSION

EXTENSION

■ Extension Injury   (Fig 16–19)

Unstable Injury

Mechanism. This mechanism results in disruption of all three complexes. The anterior and middle columns fail from tension and the posterior column from compression[13]; therefore, this is an unstable injury. Pure extension does not create spinal displacement; this requires shearing forces[12] (see shearing injuries).

Clinical Features. Although extension injuries are relatively common in the cervical region, they are extremely rare in the thoracic and lumbar spine.[3,4,12,13,23] Because these injuries are so unusual, little is known about the general setting in which they occur and whether neurologic compromise is a frequent sequelae. This situation is further complicated by the fact that some authors have misclassified shearing injuries as extension injuries. Neurologic damage is probably unusual.[13]

Associated Injuries. No specific associated injuries are known.

Radiographs (Fig 16–19). This rare injury results in disruption of the anterior longitudinal ligament and the intervertebral disc as well as varying combinations of

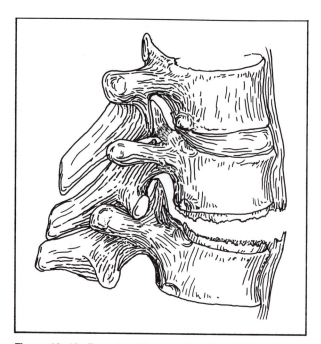

Figure 16–19. Extension injury causing disruption of the anterior longitudinal ligaments and intervertebral disc.

posterior element fractures.[3,13] The injury is difficult to appreciate in the AP view but the lateral film often shows widening of the disc space. Posterior element fractures (laminae, articular processes, pedicles) are also noted in this projection.

As with other posterior element fractures, CT will aid in determining the extent of injury.

Complications. The complications are similar to those of anterior wedge fractures. Although progressive deformity is not thought to occur,[13] acute instability with potential neurologic compromise must be anticipated due to the failure of all three columns.

Emergency Management and Referral. Similar to that for flexion–rotation injuries. As with these injuries, it is thought that spontaneous reduction of the fracture can occur, making the diagnosis difficult by standard radiography.[13]

□ SHEARING

SHEARING

■ Type A Shear Fracture   (Fig 16–21)
■ Type B Shear Fracture   (Fig 16–22)
■ Type B Shear Dislocation   (Fig 16–23)

Unstable Injury

Mechanism. Because all three ligamentous complexes are completely disrupted, these injuries are extremely unstable. The mechanism of injury in these cases is nearly always a massive direct blow to the back.[4,10,13,20,21] Type A injuries generally occur in the thoracic region when the person is struck by a heavy object such as a falling tree.[10] Type B injuries occur in the lumbar region and often result from the victim being struck from behind by a motor vehicle. Falls onto the low back may also cause these injuries (Fig 16–20).[41]

Clinical Features. Fortunately, these injuries are rare. Only 7 of 412 thoracolumbar fractures (1.7%) in the series by Denis were shear injuries.[10] As already discussed, type A injuries occur almost exclusively in the thoracic region and type B injuries in the lumbar spine. Type A injuries probably occur much more frequently than type B. Of seven shear injuries in the series by Denis,[10] only one was a type B injury (1.5% of fracture dislocations). Interestingly, De Oliveira[41] reported ten type B fractures from a series of 195 fracture–dislocations (5%).

Type A injuries generally result in severe neurologic sequelae with complete paraplegia occurring in

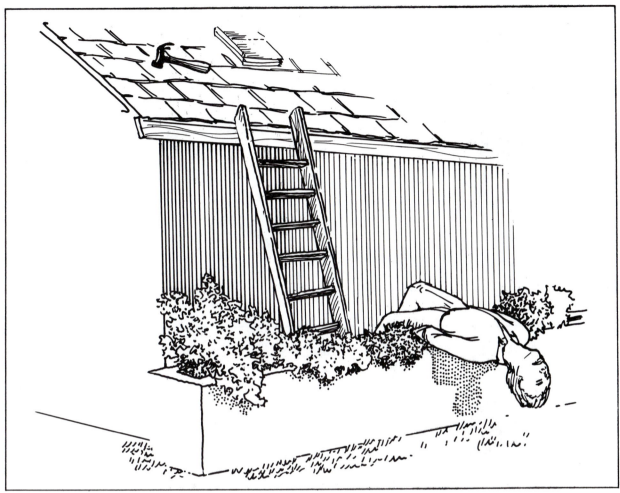

Figure 16–20. Example of a shearing mechanism.

nearly all patients.[4,10,13,15,20] Type B fractures also result in frequent neurologic signs initially, but most patients have complete resolution and seem to be free of long-term neurologic complications.[41]

The clinical presentation is similar to that of flexion–rotation injuries. One unique aspect is that all patients with type B fractures in the lumbar region present with a large contusion in the lumbosacral area due to the direct blow.[41]

Radiographs. The radiographic findings are generally not subtle as there is significant spinal displacement with these injuries. All of these injuries are easily seen in the lateral view. Type A fractures result in displacement of the superior vertebral body anteriorly with complete disruption of all three ligamentous complexes (Fig 16–21A). The vertebral bodies remain essentially intact.[4,10] The spinous process of the superior vertebra and the articular processes of the inferior segment are fractured. In addition, various posterior arch fractures may occur (Fig 16–21B).[4,10] Type B fractures were first described by De Oliveira.[41] With these injuries, the

direction of spinal displacement is opposite that of type A injuries. The superior segment is displaced posteriorly with respect to the inferior vertebra (Figs 16–22A and 16–22B). Generally, the displacement is no greater than one-third of the AP measurement of the vertebral body.[41] However, complete ligamentous disruption occurs. The lower portion of the superior vertebral body may be avulsed (Fig 16–22A) and disruption of the facet joint often occurs (Fig 16–22A). At times, the injury will include several levels and may lead to complete disruption of the pedicles from the lower vertebral body (Figs 16–22B and C).[21,41] Type B dislocations lead to complete ligamentous disruption without fracture (Fig 16–23).

CT is useful for giving detailed information on the extent of bony injury. CT myelography may be necessary as dural tears frequently occur with these injuries.[10]

Associated Injuries, Complications, Emergency Management, and Referral. Essentially the same as for flexion–rotation slice fractures.

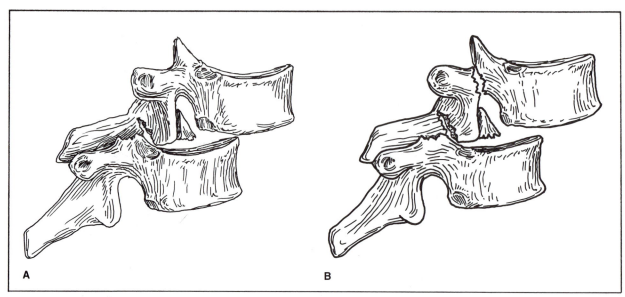

Figure 16–21. A. Type A shear fracture. **B.** Type A shear fracture with pedicle fracture of the upper vertebra.

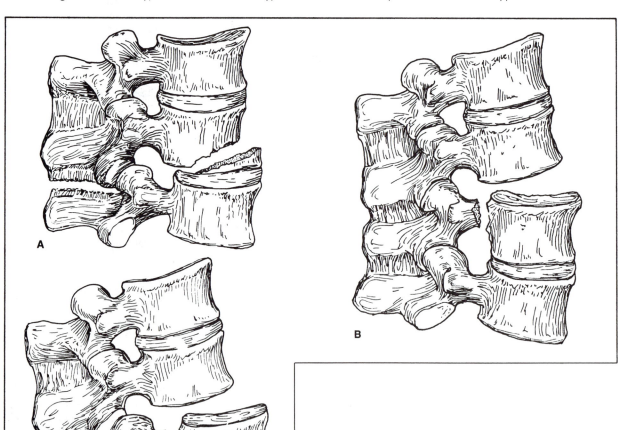

Figure 16–22. A. Type B shear fracture. The lower portion of the superior vertebral body may be avulsed. There can also be disruption of the facet joint. **B.** and **C.** Type B shear fracture. Sometimes injury may involve several levels with disruption of the pedicles from the lower vertebral body.

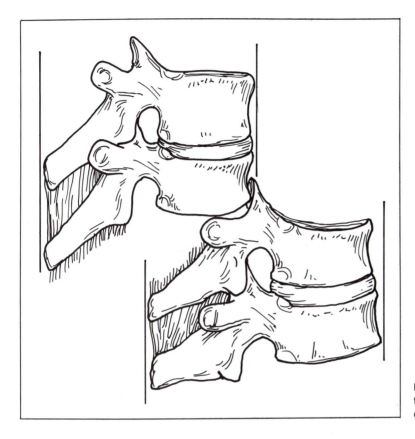

Figure 16–23. Complete ligamentous disruption resulting in type B dislocation.

□ LATERAL BENDING

PURE LATERAL BENDING

■ Lateral Wedge Fracture   (Fig 16–24)

Pure Lateral Bending

Stable Injury

Mechanism. The anterior and middle columns fail unilaterally from compression, but the posterior column is entirely intact; thus, the injury is stable.

This fracture is produced by an excessive lateral flexion force. The vast majority occur in the lumbar region probably because of the stability afforded by the rib cage.[10,33] Only 1 of 16 lateral wedge fractures (6%) in the series by Denis[10] was located in the thoracic region.

Clinical Features. This is an uncommon injury, accounting for only 4% of the 412 thoracolumbar fractures compiled by Denis.[10]

With the exception of location (lumbar rather than thoracic), the clinical features are essentially identical to anterior wedge fractures. As with these fractures, acute neurologic injury does not occur.[10]

Radiographs. The AP film reveals a wedge-shaped fracture of the vertebral body with shortening of the lateral cortex on one side (Fig 16–24B). The lateral view generally appears normal although the body may appear very slightly shortened. The posterior elements and posterior cortex of the vertebral body are intact. No displacement or increase in interspinous distance occurs.

As with anterior wedge fractures, great care must be taken to insure that the posterior cortex of the vertebral body is intact. Failure to do so may result in missing a lateral burst fracture and consequent neurologic injury (Fig 16–25).

On occasion, CT is necessary to confidently rule out a retropulsed bony fragment (burst fracture).

Associated Injuries, Complications, Emergency Management, and Referral. Essentially the same as for anterior wedge fractures. We will reemphasize that before labeling a lateral flexion fracture as a wedge rather than a burst injury, the emergency physician must be assured that the posterior cortex of the vertebral body is intact. (The in-depth discussion of this issue in the section on burst fractures caused by axial load is equally important for lateral flexion injuries.)

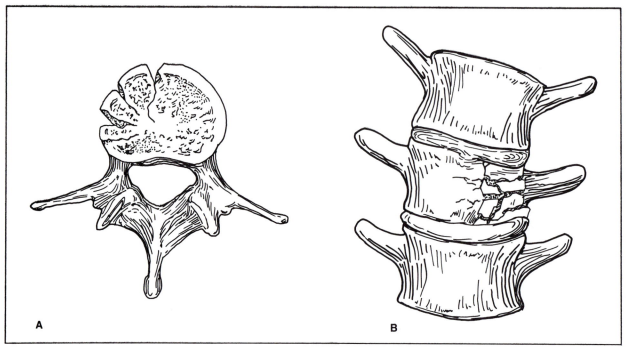

Figure 16–24. Lateral wedge fracture as viewed from above **(A)** and anteriorly **(B)**. Note the shortening of the vertebral body on one side.

LATERAL BENDING WITH AXIAL LOAD

■ Lateral Burst Fracture   (Fig 16–25)

Lateral Bending With Axial Load

Unstable Injury

Mechanism. The discussion of the instability of axial load burst fractures holds equally true for lateral burst fractures.

The mechanism is similar to the one producing burst fractures with the lateral bending component causing the injury to be unilateral in character.[10] As discussed, when the lateral bending forces are severe, there may be tension failure on the side opposite the compression failure.[13]

Clinical Features. These injuries are rare. Only 3 of 412 fractures were lateral burst injuries in the study by Denis. The clinical features are similar to those of burst fractures. Neurologic injury is common.[10,11,13]

Radiographs. The AP film appears very similar to the lateral wedge fracture (Fig 16–24B) with unilateral shortening of the vertebral body. The important differences are noted in the lateral view where a retropulsed fragment of the posterior vertebral body cortex is noted (Figs 16–25A and 16–25B). Unlike burst fractures, the vertebral body height appears essentially normal since approximately one-half of the body remains intact. As with burst fractures, posterior element fractures may be present.[10,13] Ferguson and Allen[13] have reported that tension failure of the posterior elements may occur contralaterally to the vertebral body fracture and may lead to facet dislocation on that side.

CT very nicely details these fractures and may be especially important for revealing retropulsed fragments.

Associated Injuries, Complications, Emergency Management, and Referral. Essentially the same as for burst fractures.

☐ MINOR FRACTURES

Isolated injuries to the transverse processes, spinous processes, articular processes, or pars interarticularis may occur in certain settings. Direct blows cause the majority of these fractures although powerful muscle contractions account for a few. All of these injuries are stable. In the series by Denis,[10] transverse process fractures represented 14% of all injuries with the other three types of minor fractures each accounting for only 1%. The great majority of these injuries occur in the lumbar region.[10] Neurologic complications are very unusual[10,11,13] although associated brachial plexus injury (high thoracic fractures) and lumbosacral plexus injury

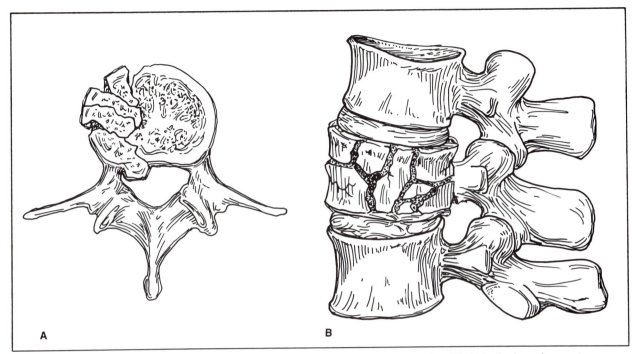

Figure 16–25. Lateral burst fracture as viewed from above **(A)** and in lateral view **(B)**. Note the bony fragment retropulsed into the neural canal on one side.

in combination with pelvic fractures have been reported.[10]

Management includes bedrest, pain relief, and referral to an orthopedist.

□ PENETRATING INJURIES

Stable Injury

Mechanism. In two large series of gunshot wounds to the spine, no cases of instability occurred as a result of the penetrating injury.[44,45] In the study by Stauffer and colleagues,[45] 6 of 185 cases were complicated by late instability. Of note was that all of these patients had undergone laminectomy and no cases of instability occurred in patients treated conservatively.

In the civilian setting, most of these injuries are caused by handguns.[44] Stabbings account for a smaller, but still significant number of cases. Rare causes, such as spearguns and projectile glass fragments, have also been reported.[46–48]

The extent of neurologic damage suffered from low-velocity gunshot wounds (handguns) does not seem to be affected by the caliber of the slug.[45]

Clinical Features. The incidence of penetrating spinal wounds is probably increasing,[45] and it may be a more frequent occurrence than is commonly thought. In fact,

at one institution that cares for a large number of patients with spinal trauma, gunshot wounds are second only to motor vehicle accidents as the cause of cord injuries.[45] Men are at much higher risk for these injuries than women, and at least two-thirds of these victims are between the ages of 15 and 29.[44,45]

There is a high incidence of associated intrathoracic and abdominal injuries that often overshadows the spinal injury early in the course of these patients. In these cases, rapid deterioration from hemorrhagic shock may preclude the careful evaluation of the spinal trauma. Most of the penetrating wounds that lead to neurologic damage occur in the thoracic spine with lumbar and cervical injuries being significantly less common.[44,45] The exact percentage of these injuries resulting in serious neurologic sequelae is not known, but it is indeed very high.[15,44,45] Although rare, major neurologic damage may be the result of a vascular injury rather than direct spinal cord trauma.[49]

Associated Injuries. A large number of associated intrathoracic and intra-abdominal injuries occur. These include pulmonary, bronchial, vascular, esophageal, and cardiac injuries in the thorax. Injury to the diaphragm, small and large intestines, liver, spleen, kidneys, retroperitoneum, and pararenal space also occur.[42,44,45,50] An interesting (and unexplained) association between gunshot wounds to the spinal cord and intracranial subarachnoid hemorrhage has also been reported.[51]

Radiographs. Penetrating injuries to the spine can produce bony injury to any of the spinal structures either alone or essentially in any combination. Determining whether a spinal injury has occurred is generally not difficult; however, evaluating the exact pattern and extent of the bony injury as well as the presence and location of metallic fragments may be very difficult by standard radiography.[42,43] CT is significantly better at making these determinations than either standard radiography or conventional tomography.[42] In addition, CT can provide valuable information regarding associated injuries of other organ systems.[42] Because of this, essentially all patients with penetrating spinal injuries should undergo CT as soon as the acute management of life-threatening injuries has been accomplished.

Myelography has little role in the evaluation of these injuries and may, in fact, cause arachnoiditis in the presence of bloody cerebrospinal fluid.[44]

Complications. Neurologic damage is the most common and most serious complication of these injuries. If complete and immediate loss of neurologic function occurs, recovery is extremely rare.[44,45] Patients with cauda equina lesions fare better and may have significant recovery of function. Rare cases of Brown-Séquard syndrome, caused by stab wounds to the spine, have been reported.[52]

Historically, meningitis was thought to be a frequent sequela.[29] Although this complication certainly does occur,[46,52] it is probably uncommon. Yashon and colleagues[44] reported no central nervous system infections in 65 cases with neurologic injuries even though 31% of them were not treated surgically. All received antibiotics. Stauffer and colleagues[45] reported only four cases of infection among 185 patients with gunshot wounds to the spine. Interestingly, all four cases occurred in patients treated operatively. No infectious complications were reported among the 84 patients managed nonoperatively.

Other relatively uncommon complications include cutaneous or pleural cerebrospinal fluid fistulae, thromboembolism, pneumonia, fecal contamination of the cerebrospinal fluid, and scoliosis.[29,45] Rarely, patients will present with late instability; however, this is probably a complication of surgical management rather than the injury.[45]

Emergency Management and Referral. The management of other life-threatening injuries takes precedence over the evaluation and treatment of the spinal injury. Although these injuries are stable, it is prudent to maintain spinal immobilization until a full evaluation of the spinal injury can be completed. As discussed previously, CT is very useful in this setting and should probably be obtained in all patients with penetrating spinal injury. Standard tetanus prophylaxis is, of course, indicated. Prophylactic antibiotics should be administered in consultation with the admitting physician.[29,44,45]

All of these patients should be admitted. The extent and severity of the patient's injuries will dictate which surgical specialist should have primary responsibility for inpatient care. In general, a trauma surgeon will probably be most appropriate.

□ REFERENCES

1. Bohlman HH: Traumatic fractures of the upper thoracic spine with paralysis. J Bone Joint Surg 56A:1299, 1974
2. Kahn EA: On spinal cord injuries (Editorial). J Bone Joint Surg 41A:6, 1959
3. Holdsworth FW: Fractures, dislocations, and fracture–dislocations of the spine. J Bone Joint Surg 45B:6, 1963
4. Holdsworth FW: Fractures, dislocations, and fracture–dislocations of the spine. J Bone Joint Surg 52A:1534, 1970
5. Bedbrook GM: Stability of spinal fractures and fracture dislocations. Paraplegia 9:23, 1971
6. Stauffer ES, Neil JL: Biomechanical analysis of structural stability of internal fixation in fractures of the thoracolumbar spine. Clin Orthop 112:159, 1975
7. Nagel DA, Koogle TA, Piziali RL, et al: Stability of the upper lumbar spine following progressive disruptions and the application of the individual internal and external fixation devices. J Bone Joint Surg 63A:62, 1981
8. Panjabi MM, Hausfeld JN, White AA: A biomechanical study of the ligamentous stability of the thoracic spine in man. Acta Orthop Scand 52:315, 1981
9. Denis F: Updated classification of thoracolumbar fractures. Orthop Trans 6:8, 1982
10. Denis F: The three-column spine and its significance in the classification of acute thoracolumbar spinal injuries. Spine 8:817, 1983
11. Denis F: Spinal stability as defined by the three-column spine concept in acute spinal trauma. Clin Orthop 189:65, 1984
12. McAfee PC, Yuan HA, Fredrickson BE, et al: The value of computed tomography in thoracolumbar fractures: The analysis of 100 consecutive cases and a new classification. J Bone Joint Surg 65A:461, 1983
13. Ferguson RL, Allen BL: A mechanistic classification of thoracolumbar spine fractures. Clin Orthop 189:77, 1984
14. Trafton PG, Boyd CA: Computed tomography of thoracic and lumbar spine injuries. J Trauma 24:506, 1984
15. Kaufer H, Kling TF: The thoracolumbar spine. In Rockwood CA, Green DP (eds): Fractures in Adults. Philadelphia, JB Lippincott, 1984
16. White AA, Panjabi MM: Clinical biomechanics of the spine. Philadelphia, JB Lippincott, 1978
17. Smith WS, Kaufer H: Patterns and mechanisms of lumbar injuries associated with lap seat belts. J Bone Joint Surg 51A:239, 1969

18. Roaf R: A study of the mechanics of spinal injuries. J Bone Joint Surg 42B:810, 1960
19. Bradford DS: Management of injuries to thoracolumbar spine. In Evarts CM (ed): Surgery of the Musculoskeletal System. New York, Churchill Livingstone, 1983
20. Angtuaco EJC, Binet EF: Radiology of thoracic and lumbar fractures. Clin Orthop 189:43, 1984
21. Connolly JF (ed): Dislocations, fractures, and fracture–dislocations of the thoracic and lumbar spine. In The management of fractures and dislocations: An atlas. Philadelphia, WB Saunders, 1981
22. Kaufer H, Hayes JT: Lumbar fracture–dislocation: A study of 21 cases. J Bone Joint Surg 48A:712, 1966
23. Dorr LD, Harvey JP, Nickel VL: Clinical review of the early stability of spine injuries. Spine 7:545, 1982
24. Campbell J, Bonnet C: Spinal cord injury in children. Clin Orthop 112:114, 1975
25. Chance GQ: Note on a type of flexion fracture of the spine. Br J Radiol 21:452, 1948
26. Rennie W, Mitchell N: Flexion distraction fractures of the thoracolumbar spine. J Bone Joint Surg 55A:386, 1973
27. Fletcher BD, Brogdon BG: Seat belt fractures of the spine and sternum. JAMA 200:167, 1967
28. Howland WJ, Curry JL, Buffington CB: Fulcrum fractures of the lumbar spine. Transverse fracture induced by improperly placed seat belt. JAMA 193:240, 1965
29. Norrell HA: Fractures and dislocations of the spine. In Rothman RH, Simeone FA (eds): The Spine. Philadelphia, WB Saunders, 1975
30. Williams JS, Kirkpatrick JR: The nature of seat belt injuries. J Trauma 11:207, 1971
31. DeWald RL: Burst fractures of the thoracic and lumbar spine. Clin Orthop 189:150, 1984
32. McAfee PC, Yuan HA, Lasda NA: The unstable burst fracture. Spine 7:365, 1982
33. Smith GR, Northrop CH, Loop JW: Jumper's fractures: Patterns of thoracolumbar spine injuries associated with vertical plunges. Radiology 122:657, 1977
34. Suomalainen O, Kettunen K, Saari T: Computed tomography of spinal and pelvic fractures. Ann Chir Gynaecol 72: 337, 1983
35. Keene JS: Radiographic evaluation of thoracolumbar fractures. Clin Orthop 189:58, 1984.
36. Post MJ, Green BA, Quencer RM, et al: The value of computed tomography in spinal trauma. Spine 7:417, 1982
37. Lindahl S, Willen J, Irstam L: Computed tomography of bone fragments in the spinal canal. Spine 8:181, 1983
38. Malcolm BW, Bradford DS, Winter RB, et al: Post-traumatic kyphosis: A review of 48 surgically treated patients. J Bone Joint Surg 63A:891, 1981
39. Frankel HL, Hancock DO, Hyslop G, et al: The value of postural reduction in the initial management of closed injuries of the spine with paraplegia and tetraplegia. Paraplegia 7:179, 1970
40. Bohlman HH, Ducker TB, Lucas JT: Spine and spinal cord injuries. In Rothman RH, Simeone FA (eds): The Spine. Philadelphia, WB Saunders, 1982
41. De Oliveira JC: A new type of fracture–dislocation of thoracolumbar spine. J Bone Joint Surg 60A:481, 1978
42. Plumley TF, Kilcoyne RF, Mack LA: Computed tomography in evaluation of gunshot wounds of the spine. J Comput Assist Tomogr 7:310, 1983
43. Yashon D: Missile injuries of the spinal cord. Proc Veterans Adm Spinal Cord Inj Conf 19:160, 1973
44. Yashon D, Jane JA, White RJ: Prognosis and management of spinal cord and cauda equina bullet injuries in 65 civilians. J Neurosurg 32:163, 1970
45. Stauffer ES, Wood RW, Kelly EG: Gunshot wounds of the spine: The effects of laminectomy. J Bone Joint Surg 61A:389, 1979
46. Tuncbay E, Ovul I, Zileli M: Unusual spinal cord injury by a speargun. Surg Neurol 20:57, 1983
47. Tsu T, Iwasaki Y, Sasaki H, et al: Spinal cord and root injuries due to glass fragments and acupuncture needles. Surg Neurol 23:255, 1985
48. Baghai P, Sheptak PE: Penetrating spinal injury by a glass fragment: Case report and review. Neurosurgery 11:419, 1982
49. Syracuse DC, Seaver PR, Amato JJ: Aortic gunshot injury and paraplegia: Preoperative definition with arteriography and computerized axial tomography. J Trauma 25:271, 1985
50. Stanley WE, Anderson DJ: Successful surgical management of stab injury of the thoracic aorta with penetration of the spinal cord. J Am Osteopath Assoc 81:531, 1982
51. Smialek JE, Chason JL, Kshirsagar V, et al: Secondary intracranial subarachnoid hemorrhage due to spinal missile injury. J Forensic Sci 26:431, 1981
52. Gentleman D, Harrington M: Penetrating injury of the spinal cord. Injury 16:7, 1984

17

Minor Injuries

□ INTRODUCTION

This chapter will discuss the assessment and management of acute strains, sprains, and contusions of the back. The complex issues regarding the syndrome of low back pain and chronic back problems and the myriad of these disorders that can lead to these are reviewed at length in Chapter 19. This discussion is limited to acute minor soft tissue injuries of the thoracic and lumbar region.

□ CONTUSIONS OF THE THORACIC AND LUMBAR REGIONS

Mechanism

Although the true incidence of soft tissue injuries to the back resulting from direct blows is unknown, they are indeed very common and account for a large number of emergency department visits. Contusions of the back occur in nearly any setting but probably most frequently result from occupational and sporting accidents. The muscles and the ligaments of the spine and the paraspinous regions can be injured in various patterns that are not well understood or anatomically defined. Due to the nonspecific nature of the physical examination, it is often impossible to determine whether the signs and symptoms are caused by injury to muscles, ligaments, deep underlying tissues and organs, or a combination of these. Fortunately, as long as associated organ or bony injury is excluded, an exact anatomic definition of the injury is not necessary for effective management.

Clinical Features

These patients present with a history of a blow to the back, usually relatively minor in nature. As with soft tissue contusions in any region of the body, pain and tenderness are the main clinical features. Ecchymosis or soft tissue hematomas may also be noted. If the blow occurred over the spine or the paraspinous tissues, differentiation of bony versus soft tissue tenderness may be difficult by examination. Pain due to contusions in both the thoracic and the lumbar regions is increased with movement of the injured area. Rotation or forward bending exacerbates the pain as does lateral bending, especially in the direction opposite the side of the injury. Contusions in the thoracic region will often have a pleuritic component to the pain. A sensation of shortness of breath may also accompany these injuries even in cases where the possibility of pulmonary injury is excluded.

Diagnosis

The clinical features define the clinical entity and the diagnosis. In some cases there is significant tenderness of the spine that will lead the physician to obtain radiographs, but in this general clinical setting, fractures are very unusual. When fractures do occur they are nearly always isolated and involve a spinous process, a transverse process, or an articular process. Blows that result in unstable fractures (shear injuries) occur nearly exclusively in the setting of massive direct spinal trauma and should be suspected by the impressive mechanism (see Chapter 16).[1-5] On the other hand, the vast majority of direct trauma to the back is minor in nature and does not warrant radiographic evaluation.

Associated Injuries

Although a contusion to the back is itself of little clinical consequence, on occasion there is significant underlying organ damage that must not be missed simply because of the otherwise minor and mundane nature of the injury. Direct blows to the lumbar region may result in renal or other retroperitoneal injuries with possible formation of a retroperitoneal hematoma. Blows to the upper back may lead to rib fractures, hemothorax, pneumothorax, or pulmonary contusion. Fortunately, these serious injuries associated with contusions of the back are quite uncommon.

Complications

Contusions of the thoracic and the lumbar region are seldom accompanied by significant complications. Probably the most serious sequelae of these injuries is their propensity to result in chronic back pain. The incidence of this complication is not known; however (at least in industrial injuries), it is probably significant.

Emergency Management and Referral

The most important aspect of management is determining (by history and physical examination) those patients with a significant risk of an associated organ injury. When the clinical setting leads to concern, appropriate work-up should be undertaken, dictated by the exact location of the blow.

Treatment includes bedrest, pain relief, and ice to the injured region. As symptoms abate, activity can be increased and range-of-motion exercises encouraged. Orthopedic referral is necessary only in those patients who still have significant symptoms after several weeks.

☐ ACUTE STRAINS AND SPRAINS OF THE THORACIC REGION

Mechanism

Surprisingly little is known about strains and sprains occurring in the region of the thoracic spine as evidenced by the paucity of literature on the subject. This is in contradistinction to the voluminous literature that exists on such injuries in the lumbar region. This is probably a result of two primary factors: first, although the true incidence is not known, these injuries occur much less frequently in the thoracic region than in the lumbar. Second, and probably more importantly, they are much less likely to result in chronic pain syndromes and disability than similar injuries in the lumbar region.

The majority of acute sprains and strains occurring in the thoracic region result from lifting a heavy object while bending over. The mechanism is similar to the one that causes acute lumbar strain. Why this mechanism leads to thoracic rather than lumbar strain in a few patients is not well understood. Other mechanisms resulting in this injury include motor vehicle accidents, sporting injuries, rapid bending or twisting of the torso, or carrying a heavy object with the hands held overhead.

Clinical Features

The primary complaint is pain although various other symptoms such as stiffness, tightness, or a "pulling"

sensation may be experienced by the patient. In some patients there is a pleuritic component to the pain, especially with coughing. In general, the onset of symptoms occurs immediately after the precipitating event. In the authors' experience, however, there is often a delay of hours or even days before the symptoms appear.

Examination reveals tenderness and spasm of the paraspinous muscles in the region of the injury. Sprains of the supraspinous, interspinous, intertransverse, and radiate ligaments will lead to the additional finding of spinous tenderness (see Chapter 13). Decreased mobility and pain with motion are also typical findings, especially with lateral bending away from the side of the injury. On inspection of the unclad patient, the shoulder on the side of the injury is often lower than the other and a mild scoliosis (concave toward the injury) may be noted due to paraspinous muscle spasm.

Diagnosis

As with contusions in this region, the diagnosis is defined by the injury mechanism and clinical features as discussed previously. Radiographs are rarely indicated unless a significant underlying structural problem, such as scoliosis, spinal tumor, infection, or severe osteoporosis, is suspected.

Associated Injuries

Associated injuries are rare but include thoracic wedge fractures in osteoporotic patients. One of the authors has also seen a case of spontaneous pneumothorax presenting primarily with the features of thoracic strain. Presumably a Valsalva maneuver occurring during the lift was the precipitating cause. The patient did not complain of shortness of breath or chest pain and had an entirely normal lung examination. The patient, however, had a respiratory rate of 24 even when resting quietly. This prompted the physician to obtain a chest x-ray, which led to the diagnosis. (Once again the importance of paying attention to vital signs regardless of patient complaint is highlighted.)

Complications

Complications rarely occur but there are a few patients who will suffer chronic pain and disability. Fortunately, the vast majority of patients have a rapid and complete recovery.

Emergency Management and Referral

Therapy is the same as for contusion of the thoracic region.

□ ACUTE STRAINS AND SPRAINS OF THE LUMBAR AND LUMBOSACRAL REGION

Mechanism

Strains and sprains of the low back are encountered very commonly in emergency medicine. The exact incidence is not known; however, the problem is widespread and the cost to society and industry in terms of medical bills and disability is truly massive. These injuries occur most frequently between the ages of 25 and 50. Men suffer this injury approximately twice as often as women,[6] primarily because of the preponderance of men in the physically strenuous labor force.

Our understanding of the exact anatomic and pathologic mechanisms involved in these injuries is still relatively primitive. This is complicated by the fact that there is no "test" that confirms or rules out the diagnosis.[7,8] Furthermore, there is great opportunity for secondary gain on the part of the patient with low back strain (i.e., monetary compensation for disability). Thus, response to treatment is not solely dependent on resolution of the pathology but on a multitude of other variables.

The lumbar and lumbosacral regions of the back are "anatomic set-ups" for straining injuries. The low back must accommodate large axial, rotatory, shear, and bending forces. The lumbosacral region endures particularly great forces due to its location at the junction of the relatively mobile lumbar spine and the sacrum, which is essentially fixed. The exact structures involved in a given injury are often difficult to delineate but may include the erector spinae, interspinales and paraspinous muscles, and the ligamentum flavum, supraspinous, interspinous, and intertransverse ligaments. The facet capsules may also be torn and lead to small facet subluxations that are too subtle for radiographic identification.

These injuries are created by forceful muscle contractions and most commonly occur while lifting from a bent position (Fig 17–1). Other mechanisms include violent sneezing, a sudden twisting motion, attempting to prevent a heavy object from falling, or attempting to regain balance after a sudden, unexpected body movement. In many of these cases the musculature is "caught off guard" and thus the entire force is sustained by the ligamentous structures of the low back.

Although these injuries may occur in anyone, there

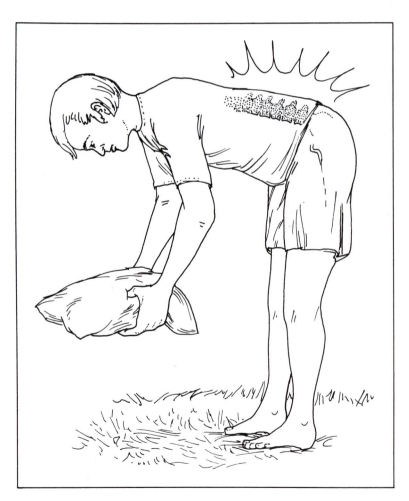

Figure 17–1. Improper lifting technique.

are several predisposing circumstances that place certain persons at particular risk. Any factor that increases the lumbar lordosis will magnify the stresses that must be endured by this region of the spine. These include obesity, pregnancy, poor abdominal muscle tone, and wearing high heels (Fig 17–2). Other predisposing factors are repetitive lifting from a bent position, increasing age, degenerative spondylosis, and an extra lumbar vertebra (Table 17–1).

Clinical Features

Pain at the site of injury is the chief complaint with various accompanying symptoms such as stiffness, increasing pain with movement, and radiation. Coughing

TABLE 17–1. PREDISPOSING FACTORS FOR ACUTE STRAINS AND SPRAINS OF THE LOW BACK

Obesity
Pregnancy
Poor abdominal muscle tone
High heels
Thoracic kyphosis with secondary increase in lumbar lordosis
Any factor causing increased lumbar lordosis
Repetitive, heavy lifting (often occupational)
Increasing age with degenerative spondylosis
Extra lumbar vertebra

and sneezing may also exacerbate the pain. Generally, the symptoms begin at the time of the injury but there may be a delay in onset. The pain is continuous and only partially relieved by rest. The radiation in this setting is generally not dermatomal but diffuse and "deep" in character. It may spread to the gluteal region and to the posterior aspect of the thigh either unilaterally or bilaterally. Apparently radiation to the lower legs or feet is unusual.[9] The etiology of the radiating pain is unclear in the setting of muscular and ligamentous injuries. It is probably different than the direct nerve root irritation that occurs in the setting of disc herniation or narrowed intervertebral foramina.

Examination reveals significant tenderness that may be diffuse or localized. If it is diffuse, there is generally a fairly discrete area of maximum tenderness. The tenderness may be spinous, paraspinous, or both. Paraspinous muscle spasm is frequently noted and when it is unilateral, a lumbar scoliosis may be present. As with this finding in the thoracic region, the curve is concave toward the side of injury (Fig 17–3). Motion in all directions is limited but extension and lateral bending away from the side of injury are particularly restricted. If the spasm is severe, any body movement may cause pain, and motion of the legs or straight leg raising may cause great distress. In most cases, however, these maneuvers are tolerated without complaint.

Examination of gait is usually normal but may reveal a limp due to pain or unilateral hamstring spasm. In severe cases, ambulation is essentially impossible due to the pain. Reflex and sensory examination are normal as is the motor examination. Pain, however, may limit a patient's ability to perform certain aspects of the motor examination.

Diagnosis

The diagnosis of acute low back strain is relatively easy in the typical case. The clinical features discussed above are present to varying degrees in different patients, but nonetheless the diagnosis is generally simple in the right setting. The syndrome of low back pain, however, has many causes, and if anything in a pa-

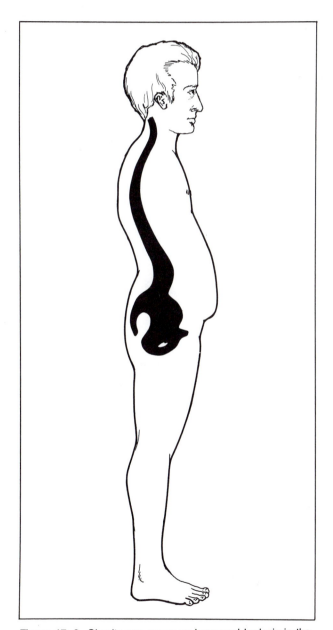

Figure 17–2. Obesity can cause an increased lordosis in the lower lumbar spine and excessive back strain.

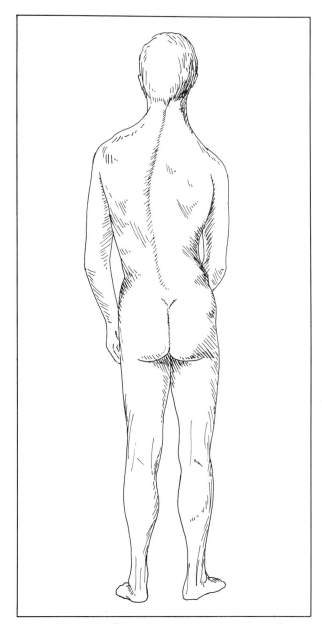

Figure 17–3. When injury to the back occurs, the spine may develop a lateral curve due to paraspinous muscle spasm with the concave side toward the injury.

gion.[8,10,12,16,17,19] In addition, radiation exposure to the gonads is by no means trivial.[8,11,15,19] Another problem is the tendency to seize on any abnormal finding as the cause of the patient's symptoms. In fact, many spinal abnormalities have been shown to be present with similar or equal frequencies in symptomatic and asymptomatic persons.[8,13,18,20]

In a study by Scavone and colleagues[10] lumbosacral spine films were obtained in 212 cases of minor trauma. Only seven patients (3.3%) had acute fractures and all of these occurred in women 70 years old or older and had stable compression fractures. Only one of these seven patients presented without significant, localized spinous tenderness. Thus, in patients with a history and physical examination typical of low back strain, a reasonable approach is to withhold radiographs unless one or more of the following circumstances apply: (1) marked spinal tenderness, (2) neurologic findings, (3) women over age 50, (4) significant likelihood of underlying pathology (tumor, infection, osteoporosis, patient's taking steroids, etc), and (5) other atypical or compelling reasons (Table 17–2). This approach is very unlikely to miss significant spinal pathology. Furthermore, if abnormalities are missed, it is unlikely that "picking them up" at the time of first presentation would alter management. Although rarely this approach may miss an acute fracture, it is exceedingly unlikely to be unstable. Medicolegal risk can be significantly lessened by discussing this small possibility with the patient and instructing him or her to return if symptoms worsen or do not improve in a reasonable amount of time.

Complications

The main complication of low back strain is the propensity to result in chronic pain and disability. This can be a tremendous problem and accounts for a large portion of occupational compensation cases. Fortunately, the typical patient experiences significant improvement within weeks[21,22] and 90% of patients have resolution

tient's presentation is unusual or if the minor traumatic event precipitating the pain is vague or atypical, then a differential diagnosis must be formulated (see Chapter 19). Having said this, it remains true that the vast majority of patients presenting with acute minor injuries of the low back present no diagnostic dilemma.

A major diagnostic issue is deciding which patients require radiographic evaluation. A host of literature exists on the use and abuse of lumbosacral radiographs.[8,10–18] The main problem centers around the fact that radiographs seldom alter management or outcome in patients with pain in the lumbar re-

TABLE 17–2. INDICATIONS FOR RADIOGRAPHS IN PATIENTS PRESENTING WITH PROBABLE LOW BACK STRAIN

Marked spinous tenderness

Neurologic findings

Women over age 50

Significant likelihood of underlying disease
 Tumor (primary or metastatic)
 Infection (patients with tuberculosis, drug abusers, etc.)
 Fever
 Osteoporosis
 Patients taking steroids

Atypical presentation or other compelling reasons (i.e., patients unable to ambulate secondary to pain)

within several months.[22,23] Unfortunately, a few patients require prolonged bedrest and thus are subject to thromboembolic complications.

Emergency Management and Referral

As with contusions to the back, treatment consists of bedrest with a firm mattress or bedboard, pain relief, and cold packs to the injured region. Some patients receive significant relief from muscle relaxants. Patients with a reproducible maximum point of muscular tenderness ("trigger point") may respond to injection with a local anesthetic. Within 3 to 7 days, as symptoms improve, activity can be increased and range of motion exercises begun. Local heat will often decrease pain and stiffness at this point.

Patient education regarding weight loss, conditioning, wearing flat rather than high-heeled shoes, avoidance of sleeping in prone position, and avoidance of improper lifting mechanics (Fig 17–1) is an important aspect of the emergency department visit. This is particularly true as this is often the only contact that the patient will have with a physician, and simple education may prevent a future recurrence.

Except in the very rare patient with immediate, severe debilitating pain who may require admission, orthopedic referral is indicated only in those patients who fail to have significant improvement after several weeks. In these patients, physical therapy may also be of benefit and can be directed by the consulting physician.

□ REFERENCES

1. Holdsworth FW: Fractures, dislocations, and fracture–dislocations of the spine. J Bone Joint Surg 52A:1534, 1970

2. Denis F: The three-column spine and its significance in the classification of acute thoracolumbar spinal injuries. Spine 8:817, 1983

3. Ferguson RL, Allen BL: A mechanistic classification of thoracolumbar spine fractures. Clin Orthop 189:77, 1984

4. Angtuaco EJC, Binet EF: Radiology of thoracic and lumbar fractures. Clin Orthop 189:43, 1984

5. Connolly JF (ed): Dislocations, fractures, and fracture–dislocations of the thoracic and lumbar spine. In The Management of Fractures and Dislocations: An Atlas. Philadelphia, WB Saunders, 1981

6. Finneson BE: Lumbosacral strain. In Low Back Pain. Philadelphia, JB Lippincott, 1980

7. Dillane JB, Fry J, Kalton G: Acute back syndrome: A study from general practice. Br Med J 2:82, 1966

8. Kelen GD, Noji EK, Doris PE: Guidelines for use of lumbar spine radiography. Ann Emerg Med 15:245, 1986

9. Brashear HR, Raney RB: Affections of the low back. In Shands' Handbook of Orthopedic Surgery, 9th ed. St. Louis, CV Mosby, 1978

10. Scavone JG, Latshaw RF, Rohrer GV: Use of lumbar spine films: Statistical evaluation at a university teaching hospital. JAMA 246:1105, 1981

11. Patrick JD, Doris PE, Mills ML, et al: Lumbar spine x-rays: A multihospital study. Ann Emerg Med 12:84, 1983

12. Hall FM: Back pain and the radiologist. Radiology 137:861, 1980

13. Torgerson W, Dotter WE: Comparative roentgenographic study of the asymptomatic and symptomatic lumbar spine. J Bone Joint Surg 58A:850, 1976

14. McGura A, Schwartz A: Relation between the low back pain syndrome and x-ray findings. Scand J Rehabil Med 10:135, 1978

15. Kaplan D: Spine problems in emergency department patients: Does every patient need an x-ray? J Emerg Med 2:257, 1985

16. Rockey PH, Tompkins RK, Wood RW, et al: The usefulness of x-ray examinations in the evaluation of patients with back pain. J Fam Pract 7:455, 1978

17. Neidre A: Low back pain—Evaluation and treatment in the emergency department setting. Emerg Med Clin North Am 2:441, 1984

18. Witt I, Vestergaard A, Rosenklint A: A comparative analysis of x-ray findings of the lumbar spine in patients with and without lumbar pain. Spine 9:298, 1984

19. Hall FM: Overutilization of radiological examinations. Radiology 120:443, 1976

20. Fullenlove TM, Williams AJ: Comparative roentgen findings in symptomatic and asymptomatic backs. Radiology 68:572, 1957

21. Kelsey JL, White AA: Epidemiology and impact of low back pain. Spine 5:133, 1980

22. Rissanen PM: The surgical anatomy and pathology of the supraspinous and interspinous ligaments of the lumbar spine with special reference to ligament ruptures. Acta Orthop Scand [Suppl] 46:1, 1960

23. White AWM: Low back pain in men receiving workmen's compensation. Can Med Assoc J 95:50, 1966

18

Scoliosis and Kyphosis

Scoliosis and kyphosis are chronic, nonemergent disorders. An understanding of their clinical presentation, however, remains important to the emergency medicine specialist for three reasons: (1) these deformities may be the sign of serious underlying disease; (2) early diagnosis and referral for proper treatment and follow-up is the key to prevention of significant deformity and disability; and (3) these disorders are common in the general population, thus providing the emergency physician the opportunity to make the diagnosis on a relatively frequent basis.

□ SCOLIOSIS

Incidence

Scoliosis is a common disorder. In a study by Shands and Eisberg[1] of 50,000 chest x-rays obtained in a survey for tuberculosis, the incidence was 1.9%. Routine screening evaluations of schoolchildren have found some degree of scoliosis to be present in 10 to 12% of those aged 10 to 14. The great majority of these curves are less than 20 degrees. Early detection and treatment have decreased the number of adolescents requiring surgical management. Interestingly, the number of adult patients seeking medical attention for scoliosis is increasing despite early detection programs.

Pathophysiology

Scoliosis is a lateral curvature of the spine of 10 or more degrees. There are two types, structural and non-structural. Structural curves are those caused by anatomic abnormalities of the spine or its supporting structures. The affected vertebrae are fixed in a rotated position and side bending demonstrates asymmetry by clinical examination and radiography. Nonstructural scoliosis, on the other hand, is caused by forces extrinsic to the spine such as a shortened extremity. In this case, lateral bending is symmetrical, and correction of

the extrinsic abnormality resolves the spinal curvature.

When spinal curvature is extreme, it may lead to cardiovascular, respiratory, or neurologic sequelae, which may lead to disability and early death.

The causes of scoliosis are legion and a comprehensive discussion of its etiologies is beyond the scope of this text. Some of the more common causes include infection, trauma, extensive burns of the torso, paralysis, cerebral palsy, poliomyelitis, neurofibromatosis, rheumatoid arthritis, congenital causes, and thoracotomy with disruption of the transverse spinous ligaments. The majority of cases, however, are idiopathic (70 to 90%). Three groups of idiopathic scoliosis are recognized according to the age of presentation: infantile, juvenile, and adolescent. Generally, prognosis improves with later onset although even in the infantile group, the majority of cases resolve spontaneously and require no treatment. Infantile scoliosis has its onset at or shortly after birth. The spinal curves are to the left in the thoracic region in most cases. Juvenile idiopathic scoliosis is defined by onset between age three and puberty with progression to a severe deformity in most cases if undetected or left untreated. The adolescent form occurs after the onset of puberty with 90% of patients being girls and the thoracic curve being to the right in 80 to 90% of cases. As implied by the name, the etiology of idiopathic scoliosis is unknown, and the mechanism by which spinal curvature is produced is unclear.

Clinical Features

In the child or adolescent, most cases of scoliosis are asymptomatic. In fact, the child is generally unaware of the presence of the deformity until it is pointed out by someone else, usually a parent. Unfortunately, a significant number of patients have been made aware of the diagnosis by their physician, but are "being followed to see how things go" without a thorough evaluation by a specialist. The past medical history is generally unrevealing, although, on occasion, a history of trauma, spinal infection, poliomyelitis, or other disorders that imply a specific etiology may be present. When symptoms are present, the most common complaint is back pain, generally in the lumbar or low thoracic region. The pain is exacerbated by strenuous activity and improved with rest. Back pain is much more common in adults than children or adolescents presumably due to secondary osteoarthritis. Other symptoms are much less common and occur only in patients with severe deformity. These include radicular pain, impingement of the ribs on the iliac crests, and dyspnea.

Because of the vast number of associated disorders, the physical examination should be complete when scoliosis is suspected. The patient must be entirely disrobed or the subtle findings of minimal deformity may be overlooked. General appearance should be noted and may reveal congenital anomalies. The skin should be carefully examined for tumors, cafe-au-lait spots, and abnormalities of pigmentation or hairy patches in the low back region. The signs of spinal deformity are numerous, but are often subtle in patients who do not already carry the diagnosis. The scapulae may be asymmetric with one side being prominent. The shoulder is higher and the hemithorax is larger on the side of the thoracic convexity. The iliac crest and the abdominal and inguinal folds are more prominent on the side of the thoracic concavity. Palpation of the spine may reveal the curve; however, the absence of this finding on palpation does not rule out mild deformity. With the patient bending forward at the hips, the posterior aspect of the thorax is examined. In patients with scoliosis, the rib cage on the side of the concavity is depressed, whereas the opposite side is elevated and prominent (Fig 18–1). Trunk alignment is evaluated by dropping a plumb line from the midline of the occiput to the gluteal cleft and measuring the horizontal distance from the cleft to the plumb line (Fig 18–2). The head will displace toward the side of the thoracic curve. Leg length (the distance from the anterior superior iliac spine to the ipsilateral medial malleolus) should be measured bilaterally and may reveal the etiology of a nonstructural curve (Fig 18–3). A complete neurologic examination should be done as there are multiple congenital and neuromuscular abnormalities associated with scoliosis. In rare cases, the findings of nerve root impingement may be present.

Complications

Scoliosis is not a benign disease. Congenital anomalies of the heart, lungs (partial pulmonary agenesis), genitourinary system, and central nervous system occur frequently. In its severe forms, life-threatening complications are common. As the rib cage impinges on the lungs, pathologic changes occur at the vascular level leading to pulmonary hypertension. The ultimate result is respiratory compromise and cor pulmonale. Once right ventricular failure ensues, the prognosis for survival is grave with death usually occurring within 1 to 2 years. Pulmonary physiology is markedly altered with significant reductions in total lung volume, residual volume, vital capacity, and functional residual capacity.[2] A study of patients with longstanding scoliosis found that the overall mortality rate was twice that of the normal population.[3] Another investigation that followed patients with untreated scoliosis found that 47% were disabled and the mean age of death was 46.6 years.[4] Paraplegia is common in congenital scoliosis, but is a result of the congenital neurologic abnormalities rather than the scoliosis. In fact, paraplegia is rarely, if ever, caused by scoliosis alone. The addition of a kyphotic angulation, however, may produce cord damage with resultant paraplegia. Thromboembolic disease also occurs more commonly than expected probably due to mechanical disability and prolonged bedrest.

One important (although uncommon) complication of treatment for scoliosis is duodenal compression by the superior mesenteric artery.[5] This may result from multiple treatment modes including traction, body casting, Harrington instrumentation, or Milwaukee brace, and is caused by correction of the spinal curvature. The patient presents with nausea, vomiting, abdominal distension, and pain. Radiographs show evidence of proximal small bowel obstruction. These patients may become very ill and, in fact, will often die. At times, surgical intervention is necessary to relieve the obstruction.

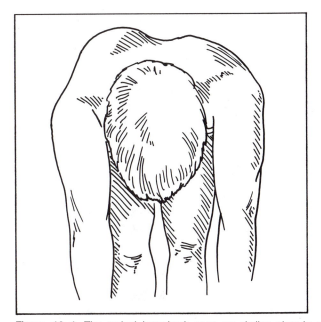

Figure 18–1. The typical humpback seen on skyline view in a patient with scoliosis.

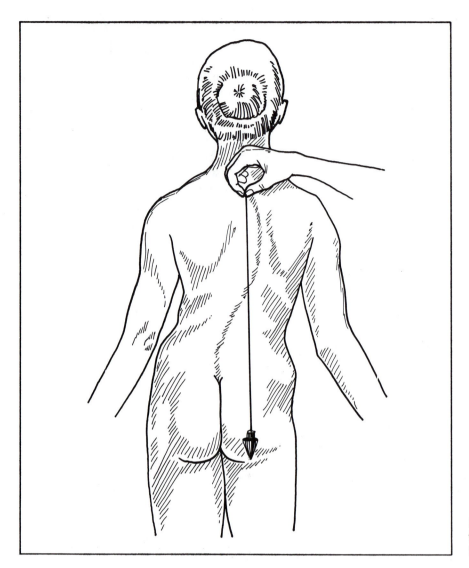

Figure 18–2. A plumb line dropped from the occiput is not on the midline in a patient with scoliosis.

In adolescent patients, the most significant complication is the deformity itself. Significant psychologic problems are common presumably due to their perception of themselves as being unsightly. Referral for this aspect of the disease (which can be severely disabling) should not be neglected.

Axiom: *Patients who have been or are being treated to correct spinal curvature that present with nausea, vomiting, or abdominal pain should be presumed to have high-grade duodenal obstruction until proven otherwise.*

Diagnosis, Emergency Management, and Referral

The radiography of scoliosis is very complex. From the perspective of the emergency or primary care physi-

cian, however, it is quite simple. X-ray of the spine reveals one or more curves. The detailed radiographic evaluation and careful measurement of spinal curvature can be left to the specialist. In fact, radiation exposure should be minimized in these patients whenever possible because many of them will have large numbers of radiographic studies during their lifetime. In the setting of trauma, great care must be taken to rule out fractures since the anatomy is altered and, therefore, may make radiographic interpretation difficult. In this situation, tomography and computed tomography may be necessary.

Most overt cases of scoliosis will have been diagnosed before their presentation to the emergency department for what is usually an unrelated urgent medical problem. The assumption, however, that those patients are being followed and managed appropriately should not be made. The approach of many primary care physicians is to "watch" their patients with scolio-

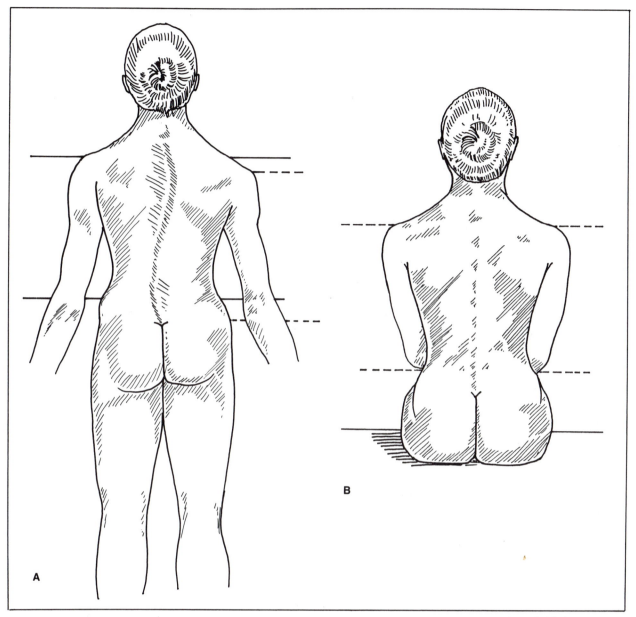

Figure 18–3. The nonstructural scoliosis secondary to a shortened leg **(A)** disappears when the patient is examined in the sitting position **(B)**.

sis to "see if they get worse." Unfortunately, many of them do and this leads to referral late in the course of the disease when the opportunity for preventive management has been lost. All patients with an abnormal curvature should be referred at the time of diagnosis, regardless of its severity.

The other group of patients who are of concern to the emergency physician are those with early, relatively minor curves who have not yet been diagnosed. In this group of patients, the diagnosis will be made in three ways: (1) confirmation of the concerns of the patient or family members that a curve exists, (2) discovery of a curve by physical examination that has been previously unnoticed, and (3) as an incidental finding on a chest x-ray obtained for other purposes. Regardless of the means of diagnosis or the severity of newly discovered scoliosis, under no circumstances should it be ignored despite the fact that it may have nothing to do with the patient's presenting complaint.

Axiom: *Every patient with abnormal spinal curvature should be referred for follow-up at the time of initial diagnosis, regardless of the severity.*

It should be noted that any abnormal curvature, regardless of its etiology, possesses the potential to progress and may lead to multiple complications and early death.

Axiom: *Every abnormal spinal curve must be considered to have the potential for progression.*

Because in nonstructural scoliosis the abnormality is located outside of the spine and its supporting structures, there is generally no treatment required for the spine itself. Rather, therapeutic measures are directed toward the actual cause.

A detailed discussion of the operative and nonoperative management of structural scoliosis is beyond the scope of this text. Suffice it to say that careful follow-up and appropriate treatment by a physician experienced in the management of these patients will nearly always lead to a significant improvement in patient outcome medically, psychologically, and vocationally.

☐ KYPHOSIS

Incidence

The true incidence of an abnormal dorsal kyphosis is unknown. Depending on the criteria for diagnosis, it is present in approximately 3 to 8% of the population. The vast majority of cases, however, are of little clinical significance and severe deformity is quite uncommon.

Pathophysiology

The normal thoracic spine has a kyphus of 20 to 40 degrees[6,7] which is maintained by muscular and ligamentous supporting structures. A large number of disease processes can lead to an abnormal increase in the dorsal kyphosis.[8] Despite a wide variety of etiologies (Table 18–1), the actual mechanisms that produce the deformity are common to nearly all of them. That is, either loss of height anteriorly with vertebral body wedging or loss of structural (ligamentous or muscular) integrity posteriorly, or both. Frequently, the kyphosis is not pure, but includes some element of rotation and lateral curvature in the upper thoracic region.

Clinical Features

With such a large number of etiologies, it is not surprising that kyphosis can present at any age. Congenital kyphosis is generally obvious at birth. Adolescent kyphosis, or Scheuermann's disease, develops gradually

TABLE 18–1. COMMON CAUSES OF KYPHOSIS

Congenital
Adolescent kyphosis (Scheuermann's disease)
Postural
Infectious (see Chapter 5)
Pyogenic bacteria
Tuberculosis
Brucella
Fungi
Parasites
Syphilis
Trauma (see Chapter 16)
Fracture
Ligamentous disruption
Surgical
Osteoporosis
Arthridities (see Chapter 3)
Neoplasm (see Chapter 6)

around the time of puberty with girls being affected twice as often as boys.[9] Kyphosis due to osteoporosis occurs predominantly in postmenopausal women. Neoplasm, infection, and trauma may lead to a kyphotic deformity in patients of all ages. Regardless of the etiology or age of onset, the symptoms caused by the deformity are similar. Pain in the lower thoracic region is generally the problem that leads the patient to seek medical attention. Gradual onset is the norm and the pain is often improved with rest. The patient may describe radiation of the pain to the inguinal region. It is uncommon for the patient to be aware of the deformity early in the course although others may have noticed it. Systemic symptoms are present only in the setting of underlying illness (i.e., infection, advanced malignancy, rheumatoid arthritis). After longstanding severe deformity, there may be symptoms of neurologic dysfunction or respiratory compromise.

Physical examination generally reveals a deformity by the time the patient presents for evaluation. Although subtle early on in the course, a hump will be present in the mid or low thoracic region. This becomes much more prominent with forward bending (Fig 18–4). There may be tenderness and spasm with forward bending. There may be tenderness and spasm noted on palpation of the paraspinous muscles in the region of the deformity. Tightness of the hamstrings and pectoralis muscles may be present. In a few patients with severe deformity, spastic paralysis will be present.

Complications

The deformity of kyphosis is often of great concern to patients as it produces an unsightly "roundback" appearance. It is felt that this plays an important causative

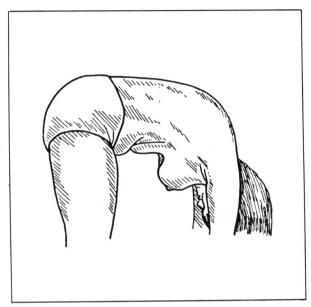

Figure 18–4. In a patient with thoracic kyphosis, the abnormal curve is accentuated on flexion.

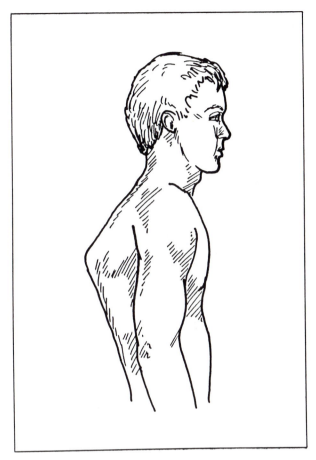

Figure 18–5. Gibbus deformity.

role in the psychologic problems that are frequently experienced by these patients. When the kyphotic angle is severe, a gibbus protrudes posteriorly, which may be painful (Fig 18–5). This creates a pressure point and leads to ulceration in some patients, particularly in those who are at bedrest. Neck and low back pain are also common sequelae, presumably due to increased lordosis in these regions. As with scoliosis, severe thoracic deformity may lead to respiratory compromise. Cord compression resulting in spastic paralysis is another complication of severe kyphotic deformity.[10] Although this occurs much more frequently with kyphosis than with scoliosis, it is still very uncommon.

Diagnosis
The history and physical examination, as previously discussed, should lead one to suspect the diagnosis. Radiographically, the hallmark is vertebral body wedging in the mid to low thoracic region with the dorsal kyphus measuring greater than 40 degrees. The specific radiographic findings, however, vary greatly and depend upon the etiology of the deformity, i.e., tuberculosis, ankylosing spondylitis, previous fracture. (The reader is referred to the appropriate chapters for a discussion of these radiographic findings.) Adolescent kyphosis has a relatively specific radiographic picture that reveals three or more thoracic vertebrae that are each wedged at least 5 degrees.[11] In addition, there is irregularity of the bony end plates and small protrusions into the vertebral body that become apparent radiographically as they calcify (Schmorl's nodes). Ultimately, the disc space becomes narrowed.

Emergency Management and Referral
Whenever possible, the goal of therapy is to treat the underlying process, i.e., infection, osteopenia, malignancy. The optimum approach may require the interaction of multiple physicians, particularly if there is a medically treatable etiology. Unfortunately, as with scoliosis patients, a significant number of young patients are "followed" by their primary care physician only to miss the period during which they would gain the most from appropriate referral and treatment.

Therapy for significant deformities generally includes analgesics, bedrest, and exercise, as well as various braces or casts. The vast majority of patients receive benefit from conservative therapy. Surgical intervention is necessary only in a small percentage of cases and then only for specific indications.[12,13]

Axiom: *As with scoliosis, in all patients with an abnormal thoracic kyphus, referral should be made at the time of diagnosis.*

□ REFERENCES

1. Shands AR Jr, Eisberg HB: The incidence of scoliosis in the state of Delaware. A study of 50,000 minifilms of the chest made during a survey for tuberculosis. J Bone Joint Surg 37A:1243, 1955
2. Caro CG, DuBois AB: Pulmonary function in kyphoscoliosis. Thorax 16:282, 1961
3. Nachemson A: A long-term follow-up study of nontreated scoliosis. Acta Orthop Scand 39:466, 1968
4. Nilsonne U, Lundgren KD: Long-term prognosis in idiopathic scoliosis. Acta Orthop Scand 39:456, 1968
5. Evarts CM, Winter RB, Hall JE: Vascular compression of the duodenum associated with the treatment of scoliosis. J Bone Joint Surg 53A:431, 1971
6. Roaf R: Vertebral growth and its mechanical control. J Bone Joint Surg 42B:40, 1960
7. Moe JH: Scoliosis and Other Spinal Deformities. Philadelphia, WB Saunders, 1978

8. Bradford DS: Editoral comment. Kyphosis. Clin Orthop 128:2, 1977
9. Bradford DS, Moe JH, Montalvo FJ, et al: Scheuermann's kyphosis and roundback deformity—Results of Milwaukee brace treatment. J Bone Joint Surg 56A: 740, 1954
10. Bradford DS: Neurological complications in Scheuermann's disease. J Bone Joint Surg 51A:567, 1969
11. Sorenson KH: Scheuermann's Juvenile Kyphosis. Copenhagen Munksgaard, 1964
12. Bradford DS, Moe JH, Montalvo JF, et al: Scheuermann's kyphosis: Results of surgical treatment by posterior spine arthrodesis on 22 patients. J Bone Joint Surg 57A:439, 1975
13. Yau ACMC, Hus LCS, O'Brien JP, et al: Tuberculous kyphosis. Correction with spinal osteotomy, halo–pelvic distraction, and anterior and posterior fusion. J Bone Joint Surg 56A:1419, 1974

19

Low Back Pain

□ INTRODUCTION

Low back pain (LBP) is the most common complaint in ambulatory and emergency medicine after the common cold and minor trauma.[1] Between 60 and 80% of the population will experience at least one episode of acute LBP, the most common cause of limitation of activity in adults less than 45 years old, the third most common cause of inactivity after heart disease and arthritis in the 45 to 65 age group.[2] Accounting for $5 billion in evaluation and treatment as well as an estimated $14 billion in workman's compensation, disability, and litigation, it is the third most expensive disease after heart disease and cancer.

The differential diagnosis of LBP is extensive, including referred pain from numerous body systems, and primary musculoskeletal disorders, the latter largely due to posttraumatic causes, but also including numerous disease processes such as infection, arthritis, and neoplasm. Only by exclusion can one consider a physiologic basis for LBP. The following discussion considers the major etiologies.

For the differential diagnosis of patients presenting with either acute or chronic low back pain we propose the following schema.

Nonmusculoskeletal causes of the referred back pain
Low back pain associated with minor trauma
Low back pain with radiation
Low back pain of insidious onset at under 50 years of age
Low back pain of insidious onset at over 50 years of age

Within each of these broad categories are a number of specific conditions. Each of the major etiologies is discussed in terms of clinical features, x-rays, and treatment.

□ NONMUSCULOSKELETAL (REFERRED) CAUSES

A number of nonmusculoskeletal disorders can be perceived as either localized or radiating to the back. Table 19–1 lists a number of more common entities that can present emergently as LBP, a thorough discussion of which is beyond the scope of this text. Given such a sizable list of serious conditions, however, it is clear that a standard evaluation of all patients presenting with LBP should include a thorough history and physical examination, including chest, abdomen, vascular, pelvis, rectum, and urinalysis.

Specifically, history and physical examination of the chest should include questions regarding recent cough, weight loss, chest pain, prior history of hypertension, or myocardial infarction. Examination should include careful inspection for venous engorgement, increased jugular venous pressure, muscular asymmetry, surgical scars, and palpation of the abdominal aorta. Examine pulses in the upper extremities and lower extremities, and take blood pressures in both arms. Careful percussion and auscultation of the heart and the lungs may reveal primary thoracic pathology. Aortic dissection, pleural effusion, or pneumonia can result in pain being referred to the back. When history or examination is suggestive, these should be evaluated with electrocardiogram, chest x-rays, and other modalities.

Primary abdominal pathology can also lead to referred pain to the low back area. History of abdominal pain, dyspepsia, epigastric pain, nausea and vomiting, anorexia, diarrhea, or constipation should all be elicited. Careful physical examination for masses, abnormal pulsations, appropriate bowel sounds, rebound tenderness or guarding, and costovertebral angle tenderness should be specifically tested. Abdominal aortic aneurysm, perforated viscus, pancreatic disease, bowel obstruction, retroperitoneal pathologies, retrocecal appendix, and primary urinary tract disease can all be referable to the lower back.

TABLE 19–1. NONMUSCULOSKELETAL CAUSES OF LBP

Thoracic aortic dissection

Pleural effusion

Abdominal aortic aneurysm

Perforated viscus

Pancreatic disease—inflammation or neoplasm

Bowel obstruction

Retrocecal appendix

Retroperitoneal bleed or neoplasm

Pelvic disease—pelvic inflammatory disease,
  ectopic pregnancy

Prostatitis

Urolithiasis or urinary tract infection

All patients require a rectal examination to check for local tenderness, occult blood, and where appropriate, prostatic disease. Primary genitourinary disease is also referable to the low back, and a detailed menstrual and sexual history is necessary as well as, where indicated, complete pelvic examination.

Specific findings in examination of the chest and the pelvis should be appropriately pursued with laboratory or radiographic examinations. Only after excluding nonmusculoskeletal causes for low back pain should the examiner proceed with the more specific functional examination of lower back and lower extremities.

☐ MUSCULOSKELETAL CAUSES

Mechanism

The precise etiology of pain due to musculoskeletal causes is not well understood, but is probably multifactorial, including morphologic, biochemical, and biomechanical factors.[2,3] Lumbosacral fascia, supraspinous and interspinous ligaments, ligamentum flavum, apophyseal joint capsules, and the outermost layers of the annulus are known to have either pain or pressure and position sensation. Biomechanical factors, either from acute trauma or chronic wear, lead to tears or microfractures in the annulus fibrosus, degenerative changes, or malalignment of facet joints. These are exacerbated by poor posture, conditioning, or excess weight. Increased lordosis, tension on the disc and posterior longitudinal ligament or facet joints produces a biochemical inflammatory reaction irritating innervated structures and thereby producing pain.

Although somewhat subtle, there is a distinction to be made between referred and radiating pain.[4] Irritation to soft tissues by trauma or inflammation results in pain that is commonly referred distally to the buttocks, hips, and lower extremities. Frequently, this has no specific dermatomal distribution. Radiating pain, on the other hand, generally refers to complaints of pain along a specific dermatomal distribution corresponding to a particular nerve root.

When humans rose up on their hind legs, they did much to change the stresses on the lower spine. Nachemson[4] has studied the various forces involved in the upright position: the abdominal musculature adjusting the trunk anteriorly, the back muscles and ligaments supporting it posteriorly, and the intervertebral discs providing shock absorbancy. By recording intradiscal pressures at L-3, he demonstrated a sevenfold increase in pressure simply by sitting upright from a supine position, and a 20-fold increase while bending forward and rotating while holding a 10-kg weight.[5] It is little wonder then that when persons partake in occasional heavy physical work or intermittent athletic endeavors, they risk a number of consequences.

Although it is often difficult to determine the exact etiology of low back pain in the emergency setting, the differential diagnosis can often be narrowed on the basis of the patient's age, initial complaints, and physical examination. Specific syndromes can be categorized according to broad clinical groupings.

☐ LOW BACK PAIN ASSOCIATED WITH MINOR TRAUMA

Low back pain associated with major trauma is discussed in Chapter 16.

Myofascial Sprain

Sudden stresses from stretching or exertion can cause inflammation and pain from partial tears to muscles and ligaments of the lower back, usually within hours of the incident.[4] These injuries generally occur in young, healthy individuals, and a history of specific injury is almost always the inciting event.

Clinical Features

History of sudden pain with exertion or strenuous exercise is elicited. It is frequently intense. Pain and weakness are usually limited to a specific vertebral muscle or muscle group, often associated with spasm. Actual weakness is frequently difficult to elicit as severe pain and muscle spasm limit appropriate testing. Trigger points, focal inflamed areas that cause pain in muscle and fascial groups when palpating, have been described.[6]

Radiographs

Indications for plain radiography are discussed later in this chapter. As this is an injury to soft tissue, x-ray findings will be normal.

Treatment*

Local cooling, bedrest, and injection of local anesthetic into the trigger point have all been routinely used. Local anesthetic with or without steroids is injected into the area of maximum tenderness. Stretch and spray techniques (described in detail later in the chapter) have been shown to be effective in relieving symptoms in the acute setting if local trigger points are present.

Symptoms of acute pain and muscle spasm generally resolve within the first few days, but a dull ache may persist for several weeks.

Posterior Facet Syndrome

Posterior facet joints are true synovial joints between superior and inferior articular processes of adjacent vertebrae, surrounded by ligamentous capsules. With sudden movements, particularly hyperextension, the capsule may be stretched or torn, allowing facet subluxation. Predisposing factors leading to injury include excessive weight, acute lumbosacral angle, degenerative changes, loss of the intervertebral disc, chronic occupational strains, and exaggerated vertical disposition of the articular facets.[7] Repeated injuries to the facet lead to degenerative changes and a greater likelihood of recurrent exacerbation. Referred pain to the lower extremities is not common; however, pain may radiate along the spine to the buttocks. In severe subluxation or with progressive degenerative changes, nerve root impingement can be seen.

Clinical Features

The history generally includes a description of acute back pain associated with hyperextension. Frequently, the patient will complain of a number of prior similar episodes. Sneezing and coughing can exacerbate the pain. In the acute setting, and frequently between attacks, even mild hyperextension can increase symptoms, as in sleeping in the prone position.

Upon inspection the patient will frequently stand in mild flexion at the hips. Motion is limited in all directions and tenderness may be elicited at the lumbosacral junction, frequently associated with severe muscle spasm. In the absence of severe muscle spasm, the facet joints can be palpated bilaterally between and immediately adjacent to (one fingerbreath lateral to) the spinous processes (Fig 19–1). Local tenderness over

*Discussion of each of the treatment modalities prescribed for the following syndromes is presented in detail in the "Treatment" section later in this chapter.

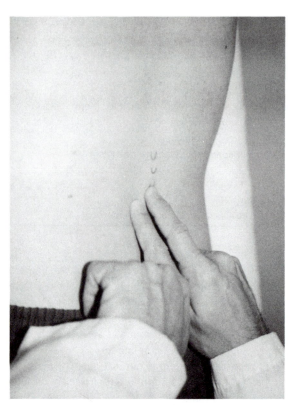

Figure 19–1. Palpation of facet joints, one fingerbreadth lateral to and between the spinous processes.

the facets, increased pain with hyperextension, and the absence of neurologic deficit are strongly suggestive of acute facet syndrome. The straight leg raising test can be positive under two circumstances. Extreme straight leg raising can stretch the facet capsule, resulting in localized pain. A true positive straight leg raising test can be elicited if true nerve root impingement exists. Leg length measurements should be done, as asymmetry can increase stresses on the facet joints.

Radiographs

Lateral plain radiography may be normal in the acute setting, or, in patients with chronic symptoms, may show degenerative changes. Oblique radiographs best demonstrate facet subluxation, with posterior displacement of the superior segment and possibly a slight narrowing of the posterior intervertebral disc. The intervertebral foramen might be narrowed.

Treatment

Conservative therapy is recommended in the acute setting, including bedrest with the knees flexed, heat, nonsteroid anti-inflammatory drugs, and antispasmodic medication in the event of severe muscle spasm. A spinal manipulation (discussed later in this chapter) is recommended for those trained to perform one. Patient education should include avoidance of maneuvers promoting hyperextension and, later, an exercise program to include the strengthening of the abdominal and gluteus muscles, increasing flexion at the lumbosacral junction. As this is a syndrome of repeated acute episodes and often chronic discomfort, referral is recommended.

Sacroiliac Sprain

The sacroiliac joint is extremely stable. Beyond age 45 the anterior capsule of the joint is ossified and thus resistant to sprain. In the younger years, significant forces are required to upset the joint, usually resulting in fracture of the pelvis. It is, therefore, relatively rare to sustain a true sacroiliac joint sprain, injury to the supporting ligament, or the structures of the sacroiliac joint.

To the contrary, pain in the sacroiliac joint region is relatively common, most frequently in the form of referred pain from disc degeneration. It is important for the emergency physician to avoid the pitfall of attributing pain in the sacroiliac area to a true sprain.

A physiologic exception to the very stable sacroiliac joint occurs during pregnancy. During the last stages of pregnancy, ligaments supporting the pelvis relax in preparation for delivery. At this time, even relatively trivial trauma can result in sacroiliac sprain.

Clinical Features

The history is usually consistent with significant trauma to the low back and pelvic region. Physical findings include tenderness over the lower one-third of the sacroiliac joint and pubic symphysis. Because the pelvis is a closed ring, injury to the sacroiliac joint must be associated with a pubic symphysis injury (Fig 19–2). As well, compression anywhere about the pelvic ring will elicit tenderness in the injured sacroiliac joint. The patient will, therefore, complain of pain with lateral manual compression of the iliac crest. Resisted abduction of the hip joint will also produce pain in the sacroiliac joint, as the gluteus medius pulls the ilium away from sacrum. Gaenslen's test, hyperextension of the hip on the affected side, is positive, but may also elicit pain due to preexisting hip disease or lumbar nerve root irritation. In addition, the patient may experience pain on the affected side with abduction of the hip, and thus tend to swing the leg on the affected side forward, known as the Trendelenburg lurch.[5]

Radiographs

Pelvic films may reveal widening of the sacroiliac joint.

Treatment

Conservative therapy is recommended with bedrest, analgesics, and anti-inflammatory medications. Some

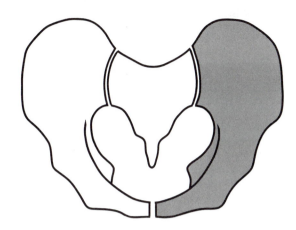

Figure 19–2. The "closed" pelvic ring.

patients obtain relief from a trochanteric belt, a strap situated circumferentially at the level between the iliac crest and the trochanteric notch.

☐ LOW BACK PAIN WITH RADIATION

Spinal Stenosis

Spinal stenosis is a condition of nerve root entrapment caused by a narrowing of the spinal canals and intervertebral foramina. Narrowing is usually secondary to developmental anomalies or degenerative changes, particularly after laminectomy. Table 19–2 is an exhaustive list of conditions leading to spinal stenosis.[8] This is a syndrome in adults rarely seen in the young without developmental abnormalities.[9] Clinical presentation is similar to that of disc herniation with radiating pain.[10] The course of spinal stenosis, however, is more chronic, generally consists of primarily back pain before leg pain develops, and appears to be worse with inactivity. Leg pain is more diffuse and somewhat less specific in localization, and although acute attacks occur less frequently than in acute disc herniation, symptoms respond less readily. The syndrome is characterized by neurogenic claudication, symptoms worsening with activity, which readily resolve with rest.

Clinical Features

Typically, patients complain of a long history of back pain, initially intermittent, but progressing to a dull ache. Radiating pain to the legs is similar to that in patients with herniated discs since the stenosis generally occurs in the lower lumbar spine. Pain extends down the back or lateral side of the thigh, the back of the calf, and onto the foot and the toe, bilaterally. Pain

TABLE 19–2. CONDITIONS ASSOCIATED WITH SPINAL STENOSIS

Congenital—Developmental Stenosis
Idiopathic
Achondroplasia
Hypochondroplasia
Morquio's mucopolysaccharidosis
Dysplasias associated with lax atlantoaxial joints (metatropic dwarfism, spondyloepiphyseal dysplasia, Kniest's disease, multiple epiphyseal dysplasia, chondrodysplasia punctata)
Down's syndrome (C1-2 instability)
Hypophosphatemic vitamin D-resistant rickets

Acquired Stenosis
Degenerative
  Spondylosis and arthrosis
  Soft tissue stenosis
  Isolated intervertebral disc resorption
  Degenerative spondylolisthesis
Combined
  Any possible combinations of congenital or developmental stenosis, degenerative stenosis, and protrusions of intervertebral disc material
Spondylolysis
  Without spondylolisthesis
  With spondylolisthesis
Iatrogenic
  Postlaminectomy
  Postfusion (anterior or posterior)
Posttraumatic, late changes
Miscellaneous
  Ankylosing spondylitis
  Calcification or ossification of the posterior longitudinal ligament
  Diffuse idiopathic skeletal hyperostosis
  Calcification or ossification of the ligamentum flavum
  Conjoined origin of lumbosacral nerve roots (relative stenosis of neural canal)
Metabolic
  Paget's disease of bone
  Epidural lipomatosis (Cushing's syndrome or long term steroid therapy)
  Acromegaly
  Fluorosis
  Calcium pyrophosphate dihydrate deposition disease (pseudogout)

From Dorwart RH, et al: Spinal stenosis. Radiol Clin North Am 41(2):301, 1981.

is frequently exacerbated by walking or standing, but symptoms will resolve with changes in posture. It is believed that increases in lumbar lordosis will exacerbate the stenosis on the nerve roots; therefore, sitting or lying down reduces the stenosis, and symptoms resolve.[9] This "neurogenic claudication," although characteristic of spinal stenosis, is not seen in all patients. Nerve root involvement is usually at L-5 to L-1 level, but frequently affects nerves at L-2 to L-3 and L-3 to L-4 in a patchy distribution. The pain is described as a numbness or dull ache. The neurologic examination is usually normal, or includes only minimal sensory motor or reflex changes. Straight leg raising is positive

due to the degree of degenerative changes and subsequent nerve compression in patients with spinal stenosis. They are more susceptible to trauma and superimposed disc herniation.

As patients are generally older, it is important to differentiate between neurogenic and vascular claudication, as symptoms of leg pain with activity that resolve with rest are similar in both. A patient with neurogenic claudication, however, has normal pulses in the lower extremity, whereas a patient with vascular claudication will have decreased peripheral pulses and evidence of chronic vascular insufficiency.

Radiographs

Plain radiographs can be normal but more typically reveal evidence of chronic degenerative changes. A narrowing of the anteroposterior (AP) or transverse diameter of the spinal canal can sometimes be seen on plain radiography, but myelography is more specific. Computed tomographic scanning, however, affords the best visualization of narrowing of the spinal canal and intervertebral lamina.[10]

Treatment

Initial treatment is conservative, including bedrest, heat, and nonsteroidal anti-inflammatory drugs in mildly symptomatic patients. Instruction on posture and an exercise regimen to strengthen the abdominal muscles thereby reducing lumbar lordosis can be helpful.[11] Degenerative spinal stenosis, however, is a progressive disease; as symptoms progress, surgical correction is warranted. All patients with spinal stenosis should be referred.

Acute Disc Herniation

Lumbar disc herniations are the most common cause of acute sciatica associated with low back pain.[12] Progressive spondylosis, recurrent episodes of acute low back pain, or conditioning in chronic stress all contribute to trauma and eventual weakness of the annulus fibrosus. Initially, small cracks develop in the annulus fibrosus due to normal wear. They begin centrally and radiate to the periphery, thus weakening the annulus fibrosus. With sudden increases in intradiscal pressure, the central nucleus pulposus can herniate and cause nerve root compression (Fig 19–3). The incidence of acute, symptomatic herniation is much greater in patients aged 30 to 50 than in others. The nucleus pulposus is bulkier and of greater turgor than in the older dessicated and fibrotic nucleus. As such, acute disc symptoms are more commonly seen in the middle-aged.[12]

Herniation usually occurs progressively as there is weakening of the posterior longitudinal ligament that acts to restrain the nucleus pulposus. The fragment can then migrate superiorly, inferiorly, or laterally into the

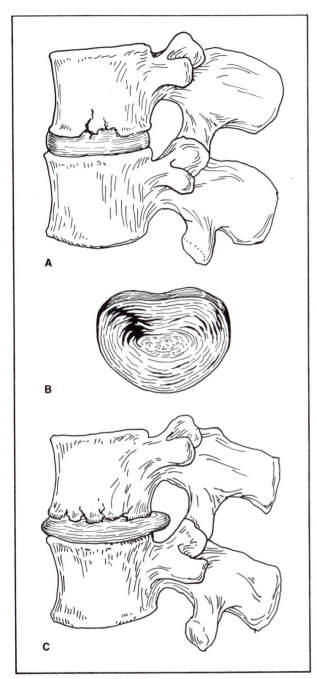

Figure 19–3. Disc degeneration: (**A**) Early degeneration with (**B**) small cracks in the annulus fibrosus; (**C**) late changes with bulging of the disc.

Clinical Features

It is important to remember that lumbar disc disease is a syndrome that can present with a variety of signs and symptoms. Although back pain and evidence of nerve root compression are classic, presentation in each patient is individual.

Axiom: *Although lumbar disc herniation is a syndrome of classic description, it is important to note that similar space-occupying lesions can present as an acute disc herniation.*

Most disc herniations are associated with degenerative disease of the lumbosacral spine. Patients give a history of chronic dull low back pain, worse with activity, episodes of mild exacerbations resolve spontaneously, and there is usually no complaint of leg pain. This picture of early disc disease is indistinguishable from other causes of low back pain, but is probably attributable to damage of the annulus fibrosus.

When a disc acutely ruptures, patients complain of severe low back pain occurring immediately or within a few hours after a particular injury. The pain is worse with Valsalva maneuver, coughing, or sneezing, and is associated with significant muscle spasm and flattening of the lumbar curve. Nerve root compression most generally occurs at the L-5 to S-1 level, and sciatic pain progresses distally in a typical dermatomal pattern. Not infrequently, patients will complain that their typical low back pain resolves once sciatica develops. This is attributed to the release in the pressure at the annulus when the nucleus ruptures; the sciatica is now due to impingement on the nerve root. With significant sciatica, the patient frequently assumes a listing posture away from the painful side. If the disc protrusion is medial to the nerve, however, patients will list toward the affected side to reduce compression (Fig 19–4). There is a decrease in the range of motion, largely due to muscle spasm. Not infrequently, the pain is so intense the patient is unable to move at all. Significant root compression can result in weakness in the lower extremity, fifth nerve root compression resulting in weakness of dorsiflexion of the toes or foot drop.

Physical examination reveals marked tenderness at the level of protrusion, particularly to one side. Pressure on examination at that point might increase sciatic pain. There is generally some degree of muscle spasm at that level. Flexion of the head by drawing up on the dura increases symptoms of sciatica. Decreased range of motion is seen in flexion, extension, and rotation. The patient maintains the painful leg flexed to reduce tension on the sciatic nerve. Generally, the patient walks with a limp to avoid weight bearing on the af-

intraverterbral foramen. Less commonly, there is mass protrusion of the nucleus with sudden neurologic compromise. Herniation can also occur through the cartilaginous plate of the superior or inferior vertebral body. Disc material ruptures through a defect in the cartilaginous plate into the cancellous bone. The herniation is generally irregular in size and shape and on x-ray is noted to be surrounded by a rim of bone sclerosis termed Schmorl's node (Fig 19–3A).

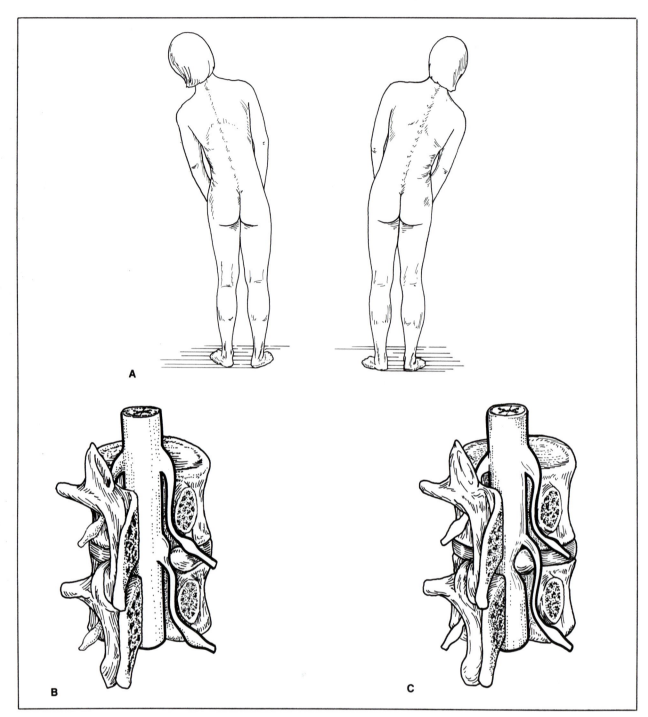

Figure 19–4. Disc herniations both lateral and medial to the nerve root.

fected side. Loss of the lumbar curve is generally attributable to paravertebral muscle spasm, which can be quite intense and unilateral. When examining the spine, the examiner should be careful not to apply direct pressure over the spastic muscle belly. Tenderness can be elicited at the level of the protrusion, slightly off the midline on the affected side. In the erect position there may be no tenderness, but palpation with the lumbar spine in slight flexion can produce marked pain. Significant deep palpation or percussion in the involved leg can increase sciatica or elicit it when only back pain is present. Palpation at the sciatic notch will increase radiating pain.

A careful neurologic examination can suggest the level of disc herniation, but is not conclusive due to variations in the disc protrusion itself and in root con-

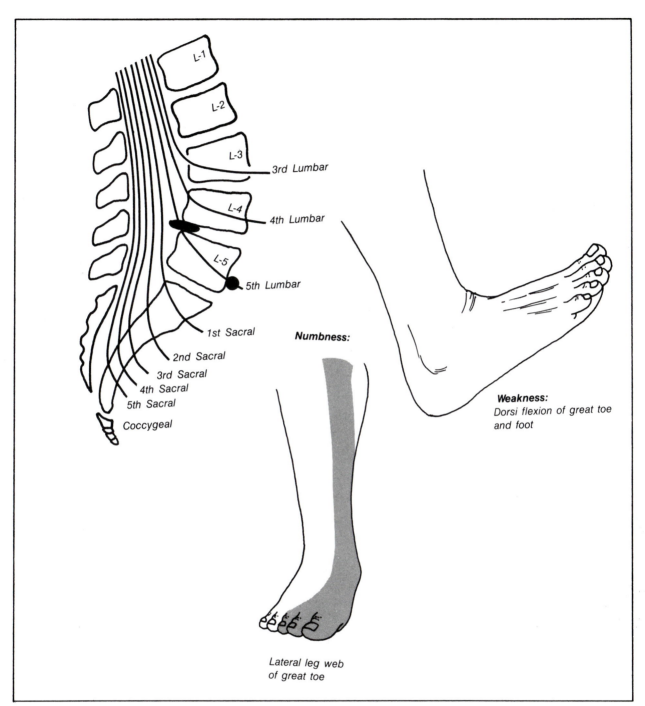

Figure 19–5. Clinical features of disc herniation at the L-5 root level.

figuration. L-4 to L-5 and L-5 to S-1 are the most common levels of disc protrusion. In general, herniation of L-4 to L-5 compresses the fifth lumbar nerve root (Fig 19–5), L-5 to S-1 will compress the sacroiliac root (Fig 19–6), and L-3 to L-4 involvement, the next most common, compresses the fourth nerve root (Fig 19–7). Table 19–3 summarizes these clinical findings.

Motor signs are seen in approximately 96% of cases.[7] Weakness or paralysis of a muscle group de-creases tone and atrophy. Compression of the fourth nerve root affects the quadriceps and results in weakness with extension of the knee and instability; fifth nerve root compression causes weakness of the toe extensors and dorsiflexors of the foot; first sacral root compression incurs only minimal weakness in flexion of the foot and the great toe. Measurement of leg circumferences will demonstrate subtle atrophic muscle changes.

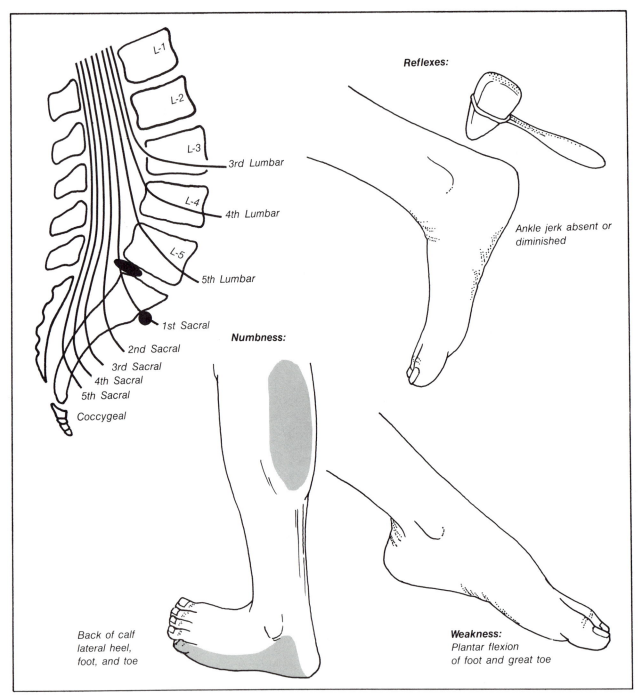

Figure 19–6. Clinical features of disc herniation at the S-1 root level.

Sensory findings are seen in approximately 80% of patients[7] and are generally of specific dermatomal distribution. Compression of the fourth lumbar nerve results in decreased sensation in the anteromedial aspect of the leg; involvement of the fifth lumbar nerve root produces decreased sensation in the anterolateral portion of the leg and the medial aspect of the foot to the great toe; compression of the first sacral nerve root results in decreased sensation in the posterior aspect of the calf and the bilateral aspect of the foot.

Deep tendon reflexes are frequently reduced as a result of nerve root compression. Compression of the fourth lumbar nerve root diminishes the patellar reflex; compression of the fifth lumbar nerve root results in no reflex change; compression of the first sacral nerve root diminishes the Achilles reflex.

Straight leg raising tests elicit or augment sciatica by stretching the sciatic nerve and pulling the lumbosacral nerve root, particularly the fifth lumbar and first sacral nerve. This is of most value in young individ-

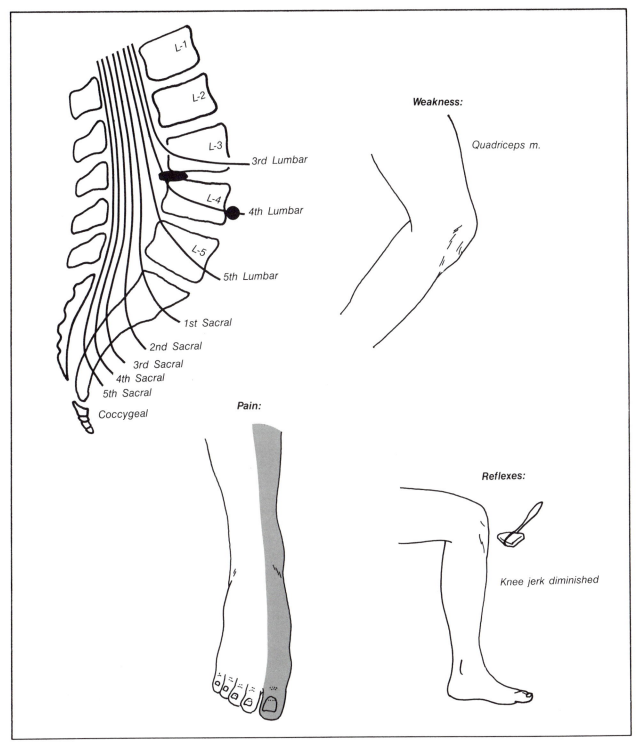

Figure 19–7. Clinical features of disc herniation at the L-4 root level.

uals. Performed with the patient in the supine position, one hand supports the ilium and the other elevates the leg from the heel with the knee straight (Fig 19–8). A positive test elicits leg pain or radicular symptoms, but back pain alone is not a positive finding. It is positive if it reproduces sciatica in the opposite extremity. A variation of straight leg raising involves flexing both the knee and the hip at 90 degrees and gradually extending the knee. A positive test reproduces or elicits leg pain. Fajersztan's test involves dorsal flexion of the foot producing radicular pain (Fig 19–9). The sitting root test is performed with the patient in the sitting position and the cervical spine flexed. When the knee is extended, a positive test will elicit leg pain.

Once again it should be emphasized that patients may present with varied complaints. With complete extrusion of the nuclear pulposus, back pain may be absent and only sciatica present; however, the examiner will usually detect the muscle spasm and limitation of motion. It is also possible the sciatic pain in the complete sciatic distribution may not be present, but rather only patchy with complaints only at the knee, calf, ankle, or heel. It is also possible to have discogenic pain limited solely to the back with no evidence of sciatica.

Large central disc herniations can result in compression of several nerve roots and this is termed cauda equina syndrome (Fig 19–10). In this instance, radicular symptoms may be limited, but back or perianal pain will be noted. Urinary symptoms including total urinary retention, chronic partial retention, bladder irritability, and loss of the desire to void are also noted with this syndrome.

It cannot be overemphasized that other entities can mimic disc herniation. Although this discussion has dealt with signs and symptoms associated with disc herniation, it is incumbent upon the emergency specialist to perform a complete physical examination on all patients complaining of low back pain.

TABLE 19–3. ROOT COMPRESSION SYNDROMES

L-5 to S-1   Disc (S-1 root)
        Pain/numbness—Posterior thigh and leg; posterolateral foot, lateral toes
        Weakness/atrophy—Plantar flexion foot, toes decreased; atrophy posterior compartment
        Reflex—Depressed Achilles reflex

L-4 to L-5   Disc (L-5 root)
        Pain/numbness—Posterior thigh, anterolateral leg, medial foot and great toe
        Weakness/atrophy—Dorsiflexion foot, toes decreased; atrophy anterior compartment
        Reflex—No change

L-3 to L-4   Disc (L-4 root)
        Pain/numbness—Posterolateral aspect of thigh, across patella, anteromedial leg
        Weakness/atrophy—Knee extension weak; quadriceps atrophy
        Reflex—Depressed patellar reflex

Radiographs

It must be noted that particularly in younger individuals, plain radiography may be normal. Similarly, abnormal findings may not be attributable to discogenic symptoms. Findings associated with disc rupture include thinning or loss of disc height, evidence of degenerative disease, including osteophytes and sclerosis

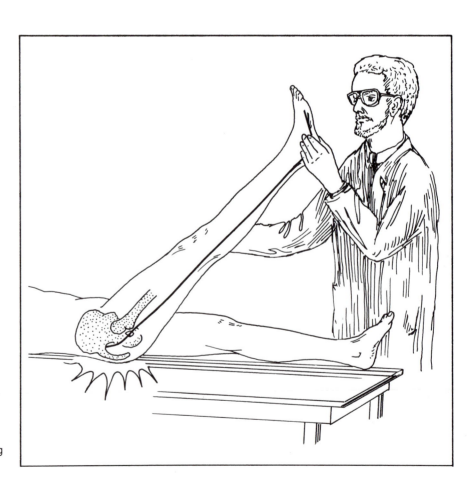

Figure 19–8. Straight leg raising test.

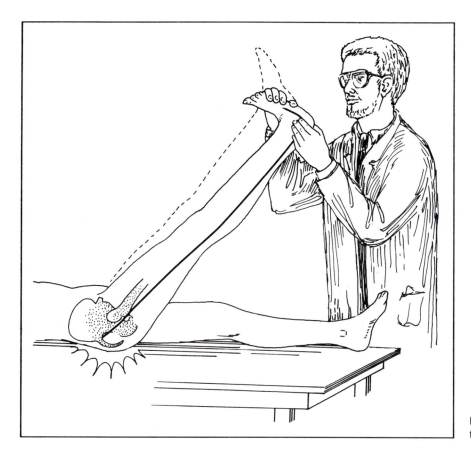

Figure 19–9. Straight leg raising test with dorsal flexion of the foot.

of the subchondral bone, Schmorl's nodes, minor malalignments of the vertebrae, calcification of the nucleus of the disc or vacuum disc phenomena, and a gas shadow in the area of the nucleus pulposus.

The diagnosis is confirmed by myleography and computed tomography.

Treatment

Initial therapy is conservative including bedrest with the knees flexed, anti-inflammatory drugs, muscle relaxants and analgesics, and local heat therapy. It should be emphasized that with conservative management the extruded disc will not entirely resorb or return to its original position; however, the acute inflammatory reaction and muscle spasm will diminish. The natural course of the disease is one of exacerbations with varying pain-free or limited painful periods. These pain-free episodes can be lengthened by a back program instituted after the pain subsides. A program of lumbar flexion exercises, physical therapy, limitation of heavy exercise and lifting, sleeping on the side or back, avoiding the prone position, sitting in a slumped position, and crossing the legs will reduce the frequency of recurrences. A number of devices have been marketed that purport to reduce the tension on the disc and serve as adjuncts to therapy. Tilt tables may be useful in selected patients although their efficacy has not been proven.

Many reports suggest that approximately 20% of patients will eventually require surgery or chemonucleolysis (injection of chymopapain) into the disc to dissolve the disc material.[12] Indications for surgery include progressive neurologic deficit, persistent or frequently recurrent sciatica, and acute neurologic deficit consistent with cauda equina syndrome with impaired bowel or bladder function, requiring immediate decompression. All patients should be referred.

☐ LOW BACK PAIN OF INSIDIOUS ONSET UNDER 50 YEARS OF AGE

Fibrositis

Fibrositis was first described by Sir William Gowers in 1904 as a nonspecific inflammatory condition of fibrous tissues. Pathologic study of the "fibrositic nodules" have proven to be nodules of fat, and the exact etiology of this entity is unknown.[4] A recent study by Campbell and colleagues[3] suggests fibrositis is a syndrome, including a constellation of symptoms including axial pain, severe aching and stiffness, and morning

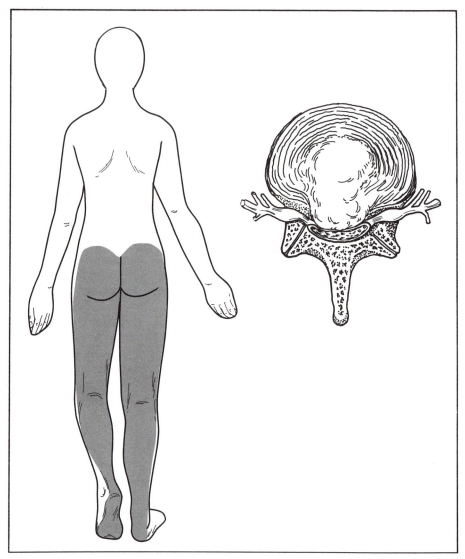

Figure 19–10. Cauda equina syndrome.

fatigue. The exact etiology and pathogenesis remain unknown.

Clinical Features
The condition is more typical in middle-aged women. Patients describe moderate to severe musculoskeletal pain and head, neck, and shoulder pain and morning aching and stiffness. Pain is more frequently axial, particularly in the neck, shoulders, and upper back, and typically is described as constant and aching. Symptoms are worse in cold, humid weather, winter, during fatigue and unusual or excessive exertion or emotional stress, and in the morning. Patients frequently complain of difficulty falling asleep, waking frequently, or waking early. Associated conditions include a tension-type headache and symptoms compatible with irritable bowel disease.

Physical examination is notable for tenderness most typically bilaterally symmetric, generally involving the paraspinous, trapezius, gluteus, and occiput. Tender points can be noted, but as described by McNab,[4] focal areas of nodules are more likely fat nodules. It is important for the examiner to rule out more specific etiologies of pain in these areas as quite frequently symptoms can be referred pain attributable to other entities. Psychologic testing of patients in this study revealed no difference between those with fibrositis and a control group.

Radiographs
This is a syndrome involving soft tissue. X-rays are indicated only when other etiologies are suspected.

Treatment
Duration of symptoms in the study by Campbell and co-workers[3] was from 18 months to 24 years with a

mean of 7.6 years. Conservative therapy of salicylates and acetaminophen, narcotics, nonsteroidal anti-inflammatory drugs, minor tranquilizers, and local physical therapy was studied. The patients reported most improvement with tricyclic antidepressants, acupuncture, and physical therapy. As this is a chronic complaint, all patients should be referred.

Infections

An in-depth discussion of this subject appears elsewhere in this text. A brief overview is presented here for continuity. If any of the following are serious considerations in the differential of your patients, the authors recommend referring to the principal discussion.

Vertebral osteomyelitis and intervertebral disc space infection are similar in clinical presentation. Although quite rare in the general population, vertebral osteomyelitis is more likely in patients with acute or chronic urinary tract infection, prostatitis, urinary instrumentation, diabetes mellitus, renal failure, and skin infection, and in intravenous drug abusers. Intervertebral disc space infections are most likely to occur after instrumentation, i.e., surgery or lumbar puncture. Previously more common in children presenting with fever or refusal to walk, 50% of pyogenic vertebral osteomyeolitis now occurs in adults most typically presenting with low back pain alone, which is insidious in onset and exacerbated with movement. The condition is associated with low-grade fever and malaise. The most common pathogen is *Staphylococcus aureus*, although the incidence of gram-negative rods (especially *Pseudomonas* species) is increasing. Tuberculous spondylitis (Potts disease) is very rare, seen in the elderly or poor, most often due to secondary spread of pulmonary *Mycobacterium tuberculosis* infection. Its presentation is similar to pyogenic spondylitis, with focal spinous tenderness and occasionally associated with constitutional symptoms or chronic illness. Because initial laboratory or radiographic findings are generally nondiagnostic, clinical suspicion, particularly in high-risk patients, warrants a radionuclide bone scan.

Sacroiliitis

Sacroiliitis is a relatively rare inflammatory condition seen most commonly in association with rheumatoid arthritis, psoriatic arthritis, ankylosing spondylitis, and chronic inflammatory bowel disease. In-depth discussions of some of these diseases appear elsewhere in the text. A brief overview is presented here for continuity. If any of the following are serious considerations in the differential of your patients, the authors recommend referring to the principal discussions.

Patients are generally young, between 15 and 40 years old, with complaints of low back pain, other joint pain, fever, fatigue, weight loss, penile discharge, diarrhea, or eye irritation (the latter three are typical of Reiter's syndrome). In ankylosing spondylitis, four out of five of the following historical criteria are 95% sensitive and 85% specific for diagnosis: age of onset at less than 40 years, gradual onset of symptoms, low back discomfort lasting at least 3 months, morning back stiffness, and improvement with mild exercise.

Helpful laboratory tests include elevations in erythrocyte sedimentation rate, serum glutamic-oxaloacetic transaminase, creatine phosphokinase, alkaline phosphatase, rheumatoid factor, antinuclear antibody, and the presence of HLA-B27. Perhaps with the exception of the erythrocyte sedimentation rate, these tests are of little help to the emergency physician.

X-ray findings of sacroiliitis range from loss of discrete margins of the sacroiliac joints to joint base narrowing eventually with complete fusion.

Spondylolysis and Spondylolisthesis

Spondylolisthesis is the anterior displacement (luxation) of the vertebra, generally accepted as L-5 slipping forward on S-1. The actual lesion allowing for the slippage is in the pars interarticularis, the section of the posterior arch between the inferior and superior articular processes. Spondylolysis is the same defect without slippage. Classification is based on etiology as presented in Table 19–4.[13] The lytic isthmic type is referred to as a true spondylolisthesis and is more common. The combination of a hereditary defect and strain on the pars interarticularis is suggested.

Clinical Features

Symptoms of spondylolisthesis vary considerably depending on severity. On presentation to the emergency department, patients complain of lumbar back ache and

---

TABLE 19–4. CLASSIFICATION OF SPONDYLOLISTHESIS

Type	Criteria
I	Dysplastic—the defect is a congenital dysplasia in the neural arch that allows subluxation
II	Isthmic—the defect is in the pars interarticularis A. Lytic type, probably a fatigue fracture with hereditary predisposition B. Elongated but intact pars, similar to type IIa, but the fatigue fractures have healed, resulting in an elongated but intact pars C. Acute fracture due to trauma
III	Degenerative—secondary to degenerative changes at the apophyseal joints (this is more frequent at L-4 on L-5 in women 40 years old or older)
IV	Traumatic—fracture of posterior elements other than pars
V	Pathologic—due to pathologic changes in posterior elements secondary to malignancy or primary bone diseases

Modified from Wiltse LL et al.: Clin Orthop 117:23, 1976.13

fatigue. Pain is also noted in the sacroiliac joints, hips, thighs, and legs. Weakness and paresthesia of the lower extremities suggestive of root irritation is uncommon as forward slippage of the vertebral body widens the intervertebral foramen. Paravertebral muscle spasm may be evident in the form of decreased range of motion. The lumbar lordosis is generally increased. Careful palpation may demonstrate a step-off of the spinous processes between L-4 and L-5. In extreme deformities, the ribs may come to rest on the pelvis and will be associated with a waddling gait. Patients tend to walk gingerly as jarring of the spinal column increases pain. The relatively uncommon nerve root irritation is suggestive of large luxation and L-4 and L-5 disc displacement with compression of the nerve roots.

Radiographs

Lateral lumbosacral radiographs in the supine position will reveal forward displacement of the L-5 vertebra. If this is further accentuated when the x-ray is taken while standing, it is highly suggestive that this finding explains the patient's symptoms. Minimal displacement of the L-5 vertebra seen both in supine and standing radiographs suggests a stable spondylolysis and is probably of little clinical significance. Oblique views may demonstrate the "Scotty dog" sign, the neck of the dog corresponding to the pars interarticularis, a "collar" typical of spondylolysis (Fig 19–11). The defect is characterized by four stages corresponding to the percent of slippage of the vertebra: 0 to 5%, 25 to 50%, 50 to 75%, and 75 to 100% (Fig 19–12).

Treatment

Initial acute painful episodes are treated conservatively with bedrest, heat, nonsteroidal anti-inflammatory drugs, and muscle relaxants in the event of significant muscle spasms.[7,14,15] This is followed by a trial of flexion exercises and abdominal muscle strenghtening. Surgical fusion is mandatory when motor deficits or incontinence is present and must be considered when slippage approaches 50% or greater.

☐ LOW BACK PAIN OF INSIDIOUS ONSET OVER 50 YEARS OF AGE

Spondylosis

Lumbar spondylosis (disc degeneration) occurs due to gradual wear and tear on the intervertebral disc. Gradual changes occur in three areas. Centrally, the nucleus become pliable and dull, small tears develop in the annulus, and the hyaline cartilage plates of the vertebral bodies rupture. As such, the smooth shock-absorber action of the disc is lost and movement becomes uneven and irregular. This stage, called segmental instability by McNab,[16] allows for excessive flexion and extension. Joint strain and subluxation allow segmental hyperextension, and as the intervertebral discs lose height, disc narrowing occurs (Fig 19–13). These changes, together with obesity, weak muscles, and poor posture put additional stresses on the posterior facet joints, leading to increased inflammation and pain. Excessive mobility leads to osteophyte formation and "traction spurs,"[16] bony horizontal projections emanating from the annulus fibers due to excessive movement of unstable segments.

With continued degeneration, calcification of the disc can occur, vacuum discs may develop (the appearance of dissolved gas from the nuclear material), and the nucleus pulposus may rupture superiorly or inferiorly through the hyaline cartilage plates of the vertebral bodies, resulting in what is seen radiographically as Schmorl's node. These chronic changes leave the disc vulnerable to acute rupture or trauma, or both.

Clinical Features

Low back pain is the patient's earliest complaint. It is frequently insidious in nature and is generally worse after prolonged activity or work. The pain lasts only a few days and generally resolves spontaneously or with limitation of activity and bedrest. It is not initially associated with sciatica. It can be made worse with standing or lifting, and is generally relieved with rest. Early symptoms are attributable to degeneration of the annulus fibrosus. At these early stages it is difficult to discern from other causes of low back pain. In time, episodes become more frequent and pain more intense. Symptoms generally do not completely resolve between acute episodes. Gradually, even minor trauma or simply coughing or stooping can bring on acute pain. In time, the patient may have referred pain, but true radicular pain in the dermatomal distribution is significant for nerve root compression and is a late finding due to disc herniation. On physical examination, there is pain to palpation of the involved area. Acute episodes will be associated with paravertebral muscle spasm. Palpation of the posterior facet joints, between and lateral to the spinous processes, can elicit tenderness due to chronic inflammation. Straight leg raising tests are generally negative, unless a bulging weakened disc causes minor compression on the nerve root. In the case of actual disc rupture, back pain and true sciatica will be present. Refer to the section on acute disc herniation for a description of this clinical entity.

Radiographs

It is important to note that evidence of chronic degenerative joint disease of the spine is often present in asymptomatic patients. As such, the emergency spe-

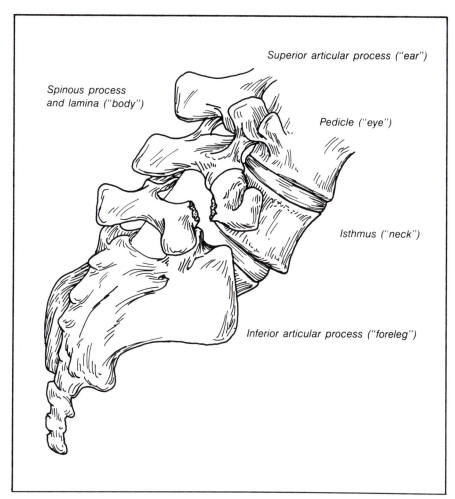

Figure 19–11. Spondylolisthesis, the "Scotty dog" sign.

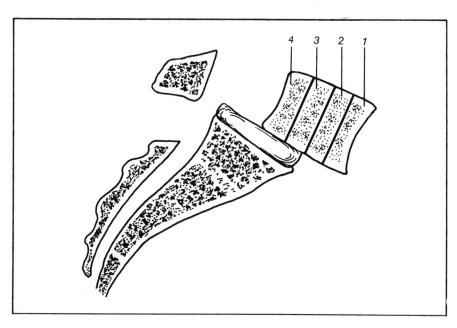

Figure 19–12. Four stages of spondylolisthesis.

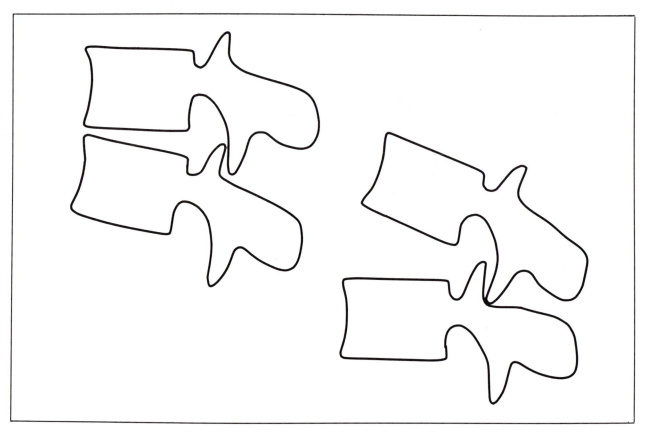

Figure 19–13. Early changes of degenerative disc disease.

cialist cannot always attribute such changes to the etiology of the patient's discomfort. Nevertheless, typical changes of spondylosis include thinning or loss of height in the disc space, sclerosis of subchondral bone, peripheral osteophytes and traction spurs, Schmorl's nodes, vacuum disc, and calcification of the nucleus.

Treatment

In the event of acute exacerbation, therapy is conservative, including bedrest with the knees flexed, nonsteroidal anti-inflammatory medications, antispasmodics in the event of significant muscle spasm, and local heat. Exercise to reduce lumbar lordosis and patient education to avoid increased lumbar strain (heavy lifting, sleeping in the prone position) are encouraged after acute symptoms resolve. Patients with evidence of acute disc herniation, particularly those with neurologic compromise, should be immediately referred.

Neoplasm

In-depth discussion of this subject appears elsewhere in the text. A brief overview is presented here for continuity. If any of the following are serious considerations in the differential of your patient, the authors recommend referring to the principal discussions.

Primary tumors of the spine are relatively rare. Benign tumors normally affect the posterior vertebral processes and occur in patients less than 30 years old. Malignant tumors most commonly involve the anterior vertebral elements in patients over 50, the most common of which is myeloma. Metastatic disease to the spine, however, is quite common with back pain being the presenting complaint in up to 25% of all malignancies. Patients are generally over 50, and low back pain has been present for over a month and is frequently associated with constitutional symptoms. Changes in all of the above are varied depending on the etiology. They include diffuse osteoporosis, osteolytic or osteoblastic lesions, or pathologic compression fractures. In all cases, the x-ray findings lag considerably behind symptoms.

Axiom: *Radiographic findings of spinal neoplasms generally lag behind symptoms by as much as four to six months or more. This is due to the fact that up to 50% of the bony matrix must be replaced by tumor before x-rays will change appearance.*

Osteoporosis

By far the most common metabolic cause of low back pain is osteoporosis. Pain is most often due to vertebral compression fractures, which usually occur between T-8 and L-1. This is due to a marked loss of trabecular bone. This condition is most commonly symptomatic in postmenopausal women, although it occurs in both sexes with advancing age. The specific clinical findings, x-ray findings, and treatment of osteoporosis are considered in detail elsewhere in this text. Refer to Chapter 4 if this is a serious consideration in the differential of your patient.

☐ HISTORY AND PHYSICAL EXAMINATION

As can be seen in the previous discussion, there are numerous causes of low back pain. Although the specific etiology in some patients may be obvious, more typically the acute presentation of several entities might be indistinguishable from others. Most important is distinguishing local musculoskeletal conditions from referred back pain due to life-threatening systemic conditions. Also, the emergency physician is commonly presented with a malingerer, that special patient whose primary objective is compensation or medication. A careful and thorough history and physical examination are indispensable in narrowing a differential diagnosis of low back pain. Elicit findings pointing toward a definitive diagnosis.

History

It is the authors' opinion that it is wise practice to ask a series of general questions of every patient regardless of their primary complaint. Although seemingly obvious and typically a part of all patient histories, specifically eliciting this information at the outset of every examination before the patient focuses on his or her primary complaint gives the examiner a general background of that particular individual. The questions include[17]:

1. Age
2. Previous medical problems
3. Previous hospitalizations or surgery
4. Drug allergy
5. Medications
6. Presently followed by a physician and when was the last time

The next obvious line of questioning involves the patient's principal complaint, that being back or leg pain. Focusing on onset and chronology can help distinguish degenerative from traumatic etiologies. Onset after exertion or trauma will point to mild facet sprain, posterior facet syndrome, or sacroiliac sprain. The sudden onset of back pain with radiation to the lower extremities is suggestive of an acute disc herniation. Gradually increasing pain with frequent exacerbations due to trauma is more suggestive of spondylosis, neoplasm, or osteoporosis in the elderly. The same type of insidious pain associated with radiation is more typical of stenosis, but can be seen also in degenerative spondylosis. Pain of insidious onset in the younger patient suggests fibrositis or spondylolisthesis. Similar complaints also associated with constitutional symptoms might suggest vertebral or disc space infection or sacroiliitis.

Frequent exacerbation of pain suggests mild facet sprain, posterior facet syndrome, fibrositis, or spondylolisthesis. Pain that resolves with rest suggests spinal stenosis or vascular etiologies. Pain from metastatic disease, on the other hand, is constant and frequently worse with rest.

Referred pain should be differentiated from radiating pain. Referred pain is more typically associated with soft tissue injuries, is more focal, and does not necessarily correspond to a specific dermatome. Radiating pain, on the other hand, suggests nerve root compression, is associated with paresthesias, numbness, tingling, and motor weakness, all corresponding to specific dermatomes. The number of dermatomes involved is significant. Multiple root involvement is more common of spinal stenosis, cauda equina syndrome, or massive disc herniation. The patient might not necessarily be aware of specific weakness of muscle groups, but might complain of an unsteady gait or instability of the knees, suggestive of an L-5 nerve root involvement.

Although unfortunately often overlooked in the emergency setting, in the case of low back pain, a social history might suggest social or psychologic problems that can amplify the patient's complaints. An occupational history, however, is mandatory and can provide valuable information regarding physical activity, heavy lifting, repetitive tasks, or significant exposures.

If not already elicited in general questioning at the outset of the examination, a more thorough general history regarding specific questions on systemic diseases, diabetes, tumors, and depression, and psychotherapy can provide valuable information. Finally, a thorough drug history, including allergies or previous adverse effects, is useful in reminding the patient of previous ailments and can help to avoid inappropriate use. It is important, as well, to specifically ask about recreational or "street" drugs.

Physical Examination

It should be stated emphatically at the outset that patients presenting with low back pain require a complete systemic physical examination. Table 19–1 lists a number of systemic conditions that can present with referred low back pain. The specific physical examination for patients with low back pain of musculoskeletal origin is comprised of four phases: standing, sitting, supine, and a separate neurologic examination. An exception to this format is the patient who presents with such severe pain that he or she is unable to stand or sit.

Standing

At the outset, the patient should be observed while standing, unclothed except for an open hospital gown, for evidence of excessive lordotic curve, scoliosis, kyphosis, gluteal asymmetry, or listing. Scoliosis or kyphosis may be a congenital anomaly. Absence of lordotic curve is suggestive of significant paravertebral muscle spasm. Gluteal asymmetry suggests neurologic involvement of the S-1 nerve group. A listing stance favoring one side can suggest weakness to the nerve root involvement and muscle atrophy. Spina bifida is not infrequently associated with a small tuft of hair in the midline of the lumbosacral area. Range of motion should be determined and measured in all directions. Generalized decreased motion in all directions is associated with muscle spasm or congenital deformities. Patients with disc degeneration when they bend forward (at the pelvis) will return to the upright position with the knees and hips slightly flexed and the pelvis tucked under the spine. As paravertebral muscle spasm is a common finding in most patients with low back pain, standing upright from the flexed position will be painful. Pain on hyperextension is evident in spinal stenosis, lumbar disc disease, and neoplasm. Lateral movement is generally unaffected in most conditions causing low back pain, with the exception of herniated discs, where the patient might purposefully list to one side and avoid either tension or compression of the involved nerve root. The stoop test, where the patient stoops to the ground in complete knee and hip flexion, is most sensitive for intermittent cauda equina syndrome, suggestive of nerve root compression from osteophytes, vertebral subluxation, malignancy, or central disc herniation. Subtle evidence of nerve compression can also be ascertained by observing the gait, which is frequently abnormal due to muscle weakness from compression of the L-5 or S-1 nerve root. Extension of the leg at the hip may produce pain in the presence of L-4 nerve root entrapment. Palpation for tenderness along the sciatic nerve can be palpated with the hip flexed at the midpoint between the ischial tuberosity and the greater trochanter. This is suggestive of nerve root compression.

Sitting

Motor examination of the quadriceps muscles should be done in the sitting position. Weakness is suggestive of L-4 nerve root compression. At this time, both patellar and Achilles reflexes can be tested; a diminished knee jerk suggests L-4 nerve root involvement; diminished ankle jerk suggests S-1 nerve root involvement. The posture in the seated position should be carefully observed. A patient with nerve root entrapment will frequently lean back involuntarily and shift the weight away from the affected side. A Valsalva maneuver in this position tests for increased intrathecal pressure and can exacerbate both back and radiating leg pain.

Supine

The patient with significant low back pain will feel more comfortable with a pillow placed under the knees. This will also help to relax the abdominal muscles and allow for deep abdominal palpation for masses or aneurysms. Careful measurements should be made of leg lengths (a difference of approximately 1 inch can significantly alter posture and place abnormal stresses on the posterior facet joints), thighs, and calves (discrepancies suggest muscle atrophy). Careful inspection, palpation, and manipulation of the hip, knee, and ankles can suggest local etiologies of pain.

Specific maneuvers in the supine position to test for spinal cord or nerve root impingement include:

Straight Leg Raising Test (Lasegue). With the leg fully extended in the supine position, the examiner uses one hand to stabilize the pelvis and with the other hand passively elevates the leg by the heel. Pain in the sciatic distribution is considered a positive test; however, back pain alone is negative (Fig 19–8).

Also attributed to Lasegue is a variation of straight leg raising with the knee and hip flexed to 90 degrees. Complaints of leg pain in the sciatic distribution when the knee is passively extended is a positive test.

Fajersztan Test. This is also a variation of the straight leg raising test involving dorsiflexion of the foot (Fig 19–9). Exacerbation of radicular pain is considered positive.

Well-Leg Straight Leg Raising Test. This is similar to the straight leg raising test except the examiner elevates the leg on the uninvolved side. Sciatic pain on the involved side is considered a positive test.

Hoover Test. This test is designed to catch the malingerer who complains of an inability to raise the leg at all. When one attempts to actively elevate an extended leg in the supine position, a downward pressure must be exerted in the opposite leg. If the examiner passively cups the heel of both legs this downward pressure can be determined if the patient is actually trying to elevate the involved leg (Fig 19–14).

Kern Test. With the patient in the supine position forceful flexion of the cervical spine can exacerbate the nerve root compression in the lumbosacral area.

Tests eliciting increased intrathecal pressure include:

Milgram Test. This is an active test requiring the patient to elevate both legs in the extended position approximately 2 inches off the table and hold that position for 30 seconds. This increases intra-abdominal and intrathecal pressure. If the patient cannot hold the position due to increased pain in the lumbosacral area,

either intrathecal or extrathecal pathology including herniated disc is suggested. Unfortunately, this manuever is difficult for most patients with low back pain due to paravertebral muscle spasm.

Pelvic Rock Test. With the hands placed bilaterally over the iliac crest, the thumbs over the anterior superior iliac spines, the examiner compresses the pelvis toward the midline. A positive test elicits sacroiliac joint pain (Fig 19–15).

Gaenslen's Sign. In the supine position, the patient is asked to hold both legs to the chest, while one buttock extends over the edge of the table, and the unsupported leg is allowed to drop over the edge of the table. The patient with sacroiliac joint disease will complain of pain in the sacroiliac joint (Fig 19–16).

FABERE (Patrick) Test. With the patient in the supine position, the foot on the involved side is placed over the opposite knee and the knee is abducted (Fig 19–17). Pain in the inguinal area suggests hip joint in-

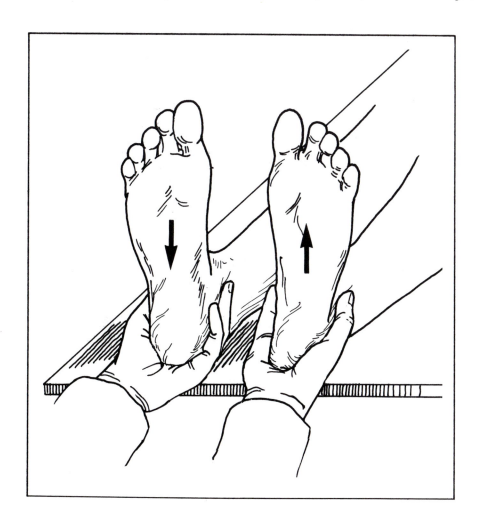

Figure 19–14. The Hoover test.

volvement. Gentle downward pressure on the knee while stabilizing the pelvis over the opposite anterior iliac spine will elicit sacroiliac joint pain.

A test to assist neurologic segmentation innervation of L-1 can be done in the supine position and is called Beevor's sign. In the supine position with the knees flexed and the arms folded across the chest, the patient is asked to do a one-quarter sit-up. Normally, the umbilicus should not move; movement to either side suggests weakness of the rectus abdominus muscles on the involved side (Fig 19–18).

Neurologic Examination

A complete motor, sensory, and reflex examination should be done on all patients who complain of acute back pain. Table 19–3 concisely reflects all of the positive findings of the various nerve root levels.

At the risk of deception, or even voyeurism, it is often instructive to observe the patient dressing or moving about the examination room without his or her knowledge. Abnormal movement suggestive of discomfort or neurologic involvement may further support your diagnosis. Inconsistencies or even complete resolution of symptoms and signs may prove fascinating. Although diagnostic in the setting of underlying malignancy metastatic to bone, unless patients present with neurologic deficits (when CT and myelography are indicated), emergency bone scans are not warranted.

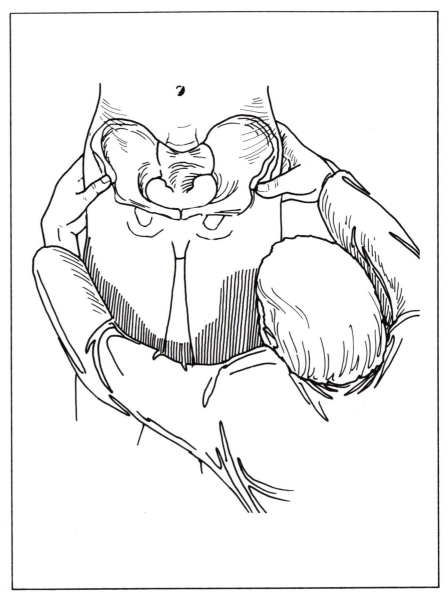

Figure 19–15. The pelvic rock test.

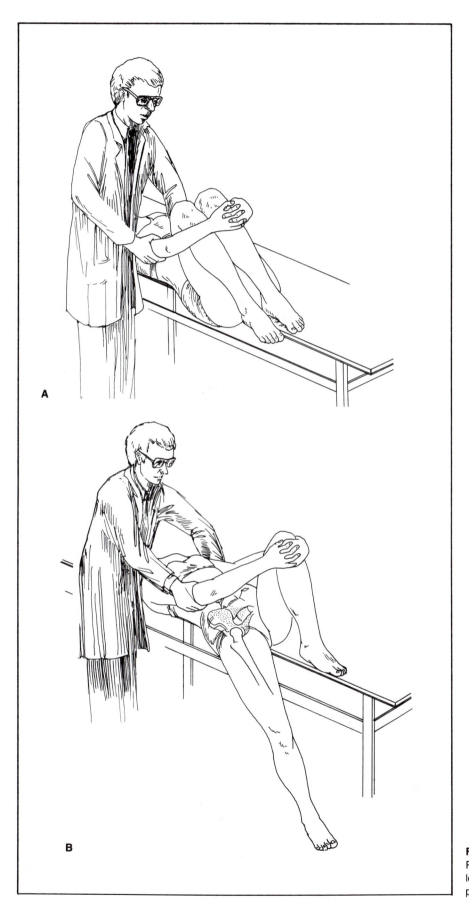

Figure 19–16. Gaenslen's test. **A.** Patient on edge of bed. **B.** Leg allowed to drop causing sacroiliac joint pain. (See text for discussion.)

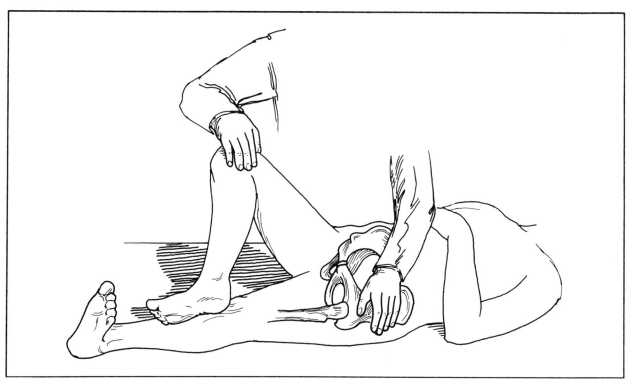

Figure 19–17. Patrick or FABERE test.

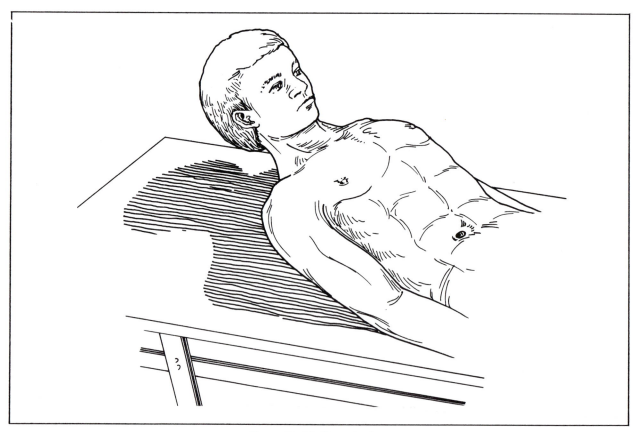

Figure 19–18. Beevor's sign.

□ LUMBAR SPINE RADIOGRAPHY

As early as 1976, Hall[18] demonstrated that approximately 7 million lumbar spine x-rays were done annually at an estimated cost of $500 million. Each series of films (AP, lateral, and oblique views) subjects the patient to a gonadal radiation exposure of approximately 392 millirads in women, 71 millirads in men. Although certain specific x-ray findings have been associated with LBP, numerous studies that compare LBP sufferers with controls have found a similar incidence of the same radiographic abnormalities in controls.[19–22]

Most studies suggesting specific criteria for lumbosacral films predict significant reductions in their use based on primary care office visit complaints of LBP. Although not necessarily always the case, patients presenting with LBP to the emergency room are more likely to have sustained either acute onset or exacerbation of pain. Studies suggest[1,9,15,18,23] that appropriate indications for emergency radiography for these patients include:

1. History of significant major trauma or certain instances of minor trauma in patients with known or suspected underlying pathology
2. History or physical examination consistent with underlying pathology
3. Presence of neurologic deficit
4. Inability to appropriately clinically evaluate, i.e., altered mental status, severe pain

Diagnostic studies beyond plain radiographs include computed tomography (CT) scanning and myelography. For numerous reasons, CT scanning is a study of choice for emergent evaluation of LBP with associated neurologic deficits. CT is safer, cheaper, and provides more specific information regarding vertebral bodies, posterior elements, paravertebral soft tissue masses, spinal stenosis, and actual bulging discs, particularly in lateral herniations. In many centers, a stepwise approach is used. Unequivocal CT findings are considered diagnostic. Myelography or CT with metrizamide myelography are used if initial studies are equivocal or do not correspond with the clinical findings.

Patients with suggestive history and physical examination consistent with vertebral osteomyelitis or disc space infection require radionuclide bone scanning in the emergent setting. Although diagnostic in the setting of underlying malignancy metastatic to bone, unless patients present with neurologic deficits (when CT and myelography are indicated), emergency bone scans are not warranted.

□ TREATMENT

Because most LBP is regional in occurrence, secondary to minor trauma or strain, the vast majority of pain syndromes completely resolve regardless of therapy, 50% within 1 week, 80% by 2 weeks, 90% by 2 months.[23] Evaluating specific therapeutic modalities has proved difficult due to the many causes of LBP, poor specific diagnosis, and subjective nature of the pain. Studies that are available have been discredited for these and methodologic reasons.[24] Nevertheless, except in circumstances of neurologic deficits or underlying pathology, the authors recommend the following conservative regimen.

Bedrest
Patients uniformly report symptomatic improvement after strict bedrest, allowing only bathroom privileges. Intradiscal pressures are reduced to one-fifth that of standing by lying on a flat surface or with hips and knees slightly flexed with a pillow placed under the knees (Fig 19–19). Weisel and colleagues[25] demonstrated that military recruits could return to full activity after acute low back injury 40 to 50% sooner than those who remained ambulatory. More recently Deyo and colleagues[26] concluded from the results of a randomized clinical trial that patients without neuromotor deficits responded well and were able to return to functional activity after 2 days of bedrest rather than the previously described 1 to 2 weeks. Although traction theoretically reduces intradiscal pressure further, 25% of the body weight is required to adequately distract vertebrae,[6] yet controlled studies showed no subjective benefit to bedrest alone.[18]

Stretch and Spray
Myofascial trigger points, hyperirritable foci located in skeletal muscle or fascia, frequently respond to stretch and spray techniques. Trigger points result in referred pain, are palpable fibers with a nodular consistency, and are areas of maximal tenderness that frequently elicit a jump sign when palpated, literally causing the patient to jump on palpation.

The muscle to be stretched should be pretreated by a stream of vapocoolant spray (a fluoromethane spray mixture of 15% dichlorodifluoromethane and 85% trichloromonofluoromethane, and therefore preferable to ethyl chloride, although both are effective), which is sprayed in one direction to the skin overlying the involved muscle until the skin appears pale. The muscle is then stretched. This should be immediately followed by the application of moist heat to rewarm the skin and prevent posttreatment soreness. Patients may complain of residual soreness for 1 or 2 days.[6]

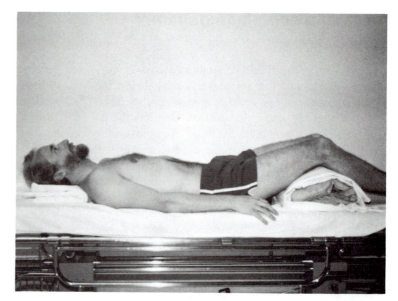

Figure 19–19. Position of rest in acute LBP syndromes.

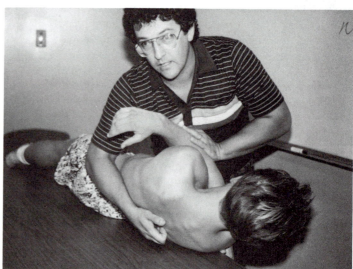

Figure 19–20. Technique for reduction of costovertebral facet subluxation.

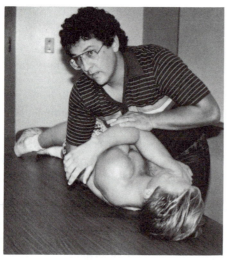

Figure 19–21. A rapid thrust with a short excursion is applied.

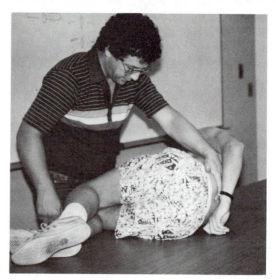

Figure 19–22. Various positions of flexion of the hip and the knee will determine which facet is manipulated.

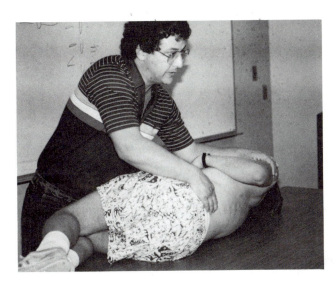

Figure 19–23. Rotate the patient's spine as shown.

Spinal Manipulation

There are limited indications for manipulation to be used in the emergency center. These include facet subluxation or "facet syndrome" in the lower back and costovertebral facet subluxation.

Both facet syndrome and costovertebral facet subluxation present to the emergency center with sudden onset of acute, severe incapacitating pain. The pain is sharp and well localized. In costovertebral subluxation the pain is localized in the thoracic spine usually over the region of T-5 to T-8 directly over the involved rib articulation with the vertebra. In facet syndrome facet pain is localized in the lumbar region either at L-2 or L-4.

When patients present with either of these syndromes a simple manipulation properly carried out can bring significant pain relief.

Costovertebral Facet Subluxation

Place the hand in a cupped position over the involved articulation with the fingers over the spinous processes and the base of the hand over the involved rib. Place the patient supine with the arms over the chest (Fig 19–20). A rapid thrust with short excursion but significant force is then applied (Fig 19–21), while the cupped hand displaces the rib inferiorly.

Facet Syndromes

Place the patient in the position indicated in Figure 19–22. The amount of bend in the knee will determine which facet will be manipulated. Rotate the patient's spine as shown in Figure 19–23 to the physiologic point of maximum bend, then a rapid thrust is applied with short excursion.

Drugs

Common to all of the acute musculoskeletal causes of low back pain and exacerbations of more chronic syndromes is an inflammatory response of pain-sensitive structures. Thus, an anti-inflammatory medication is recommended. So far, none of the nonsteroidal anti-inflammatory drugs (NSAIDs) has been proven to be more effective than aspirin. Although considerably more expensive, NSAIDs are effective, many have fewer gastrointestinal side effects, and are more convenient; therefore, they can be considered when circumstances warrant. When acute pain is severe, narcotics (i.e., aspirin with codeine) might be required, although these are discouraged when not necessary as resultant constipation leads to straining.

When acute injury leads to significant muscle spasm, the use of muscle relaxants appears to bring symptomatic relief to many patients, although clear experimental evidence is lacking. Diazepam (inexpensive, but potentially abused) and cyclobenzaprine (more expensive, causes drowsiness) are recommended, their sedative effects promoting bedrest.

Heat and Cold Applications

The efficacy of applications of heat and cold in the acute setting has not been established. Cold application after acute ligamentous injury theoretically diminishes blood flow and, hence, local bleeding and inflammation at the site. Application of cold packs (ice bag or wet towel placed in the freezer) for 10 to 15 minutes, as frequently as every hour while awake for the first 24 to 48 hours, often provides relief.

Application of heat theoretically increases blood flow, relaxes muscle spasm, and improves healing, although symptomatic relief is individual. In cases where muscle injury is primary and after a course of cold therapy in ligamentous injuries, we recommend the use of a hot towel wrapped in plastic for 10 to 15 minutes as frequently as every hour while awake. Electrical heating pads are discouraged as patients on sedative medications can sustain significant burns.

After 7 to 10 days of the above therapy, most

patients achieve significant relief. All patients should be referred to an orthopedist for follow-up at that time when, depending on the symptoms, other treatment modalities can be considered, including exercises, ultrasound, diathermy or, in the case of disc herniation, surgery or chymopapain therapy. All of these, particularly surgical intervention or chymopapain, are non-emergent considerations, discussion of which is beyond the scope of this text.

□ REFERENCES

1. Hockberger RS: Low back pain. The Digest of Emergency Medical Care, March 1986
2. Kelsey JL, et al: The impact of musculoskeletal disorders on the population of the United States. J Bone Joint Surg 61A:959, 1979
3. Campbell RM, et al: Clinical characteristics of fibrocytis: A 'blinded' controlled study of symptoms and tender points. Arthritis Rhum 26:817, 1983
4. McNab I: Spondylogenic backache: Soft tissue lesions. In McNab I (ed): Backache. Baltimore, Williams & Wilkins, 1977, p 80
5. Nachemson A: Toward a better understanding of low back pain: A review of the mechanics of the lumbar spine. Rheumatol Rehabil 14:129, 1975
6. Simons DG, Travell JG: Myofascial origins of low back pain. Postgrad Med 73(2):66, 1983
7. Turek SL: Lumbosacral sprain. In Orthopedics: Principles and Application, 4th ed. Philadelphia, JB Lippincott, 1984, p 1512
8. Dorwart RH, et al: Spinal stenosis. Radiol Clin North Am 41(2):301, 1981
9. Paine KWE: Clinical features of lumbar spinal stenosis. Clin Orthop 115:77, 1976
10. Epstein NE, Epstein JA: Lumbar spinal stenosis. In Camins M, O'Leary P (eds): The Lumbar Spine. New York, Raven Press, 1987, p 149
11. Kirkaldy-Willis WH, et al: Lumbar spinal stenosis. Clin Orthop 99:30, 1974
12. Rothman RH, Simeone FA: Lumbar disc disease. In Rothman RH, Simeone FA (eds): The Spine. Philadelphia, WB Saunders, 1982, p 443
13. Wiltse LL, et al: Classification of spondylolysis and spondylolisthesis. Clin Orthop 117:23, 1976
14. Gramse RR, et al: Lumbar spondylolisthesis: A rational approach to conservative treatment. Mayo Clin Proc 55:681, 1980
15. Magora A: Conservative treatment of spondylolisthesis. Clin Orthop 117:74, 1976
16. McNab I: Disc degeneration. In McNab I (ed): Backache. Baltimore, Williams & Wilkins, 1977, p 84
17. Baraff LJ: Personal instruction
18. Hall FM: Overutilization of radiologic examinations. Radiology 120:443, 1976
19. Scavone JG, et al: Use of lumbar spine films: Statistical evaluation at a university teaching hospital. JAMA 246:1105, 1981
20. Splithoff CA: Lumbosacral junction in patients with and without backache. JAMA 152:17: 1610, 1953
21. Rowe ML: Low back pain in industry: A position paper. J Occup Med 11:161, 1969
22. Torgerson WR, Dotter WE: Comparative roentgenographic study of the asymptomatic and symptomatic lumbar spine. J Bone J Surg 58A:850, 1976
23. Quinet RS, Hadler AM: Diagnosis and treatment of backache. Semin Arthritis Rheum 8:261, 1979
24. Deyo BA: Conservative therapy for low back pain: Distinguishing useful from useless therapy. JAMA 250:1057, 1983
25. Weisel SW, et al: Acute low back pain: An objective analysis of conservative therapy. Spine 5(4)324, 1980
26. Deyo RA, et al: How many days of bedrest for acute low back pain? N Engl J Med 315(17):1064, 1986

□ Bibliography

Brown MD: Diagnosis of pain syndromes of the spine. Orthop Clin North Am 6(1):233, 1975

Kein HA: Low back pain. In Clinical Symposium, No. 25, CEBA Series, 1973

Lankorst G, et al: Natural history of idiopathic low back pain. Scan J Rehab Med 17:1, 1985

Lechtenberg R: Nonsurgical treatments of low back pain. In Camins MB, O'Leary PF (eds): The Lumbar Spine. New York, Raven Press, 1987, p 393

Levine RL, Schutta HS: Lumbosacral root syndromes. In Camins MB, O'Leary PF (eds): The Lumbar Spine. New York, Raven Press, 1987, p 136

Leang M, Komaroff AL: Roentgenograms in primary care patients with acute low pack pain: A cost effectiveness analysis. Arch Intern Med 143:1108, 1982

Nachemson AL: The lumbar spine: An orthopedic challenge. Spine 1(1):59, 1976

Nachemson AL: Recent advances in the treatment of low back pain. Int Orthop 9:1, 1985

Neidra A: Low back pain: Evaluation and treatment in the emergency department setting. Emerg Med Clin North Am 2(2):441, 1984

Paris SV: Anatomy as related to function and pain, Symposium on Evaluation and Care of Lumbar Spine Problems. Orthop Clin North Am 14(3):475, 1983

Reuler JB: Low back pain. West J Med 143(2):259, 1985

Schellinger D: The low back pain syndrome, Symposium on Radiolgy. Med Clin North Am 68(6):1631, 1984

Simeone FA, Rothman RH: Clinical usefulness of CT scanning in the diagnosis and treatment of lumbar spine disease, Symposium on CT of the Lumbar Spine. Radiol Clin North Am 21(2):197, 1983

Smallberger GG: History and physical examination of the lumbar spine. In Camins MB, O'Leary PF (eds): The Lumbar Spine. New York, Raven Press, 1987, p 35

Tepperman PS, Devlin M: Therapeutic heat and cold—A practitioner's guide. Postgrad Med 73(1):69, 1983

Waddell G, Main CJ: Assessment of severity in low back disorders. Spine 9(2):204, 1984

Yong-Hing K, Kirkaldy-Willis WH: The pathophysiology of degenerative disease of the lumbar spine, Symposium on Evaluation and Care of Lumbar Spine Problems. Orthop Clin North Am 14(3):491, 1983

Index

Abdominal aortic aneurysm, 180
Abdominal breathing, 4
Abdomen
  examination, misleading, 221
  injuries, 8, 235
    distraction injury with, 222
  muscle tone, 167, 241
  musculature, innervation, 184, 196, 197
  pain, 246
  pathology, low back pain referred from, 252–253
Abdominal reflex, 184
Achilles reflex, 260
Acupuncture, fibrositis, 265
Adson maneuver, 93, 144, 145, 147
Age
  ankylosing spondylitis, 25
  central cord syndrome, 15
  chondrosarcoma, 51
  eosinophilic granuloma, 49
  Ewing's sarcoma, 53
  giant cell tumor, 49
  intervertebral disc infection in children, 44
  lumbosacral strains and sprains, 240–243
  malignant lymphoma, 51
  multiple myeloma, 51
  muscles of neck, 131
  osteoarthritis of spine, 29
  osteochondrome, 47
  osteoid osteoma, 48
  osteoporosis, 34
  pyogenic osteomyelitis, 38
  spinal cord injury, 2
Airplane accidents, 222
Airway, 4, 6
  maintenance, 4
  management, 6
Alcoholism, 34
Allen test, 144–145
Aminoglycoside, 39
Amyloidosis, 27
Anabolic steroids, 36

Anal pain, 53
Anal wink, 184
Analgesia, 36
Anemia, 51, 54
Aneurysmal bone cysts, 50, 51
Aneurysmal dilatation of arteries, 147
Ankle fractures, 226
Ankle jerk, 183
Ankylosing spondylitis, 24–29, 167, 171, 198, 265
  cervical spine, 26
  clinical course, 26
  clinical features, 25
  complications, 26–27
  diagnosis, 27–28
  exercise in, 25, 29
  incidence, 24–25
  insignificant trauma and, 26
  lumbar spine in, 26
  management and referral, 28–29
  pathophysiology, 25
  peripheral joint involvement, 26
  physical examination, 25–26
  prognosis, 26–27
  sacroiliac joint, 27
  symptoms, 26
  thoracic spine in, 26
Anterior cord syndrome, 14–15, 16, 114, 115
Antibiotic therapy, 39, 43, 45, 236
  prophylactic, 236
Anti-inflammatory drugs, 23, 31, 36, 277
  low back pain, 277
  nonsteroidal (NSAIDs), 23, 31, 36, 277
Antimicrobial therapy, 42
Aortic aneurysm, abdominal, 180
Aortic insufficiency, 180
Aortitis, 27
Arachnoid, 66
Arachnoiditis, 103, 236
  myelography and, 236
Arms. See Upper extremities
Arteries, cervical spine, 71, 74

Arteriography, 152
Arthridities of spine, 20–32
  ankylosing spondylitis, 24–29
  osteoarthritis of spine, 29–32
  rheumatoid arthritis, 20–24
Arthritis of spine. See Arthridities of spine
Articular processes, 60–61
Aspergillosis, 27
Aspirin, 28, 30, 31, 48, 49
Ataxia, 22
Athletic accidents. See Sports injuries
Atlantoaxial complex, 61
Atlantoaxial disassociation, 107
Atlantoaxial dislocation, pediatric, 132–133
Atlantoaxial disruption, 127, 128, 132
  pediatric, 132
Atlantoaxial joint
  greater occipital nerve syndrome, 151
  osteoarthritis and, 29
  rheumatoid arthritis, 20–21, 22, 23
Atlantoaxial ligaments, 61
Atlantoaxial subluxation, 20, 21, 22, 23, 24, 27, 132
  ankylosing spondylitis, 27
  pediatric, 132–133
Atlanto-occipital disruption, 127–128
Atlanto-occipital dissociation, 107
Atlanto-occipital fusion, 102
Atlas, 60, 61, 62, 63, 78
  distance to dens, 109, 112
  fracture, 125
  fractures, 108, 111, 124–125, 133
    avulsion fracture, 124
    burst fractures, 133
    of ring, 108, 111
  rheumatoid arthritis and, 109
Auscultation, 180
Automobile accidents. See Motor vehicle accidents
Automobile head rests, 136, 138
Automobile riding, cervical disc patients, 142

Avulsion fracture, 102, 124, 138
  atlas, 124
Axial compression, 107, 110
Axial compression test, 199, 200
Axial traction, 118, 119
Axillary artery, 144
Axillary nerve, 90–92
Axis, 60, 62, 63, 109, 112, 113,
      125–126
  extension teardrop fracture, 124
  spondylolisthesis, 109–112, 113,
      125–126

Babinski sign, 12, 21, 184, 188
Back pain, 249. See also Low back
      pain
  abdominal examination, 178
  chronic, 228, 239
  functional (nonorganic) pain, 198–
      200
  leg length and, 167
  scoliosis, 245
Backboard, half and long, 4
Bamboo spine, 27, 28
Bedrest, 36, 43, 45, 223, 275, 276
  low back pain, 275, 276
  prolonged, 223
Beevor's sign, 196, 272, 274
Biceps, 87, 88
Birth trauma, 150
Bladder, 16, 18, 30
  control, 30
  dysfunction, 16, 18
    Cauda equina syndromes, 18
    central cord syndrome, 16
Blunt trauma, spinal cord injury, 17
Blurred vision, 139, 151
Bones, 99, 101, 174–178
  palpation, 174–178
  radiography, 99, 101
Bowel control, 30
Brachial plexus injuries, 67, 72, 73,
      144, 149–151, 234–235
  clinical features, 150
  mechanisms, 150
  postfixed plexus, 149
  prefixed plexus, 149
Brachioradialis reflex testing, 88
Bracing, 51, 54
  metastatic disease, 54
  multiple myeloma, 51
Brain damage, 137
Breathing, 4, 6. See also Respiration
  abdominal, 4
  spinal injury, 6
Brown-Séquard syndrome, 17, 129,
      236
Brudzinski's sign, 191, 192
Bruits, 80, 93, 144

carotid arteries, 80
  costoclavicular maneuver, 93, 144
Bulging fontanelle, 132
Burners, 151
Burns of torso, 244
Burst fractures, 15, 121–122, 133,
      202, 203, 207, 209, 216, 225,
      226, 227, 228, 229, 233, 235
  atlas, 133
  clinical features, 122
  complications, 122
  computed tomography, 207, 209
  emergency management and referral,
      122
  Jefferson, 121–122
  lateral, 235
  mechanism, 122
  radiography, 122
  thoracolumbar axial load injuries,
      225, 226, 227, 228
  type D, 229
  wedge fractures vs, 216

Cafe-au-lait spots, 245
Calcaneal fractures, 216, 226
Calcification of ligament, 101–102
Calcitonin, 36
Calcitrol, 36
Calcium deficiency, 4
Calcium therapy, 36
Callus formation, 150
CAM (computer-assisted myelography),
      103–104
Capsules, 84
Cardiovascular abnormalities, spinal
      cord trauma, 6–7
Carotid arteries, bruits, 80
Carotid endarterectomy, 152
Carotid pulses, palpation, 79–80
Carpi radialis muscle, extensor, 88
Cartilage, radiography, 99, 101
Catecholamines, 7
Cauda equina injuries, 163, 214, 236.
      See also Cauda equina
      syndrome
Cauda equina syndrome, 18, 27, 220,
      262, 263
Central cord syndrome, 15–17, 115
  age, 15
  clinical features, 16
  management, 17
  mechanisms, 15
  prognosis, 17
Cephalosporin, 39
Cerebral injury, 132
Cerebral palsy, 244
Cerebrospinal fluid, 236
  fecal contamination, 236
  fistulae, 236

Cerebrovascular accidents, 30
Cervical collars, 4, 31, 151, 152
  rigid, 4
  soft, 4, 31, 152
Cervical disc disorders, 140–142
  clinical features, 140–141
  complications, 142
  emergency management and referral,
      142
  hard disc, 140
  radiography, 141
  soft disc, 140
Cervical spinal cord, normal, 15
Cervical spine
  anatomy, 60–71
    anterior structures in neck, 78
    arteries, 71, 74
    brachial plexus, 67, 72, 73
    intervertebral discs, 62–64, 65
    ligaments, 62–64, 65
    muscles, 82–83
    nerve roots, 66–67, 71
    nerve supply, 82–83
    spinal cord, 66–67, 71
    stability and mobility, 61–62
    topical landmarks, 81
    veins, 71, 75
    vertebrae, 60–61, 62
  ankylosing spondylitis, 26
  avulsion fractures, 138
  brachial plexus injuries, 149–151
  children, 130–133. See Children,
      cervical spine
  classification of injuries, 106, 107
  extension injuries, 66, 107, 111,
      122–126, 136–138
  extension–rotation injuries, 107,
      110, 121
  facet dislocation, 107, 109
  flexion injuries, 17, 66, 107, 108,
      114, 116–120, 138–140
  flexion–rotation injuries, 107, 109,
      120–121
  fracture–dislocation, 39, 126
  fractures, 39, 106–133, 151
    atlas, 108, 111, 124–125
    axial compression, 110
    axis, 124
    burst fracture, 122
    clay-shoveler fracture, 117–118
    extension teardrop fracture of
        axis, 124
    flexion teardrop fracture, 118–120
    fracture–dislocation, 39
    hangman's fracture, 109–112,
        113, 124, 125, 126
    Jefferson fracture, 102, 121, 133
    laminar fracture, 125
    odontoid fracture, 107, 109, 129–
        130, 132

pedicle fracture, 125, 133
pillar fracture, 120–121
simple wedge (compression)
    fractures, 116, 117
uncinate process fracture, 126–127
fractures, dislocations, and sublux-
    ations, 106–133, 151. *See also*
    fractures, *above*
anterior dislocations, 114
associated fractures of lower
    cervical spine, 125
atlantoaxial disassociation, 107
atlantoaxial dislocation, 132–133
atlantoaxial disruption, 12, 127–
    128, 127
atlanto-occipital disassociation,
    107
atlanto-occipital disruption, 127–
    128
atlas, 108, 111, 124–125
    fracture, 108, 111, 124–125
    ring, 108, 111
    spondylolisthesis, 124, 125, 126
axial compression, 110
axis, spondylolisthesis, 109–112,
    113
burst fracture, 122
classification by mechanism of
    injury, 106–107
clay-shoveler fracture, 117–118
extension injuries, 122–126
extension–rotation injuries, 107,
    110, 120–121
facet dislocation, 113, 114, 117–
    118, 120
flexion–extension views, 109,
    114, 126, 127, 129
flexion injuries, 17, 107, 108,
    114, 115–120, 138–140
flexion–rotation injuries, 107,
    109, 120–121
flexion teardrop fracture, 118–120
hangman's fractures, 109–112,
    113, 125–126
Jefferson burst fracture, 102, 121,
    133
laminar fracture, 125
lateral flexion, 107, 127
lower cervical spine, 112–114,
    133
neurologic injury, 114
odontoid fractures, 107, 109, 129–
    130, 132
    odontoid process fractures, 109
pediatric, 130–133. *See also*
    Children, cervical spine
pedicle fracture, 125, 133
pillar fracture, 120–121
radiography, 9, 96–103. *See also*
    Radiography, cervical spine

simple wedge (compression)
    fractures, 116–117
spondylolisthesis of axis, 124,
    125, 126
sprain, hyperflexion, 116
stability and, 107–114, 116
    delayed instability, 116
treatment, 115–116
uncinate process fracture, 127
upper cervical spine, 108–112,
    132
vertical compression, correction,
    121–126
intervertebral discs, 62–64, 65
Jefferson fractures, 102, 121, 133
lateral flexion, 107
ligaments, 62–64, 65, 66, 70
mechanisms of trauma, 3
    classification of injury by, 106,
    107
muscles, 66, 67, 68, 69, 70
neurologic injury, 114
osteoarthritis, 29
physical examination, 76–93
    inspection, 76
    neurologic examination, 86–92
    palpation, 76–80
    range of motion, 84–85
radiography, 9, 96–103
rheumatoid arthritis, 20, 21
shortening, 21
spondylosis, 15, 29–30, 31
stability, 107–114
strains and sprains, 136–142
    cervical sprain, 136
    disc disorders, 140–142
    hyperextension injury, 136–138
    hyperflexion injury, 138–140
thoracic outlet syndromes, 144–149
topical landmarks, 81
treatment, 115–116
vertical compression, 121–122
Chaddock test, 184
Chance fractures, 221, 222, 225
Chest, inspection, 76
Chest, 25, 26, 76, 198
    expansion, 26, 198
    inspection, 76
    pain, 25
Chest film, multiple trauma, 202
Chiari malformation, 104
Child abuse, 131–132
Children, 44, 130–133, 152, 153, 244
    cervical spine, 130–133
        atlantoaxial dislocation, 132
        clinical evaluation, 130
        first cervical vertebra, 130
        incidence of fractures and
        dislocations, 130
        ligament disruption, 132

lower spine, 133
newborn, 131–132
odontoid fracture, 132
other injuries, 133
second cervical vertebra, 131
third cervical vertebra, 131
upper spine, 132–133
vertebral arches C-1 through C-3,
    132
x-ray evaluation, 130–131
child abuse, 131–132
infantile scoliosis, 244
intervertebral disc infection, 44
juvenile scoliosis, 244
torticollis in, 152, 153
Chin, 76
Chiropractic manipulation, 152
Chondrosarcoma, 51
Chordoma, 54, 56
Circulation, assessment, 4
Clavicle, 76, 146, 150
    deformity, 76
    fracture, 146, 150
Clay-shoveler fracture, 117–118
Clonidine for spinal injury, 10
Clunk test, 21
Coccyx, 60, 177–178
    palpation, 177–178
Codfish vertebrae, 36
Cold applications, low back pain,
    277–278
Collar, cervical. *See* Cervical collars
Comatose patients, 4, 127
Complete cord syndrome, 12–14, 17
    early clinical picture, 12
    etiologies, 12
    neurologic examination, 17
    neurologic symptoms, 12
    prognosis, 12–14
Compression fractures, 15, 36, 51,
    116, 117
Compression injuries, 2
    fractures, 15, 36, 51, 116–117
    spine, 2
    vertebral body evaluation, 228
Compression test, 92, 93
Computed tomography (CT), 27, 103,
    207–209
    burst fracture, 207, 209
    facet fracture, 208
    injuries diagnostic for, 207
    laminar fracture, 125, 208
    low back pain, 275
    neoplasms of spine, 47
    pedicle fracture, 207
    pitfalls, 210
    pyogenic spondylitis, 39
    spinal stenosis, 256
    thoracolumbar spine, 207, 208, 209
        axial load injuries, 226–228

Computed tomography (CT) (*cont.*)
thoracolumbar spine (*cont.*)
distraction injuries, 223, 225
flexion injuries, 216
flexion–rotation injuries, 220
lateral bending, 233, 234
with axial load, 234
penetrating injuries, 236
shearing injuries, 230–231, 232, 233
tomography vs, 210
vertebral body, 209
Computer-assisted myelography (CAM), 103–104
Concussion, 129, 130
Conduction defects, 27
Congenital abnormalities, 102, 103, 152
block vertebrae, 102
magnetic resonance imaging, 103
torticollis, 152
Congenital anomaly, 102
Consciousness, 4, 22, 125
loss, 22
comatose patient, 4, 125
Constipation, 53
Contusio cervicalis posterior, 17
Contusions, 18, 238–239
spinal cord, 18
thoracolumbar, 238–239
Convulsions, 132
Cor pulmonale, 246
Cord, spinal. *See* Spinal cord
Corticosteroids, 10, 34
in spinal injury, 10
Costoclavicular maneuver, 93, 144
Costoclavicular syndrome, 144, 146–147
Costovertebral facet subluxation, 276, 277
Costovertebral joints, 26
Costs, 2, 34
osteoporosis, 34
spinal cord injury, 2
Coughing, 216, 239, 241, 254, 257
acute disc herniation, 257
posterior facet syndrome, 254
Cranial nerve abnormalities, 53
Cremasteric reflex, 184, 188
Crick in neck, 152
Cricoid ring, 78–79
Cricothyrotomy, 6, 120
CT. *See* Computed tomography
CT myelography, 220, 231
Cutaneous reflexes, 184
Cyclobenzaprine, 277

Deep tendon reflexes, 183–184, 260
acute disc herniation, 260
Degenerative disease, 102, 103, 151

joint disease, 151
radiography, 101–102
Dens, 61, 102, 109, 112, 124, 129
congenital abnormalities, 102
distance to atlas, 109, 112
fractures, 124, 129
type II, 124
rheumatoid arthritis and, 109
tomography, 102
Dentate ligaments, 66, 70
Dexamethasone in spinal injury, 10
Diabetes mellitus, 38
Diaphragm, 235
Diazepam, 277
Diet, 34
osteoporosis and, 34
phosphate in, high, 34
protein calorie malnutrition, 34
vitamin D deficiency, 34
Dimethyl sulfoxide for spinal injury, 10
Direct blow, 15, 150, 231
to neck, 15
Disc space infection, 103
Discs, intervertebral. *See* Intervertebral discs
Dislocations, 202
cervical spine. *See* Cervical spine, fractures, dislocations, and sub-luxations
facet, 15, 18, 107, 109, 113, 114, 117–118, 120, 218
pediatric atlantoaxial, 132–133
shoulder, 150
type B, 233
Distraction test, 92–93
Diuretics for spinal injury, 10
Diving injuries, 4, 16, 119–120
Dizziness, 116, 151
Dowager's hump, 35
Drowning, 119, 120
Drug abuse, intravenous, 38
Drugs/medications, low back pain, 277
Duodenal compression, 246
Dura, 66, 184, 191
Dysphagia, 31, 116, 123, 137, 141, 142
Dysphonia, 22
Dyspnea, 42

Elastic stretch, 84
Electric shocks, 30
Electrical heating pads, low back pain, 277
Embolism, 147, 217, 236
pulmonary, 217
thromboembolism, 236
Empyema, 39, 42
End feel, 84
Endocrinopathies, 3
Endotracheal intubation, 4

Eosinophilic granuloma, 49
Epidural abscesses, 17, 39, 42
Epidural hematomas, computed tomography of, 103
Epigastric reflex, 184
Erb plexus injuries, 150
Erector spinae muscles, 80
Erythrocyte sedimentation rate (ESR), ankylosing spondylitis, 28
Esophageal obturator, 4
Esophageal tears, 137
Estrogen deficiency, 34
Estrogen replacement therapy, 36
Ethambutol, 42
Ewing's sarcoma, 53, 55
Exercise, 25, 29, 31, 36
ankylosing spondylitis, 25, 29
osteoarthritis, 31
osteoporosis and, 36
Extension injuries, 2, 84, 85, 107, 111, 136–138
associated injuries, 137
causes, 136
cervical spine, 31, 66, 107, 110, 111, 122–126, 136–138
clinical features, 136–137
degenerative disease vs, 101
emergency management and referral, 138
extension teardrop fracture of axis, 124
fracture–dislocations, 99, 126
neck, 15
odontoid process, 99
radiography, 101, 137–138
range of motion, 84, 85
rotation simultaneous with, 107, 110, 121
sprain, cervical spine, 122–124. *See also* Hyperextension sprain
thoracolumbar spine, 170, 230
Extension–rotation injuries, 107, 110, 121
Extension teardrop fracture of axis, 124
Extremities, 42, 76, 139, 140, 181–182, 226
circumference, 181–182
lower, 42, 226
fractures, 226
referred pain, 42
upper, 76, 139, 140
pain radiating to, 140
symmetry, 76
weakness in, 139
Eyes, pain in, 20

FABERE (Patrick) test, 194–196, 271–272, 274
Facet joints, 29, 60, 78, 79, 159, 161,

170, 254–255
osteoarthritis, 29
palpation, 78, 79, 254
posterior facet syndrome, 254–255
subluxation or dislocation, 78
thoracic, 159, 161
Facet syndrome, 254–255, 276, 277
posterior, 254–255
Facets, 60. *See also* entries beginning
Facet
dislocations, 15, 18, 78, 107, 109,
113, 114, 117–118, 120, 218
fractures, 209, 218
interlocking, 100
locked, 118, 119, 120
osteoarthritis, 29
palpation, 78, 79, 254
perched, 118
posterior facet syndrome, 254–255
subluxations, 78, 240
Facial fracture, 126
Fajersztan test, 261, 270
Falling asleep in forearm or arm, 145,
146
Falls, 216, 226
tuck-and-roll landing, 218, 219
Femoral head and neck fractures, 35
Femoral nerve and root injuries, 184
Femoral nerve and root tests, 196
Femoral stretch test, 196
Fibrositis, 263–265
clinical features, 264
as syndrome, 263
treatment, 264–265
Flexion injuries, 2, 15, 17, 80, 84, 85,
107, 108, 115–116, 138–149.
See also Flexion teardrop
fracture
cervical spine, 17, 66, 107, 108,
109, 114, 115–120, 138–140
clinical features, 139
emergency management and referral,
140
lateral, 107
radiography, 140
range of motion, 84, 85
rotation simultaneous with, 107,
109, 120–121, 217, 218–221,
229
cervical spine, 120
slice fracture, 229
sprain, 100, 116
thoracolumbar spine, 107, 216–221
Flexion teardrop fracture, 119–120
clinical features, 119
complications, 119–120
emergency management and referral,
120
mechanism, 118
radiography, 119
Flexion–rotation injuries, 107, 109,

120, 217, 218–221, 229
cervical spine, 120–121
slice fracture, 229
Fontanelle, bulging, 132
Football, 151
Foramenal compression test, 93
Forehead, 16
pain in, 20
Fracture–dislocations, 39, 162–163
cervical spine, 39, 99, 126
hyperextension, 99
thoracic spine, 162–163
Fractures
ankle, 226
anklyosing spondylitis, 26
atlas, 108, 111, 123–124, 125, 133
avulsion fracture, 124
burst fracture, 133
ring, 108, 111
avulsion, 101, 102, 124, 138
burst, 15, 122, 133, 202, 203, 207,
209, 216, 225, 226, 227, 228,
229, 233, 235. *See also* Burst
fractures
calcaneal, 216, 226
cervical spine, 39, 106–133, 151.
See also Cervical spine,
fractures
Chance, 221, 222, 225
classification of, three-column
concept used in, 162
clavicle, 146, 150
clay-shoveler, 117–118
compression, 15, 36, 51, 116, 117
computed tomography, 208–210
dens, 129
displaced, 202
extremities, 130
facet, 209, 218
facial, 126
femoral head and neck, 35
flexion teardrop, 119–120
hangman's, 109–112, 113, 124,
125, 126
horizontally oriented, 102
iliac wing, 222
inaudible, 130
Jefferson, 102, 121, 133
laminar, 125, 209
lower extremity, 226
mandible, 129
minor, 234–235
multiple myeloma and, 51
odontoid, 99, 107, 129–130, 132
odontoid process, 109
osteoporosis, 36
osteoporosis and, 35
osteoporotic wedge, 167
pedicle, 25, 133, 208, 232
pelvic, 226, 235
pillar, 120–121

radial, 35
sacral, 226
shear, 232
skull, 126
slice, 218, 219, 220, 229
spinal, 2, 18, 26, 39, 106–133,
155, 212–236
thoracic spine, 203. *See also*
Thoracolumbar spine, *below*
thoracic vertebral body, 170
thoracolumbar spine, 207, 212–236.
See Thoracolumbar spine,
fractures
tomography, 102
vertebral body, 35, 98–99, 170
thoracic, 170
wedge, 116–117, 167, 202, 203,
216, 220, 221, 234, 239.
See also Wedge fractures

Gaenslen's sign, 194, 195, 271, 273
Gaenslen's test, sacroiliac sprain, 255
Gait, 76, 141, 200, 241
lumbar and lumbosacral strains and
sprains, 241
physical examination, 76
toe walk/heel walk, 200
wide-based or jerky, 141
Gardner-Wells tongs, 115, 118, 120
Gastrointestinal injuries, spinal injury
and, 8
Gender. *See* Sexual gender
Genitourinary disease, low back pain,
253
Genitourinary injuries, spinal injuries,
8
Giant cell tumor, 49
Giant osteoid osteoma, 48
Gibbus deformity, 167, 168, 219, 249
Glass fragments, projectile, 235
Gluteal region, 25, 179, 197
gluteal skyline test, 197
pain, 25
palpation, 179
Gluteal skyline test, 197
Gonads, radiation, 242
Greater occipital nerve, palpation, 80,
81
Greater occipital nerve syndrome, 80,
151
Greater trochanter, 179
Grisel's syndrome, 132–133
Gunshot wounds, 15, 150, 235, 236

Hairy patches on lower back, 245
Halo device, 132
Hamstrings, 248
Hand-Schüller disease, benign variant,
49

Hangman's fracture, 109–112, 113, 125, 126

Hard disc, 140

Head injuries, 6–7, 226
  spinal cord injuries and, 6–7

Head rests, 136, 138

Headaches, 20, 80, 139, 151
  migraine, 80, 151
  occipital, 30

Hearing defects, 132

Heart failure, 27

Heat applications, 30, 277–278
  heating pads, 277
  local, 30
  low back pain, 277–278

Heating pads, low back pain, 277

Heel walk, 181, 182, 200

Helmets, removal, 5

Hemangiomas, 49–50

Hematomas, 178, 207
  paraspinal, 207

Hemiparesis, 127

Hemorrhage, 132, 137, 150, 226, 235
  intracranial subarachnoid, 235
  intraocular, 132
  retroperitoneal, 226

Hemorrhagic shock, 235

Herniated discs, 103, 170, 173, 179
  cervical discs, 103
  computed tomography, 103
  imaging modalities, 103
  with radiating pain, 255, 256–263
    clinical features, 256–272
    radiography, 262–263
    treatment, 263
  sciatic nerve, 179
  thoracolumbar, 170, 173, 179

High heels, 241

Histocompatibility antigen HLA-B27, 25, 27

History, patient. *See* Patient history

Hoarseness, 116, 123, 137

Hoover test, 199, 200, 271

Horner's syndrome, 150

Humpback, 170, 172, 246

Hunched over posture, 26

Hyperabduction maneuver, 93, 144, 148–149

Hyperabduction syndrome, 93, 144, 148–149

Hypercalcemia, 54

Hyperextension fracture–dislocation, 99, 126

Hyperextension injuries. *See* Extension injuries; Hyperextension sprain

Hyperextension sprain, 122–124
  clinical features, 123
  complications, 123
  emergency management and referral, 123–124

mechanism, 122–123
  radiography, 123

Hyperflexion injuries. *See* Flexion injuries

Hyperirritability, 132

Hypermobility, 131

Hyperreflexia, 21

Hyperthermia, 8

Hypogastric reflex, 184, 188

Hypotension, 4, 7, 220–221

Hypothermia, 8

Hypovolemic shock, 7

Ice, 36

Ileus, 36, 217

Iliac wing fractures, 222

Immobilization, 4–5, 6, 34
  osteoporosis, 34, 36
  strict spinal, 223–225, 228

Incontinence, 21, 27

Industrial injuries, 239

Infant abuse, 131–132

Infantile scoliosis, 244

Infections, 38–45, 80, 152, 236, 244, 265
  infectious complications, 236
  low back pain, 265
  spine, 38–45
    intervertebral disc infection, 43–45
    morbidity and mortality, 38
    pathogens responsible, 38
    pyogenic spondylitis, 38–39, 40, 41
    tuberculous spondylitis, 40–43
  torticollis, 152

Inflammatory bowel disease, chronic, 265

Inguinal region pain, 248

Inion, palpation, 77

Interlocking facets, 100

Intermittent claudication test, 93, 144, 146

Intervertebral disc space infection, 103, 265

Intervertebral discs
  cervical spine, 62–64, 65
  disc space infection, 103, 265
  degeneration, 256, 257, 266–268
  fracture–dislocation through, 219
  herniation, 30, 103, 170, 173, 179, 255, 256–263
    cervical, imaging modalities, 103
    computed tomography, 103
    imaging modalities, 103
    with radiating pain, 255, 256–263
      clinical features, 257–262
      radiography, 262–263
      treatment, 263
  sciatic nerve, 179

thoracolumbar spine, 170, 173, 179
  infection, 43–45
    children, 44–45
    laboratory data, 43
    management, 45
    pain, 43
    prognosis, 44
    signs and symptoms, 43
    treatment, 43–44
  lumbar spine, 256–263
    disease, 257
    herniated, 256–263. *See also* Herniated discs, radiating pain
  protrusion, 17
  spondylosis, 266–268

Intervertebral foramen, 60, 179
  narrowed, 179

Irritable bowel disease, fibrositis, 264

Ischial tuberosity, 179

Isometric tests, 85

Isoniazid, 42

Jefferson burst fracture, 102, 121–122, 133
  clinical features, 121
  complications, 122
  emergency management and referral, 122
  mechanism, 121
  radiography, 121–122

Joint disease, degenerative, 151

Joints, 25, 26, 151
  ankylosing spondylitis, 25, 26
  costovertebral, 26
  degenerative disease, 151
  rheumatoid arthritis, 25

Juvenile scoliosis, 244

Kern test, 271

Kernig's sign, 191

Kidney, 235. *See also* entries beginning Renal

Klumpke plexus injuries, 150

Knee hyperflexion test, 196, 197

Knee jerk, 183

Kyphosis, 19, 26, 35, 39, 42, 170, 216, 217, 219, 244, 248–249
  ankylosing spondylitis, 26
  causes, 248
  complications, 248–249
  clinical features, 248
  diagnosis, 249
  emergency management and referral, 249
  importance in emergency medicine, 244
  incidence, 248
  osteoporosis, 35

pathophysiology, 248
tuberculous spondylitis, 42

Laboratory tests, 10, 39, 43, 44, 51
  intervertebral disc infection, 43, 44
  multiple myeloma, 51
  multiple trauma, 10
  neurologic deficit, 10
  pyogenic spondylitis, 39
Lacrimation, 151
Laminar fractures, 125, 209
Large intestines, 235
Lasegue sign, 189
Lasegue test, 270. *See also* Straight
    leg raising test
Lateral bending, thoracolumbar spine,
    170, 172, 233–234
Lateral flexion, 84, 85, 126–127
  range of motion, 84, 85
  uncinate process fracture, 126–127
Leg length, 29, 166–167, 168, 246,
    247, 254
  posterior facet syndrome, 254
  scoliosis and, 166–167, 168, 246,
    247
  unequal, 29
Legs. *See* Leg length; Lower extremi-
    ties
Leukemia, myelogenous, 27
Lhermitte's sign, 94
Lidocaine, 31
Lifting, 239, 240, 241
  improper, 240
  repetitive, 241
  Valsalva maneuver during, 239
Ligamenta flava, 64
Ligamenta nuchae, 64
Ligaments. *See also* entries beginning
    Ligamenta
  ankylosing spondylitis, 25
  atlantoaxial, 61
  axial traction and, 115
  calcification, 101–102
  cervical spine, 62–64, 65, 66, 70
  cervicocranium, 61, 62
  dentate, 66, 70
  disruptions, 18, 132, 220, 221, 223,
    224, 233
    pediatric, 132
    thoracolumbar distraction
      injuries, 223, 224
    type B dislocation, 233
    wedge fracture with, 220, 221
  interspinous, strain, 170
  laxity, pediatric, 131
  lumbar longitudinal, 170
  painful, 84
  palpation, 174, 176, 178, 179
    spinous ligament, 174, 176
    supraspinous ligament, 178, 179

pediatric, 131, 132
  rupture, 128
  spinal injury, 2
  supraspinous, palpation, 178, 179
  thoracolumbar spine, 156, 159, 161,
    215
  transverse, rupture, 109
Ligamentum nuchae, 80, 81
Lipomas, 103
Liver, 235
Locked facets, 118, 119, 120
Longus colli muscle, 123
Lordosis, 26, 30, 167, 169, 179, 241,
    258
  ankylosing spondylitis and, 26
  disc herniation, 258
  increased, 167, 169
  loss of normal, 26, 167, 179, 258
  lumbar spondylosis, 30
  obesity and increased, 241
Low back pain, 25, 252–278
  ankylosing spondylitis, 25
  bedrest, 275, 276
  causes, 253–253
    musculoskeletal, 253
    referred nonmusculoskeletal
      causes, 252–253
  cost, 252
  differential diagnosis, 252
  disc herniation, 256–263. *See also*
      Herniated discs, with radiating
      pain
  fibrositis, 263–265
  heat and cold applications, 277–278
  history, 269
  incidence, 252
  infections, 265
  of insidious onset over 50 years of
      age, 266–269
  of insidious onset under 50 years of
      age, 263–266
  lumbar spine radiography, 275
  mechanism, 253
  minor trauma, associated with, 253–
    255
  musculoskeletal causes, 253
  myofascial sprain, 253–255
  neoplasm, 268
  neurologic examination, 272
  nonmusculoskeletal (referred) causes,
    252–253
  osteoporosis, 269
  physical examination, 270–272
  posterior facet syndrome, 254–255
  radiating pain, 255–263
    acute disc herniation, 256–263.
      See also Herniated discs, with
      radiating pain
    spinal stenosis, 255–256
  sacroiliac sprain, 254
  sacroiliitis, 265

spinal manipulation, 276, 277
spondylolisthesis, 265–266
spondylolysis, 265–266
spondylosis, 266–268
stretch and spray, 275
traction, 275
treatment, 275–278
Lower extremities, 42, 226. *See also*
    Leg length
  fractures, 226
  referred pain in, 42
Lumbar discs, 256–263
  disease, 257
  herniation, low back pain and, 256–
    263.
Lumbar lordosis. *See* Lordosis
Lumbar spine. *See also* Thoracolumbar
    spine; entries beginning
    Lumbar; Lumbo
  ankylosing spondylitis, 26
  bony palpation, 175
  innervation, 185, 186
  mechanism of trauma, 3
  mixed injuries, 164
  mobility and stability, 159–162
  nerve roots, 163, 212, 214
  normal x-rays, 204, 205
  osteoarthritis, 29
  radiography, 275
  rheumatoid arthritis, 21, 23
  spondylosis, 30, 31, 266–268. *See
    also* Spondylosis
  vertebra, 160
Lumbosacral plexus injury, 234–235
Lungs. *See* entries beginning Pulmo-
    nary
Lymph nodes, anterior, 79
Lymphoma, malignant, 51, 53

Mach effect, 102
Magnetic resonance imaging, 104
Malignant lymphoma, 51, 53
Mandible fractures, 129
Mannitol for spinal injury, 10
Marfan's syndrome, 180
Mastoid processes, palpation, 77
Median nerve examination, 90
Mediastinitis, 39, 42
Medications. *See* Drugs/medications
Medicolegal risk, lumbosacral spine
    films, 242
Meninges, 184, 191
Meningiomas, calcified, 103
Meningitis, 39, 236
  bacterial, 39
Metrizamide, 103
Migraine headache, 80, 151
Milgram test, 191, 193, 271
Minerva jacket, 132
Mobility, 61–63, 131, 156–162

Mobility (*cont.*)
  cervical spine, 61–63
  pediatric, hyper-, 131
  thoracolumbar spine, 156–162
Motor examination, 9. *See also* Motor
    testing
Motor innervation, 14, 183
Motor signs, acute disc herniation, 259
Motor testing, 86–92
  axillary nerve, 90–92
  C-1, 86, 87
  C-2, 86, 87
  C-3, 86–87
  C-4, 87
  C-5, 87
  C-6, 87–88
  C-7, 88
  C-8, 88–89
  median nerve, 90–92
  musculocutaneous nerve, 92
  radial nerve, 90
  T-1, 89
  thoracolumbar spine, 181–182
  ulnar nerve, 90
Motor vehicle accidents, 2, 16, 125,
    136, 138, 150, 216, 222, 235
Motor weakness, nerve root compres-
    sion, 141
Movement, 3, 4, 5, 76, 85
  against resistance, 85
  extrication and movement of patient,
    3, 4
  normal, 76
  transport of patient, 5
MRI. *See* Magnetic resonance imaging
Multiple myeloma, 50–51, 52
Multiple sclerosis, 103
Multiple trauma, 10, 202
  laboratory tests, 10
  radiography, 202
Mumps, 80
Muscle relaxants, 36, 243, 277
  acute vertebral body compression,
    36
  low back pain, 243, 277
Muscle tone, abdominal, 167, 241
Muscle wasting, unilateral, 76
Muscles. *See also* entries beginning
    Muscle
  abdominal, innervation, 184, 196,
    197
  atrophy, 141
  biceps, 87, 88
  cervical area, 66, 67, 68, 69, 70
  cervical spine, 82–83
  erector spinae, 80
  extensor carpi radialis, 88
  hamstrings, 248
  innervation by cervical nerve root,
    150

longus colli, 123
newborn, 131
palpation, 79–80, 178–179, 180,
    248
paraspinous, 26, 170, 178–179,
    180, 239, 248
  palpation, 178–179, 180
  spasm, 239
paravertebral, 167, 169
pectoralis, 248
scalene, 23, 80
sternocleidomastoid, 79, 123, 152
trapezius, 80
triceps, 88, 89
Muscular atrophy, 141
Musculocutaneous nerve examination,
    92
Myelocele, 178
Myelography, 47, 57, 103–104, 103,
    210, 220, 231, 236, 275
  arachnoiditis caused by, 236
  computer assisted (CAM), 103–104
  CT, 220, 231
  low back pain, 275
  penetrating injuries, 236
  spinal cord compression, 57
  thoracolumbar, 210
Myeloma, multiple, 51, 52
Mylogenous leukemia, 27
Myofascial sprain, 253–254
  clinical features, 253
  radiographs, 254
  treatment, 254
Myofascial syndromes, 170
Myofascial trigger points, stretch and
    spray, 275
Myositis, 152, 153

Naffziger test, 191, 192
Naloxone for spinal injury, 10
Narcotics, 31, 277
  addiction, 31
  low back pain, 277
Nasotracheal intubation, contraindica-
    tions, 6
Nausea, 139, 151, 246
Near-drowning, 119, 120
Neck. *See also* Cervical spine
  asymmetry, 76
  direct blow to, 15
  gunshot wounds to, 15
  hyperextension injury to, 15
  pain, 21, 29–30, 249
Neonatal cervical spine, 131–132
Neoplasms, 46–56, 268
  low back pain, 268
  spine, 46–56
    aneurysmal bone cysts, 50, 51
    chondrosarcoma, 51

chordoma, 53, 56
classification, 47–54
  metastatic disease, 54, 57
  primary benign, 47–50
  primary malignant, 51–54
clinical examination, 46
eosinophilic granuloma, 49
Ewing's sarcoma, 53, 55
giant cell tumor, 49
hemangioma, 49–50
history, 46
laboratory studies, 46–47
malignant lymphoma, 51, 53
metastatic, 54–57
multiple myeloma, 50–51, 52
osteoblastoma, 48–49
osteochondroma, 18, 47
osteoid osteoma, 48
osteosarcoma, 51, 54
physical examination for, 46
primary malignant, 50–53
radiography, 47
sarcomatous transformation, 47
spinal cord compression, 54–57
Nerve roots, 18, 39, 66–67, 71, 140–
    141, 162–163, 184, 185, 186,
    187, 191, 212–214
  cervical, 66–67, 71, 140–141
    compression, 140–141
  compression, 39, 140–141
    cervical, 140–141
  innervation, 185, 186, 187
    lumbar, 185, 186
    sacral, 187
  lumbar, 163, 185, 186, 187
  lumbosacral, 212–214
  neurologic examination for, 184, 191
  sacral, 163
  spinal cord injury vs, 214
  thoracolumbar, 162–163
Nerve supply, 14, 15, 82–83, 150,
    183
  cervical spine, 82–83
  lumbar spine, 185, 186
  motor, 183
  motor innervation, 14
  pathway crossing, function and
    level, 15
  reflexes, 14
  sacral spine, 187
  sensory, 183
Neuralgia, 42, 125
  occipital, 125
Neuritis, 80, 151, 152, 153
  greater occipital, syndrome, 80, 151
  spinal accessory nerve, 152, 153
Neurofibromas, 103
Neurofibromatosis, 244
Neurogenic claudication, 256
Neurologic deficit, 10, 14, 17, 114.

See also Neurologic examina-
tion; Neurologic injuries
central cord syndrome, 17
instability of cervical spine and, 114
laboratory tests, 10
recovery from, 14, 17
Neurologic examination, 86–92, 181–
182. See also Motor testing;
Reflex testing; Sensory testing
abdominal musculature, 184, 196,
197
acute disc herniation, 258–259
Adson maneuver, 93
axial compression test, 199, 200
axillary nerve, 92
Beevor's sign, 196
Brudzinski's sign, 191, 192
Bulbocavernosus
C-1, 86, 87
C-2, 86, 87
C-3, 86–87
C-4, 87
C-5, 87, 88
C-6, 88, 89
C-7, 88–89, 90
C-8, 89, 91
compression test, 92, 93
contralateral (well-leg) straight leg
raising, 189
costoclavicular maneuver, 93
distraction test, 92–93
dura, 184, 191
FABERE (Patrick) test, 194–196,
271–272, 274
femoral nerve and root, 184, 196
femoral stretch test, 196
foramenal compression test, 93
functional pain, 184
Gaenslen's sign, 194, 195
gluteal skyline test, 197
heel walk, 181, 182, 200
Hoover test, 199, 200
hyperabduction maneuver, 93
intermittent claudication test, 93
Kernig's sign, 191
Lasegue sign, 189
Lhermitte's sign, 94
low back pain, 272
medial nerve, 92
meningeal, 184, 191
Milgram test, 191, 193
musculocutaneous nerve, 92
Naffziger test, 191, 192
organ systems and, 198
Patrick (FABERE) test, 194–196,
271–272, 274
pelvic compression test, 194
pelvic rotation test, 200
pelvic splay test, 191–193
peripheral nerves, 90, 91

popliteal pressure test, 189, 190
radial nerve, 90
reflex testing, 183–184
related examination, 198
root pathology, 191
sacral pressure test, 194
sacroiliac joint, 184, 191–196
scapular approximation test, 198
sciatic nerve and root, 184, 189,
190
shoulder depression test, 93, 94
sitting straight leg raising test, 199
Soto-Hall test, 196–197, 198
squat test, 181, 182
straight leg raising, 189, 190
superficial pinch test, 199–200
swallowing test, 93
T-1, 89, 92
T-1 root stretch test, 197
thoracolumbar spine, 180–200
motor testing, 181–182
reflex testing, 183–184
sensory testing, 182
toe walk, 181, 182, 200
Trendelenburg test, 197, 198
ulnar nerve, 90
Valsalva maneuver, 93, 191
vertebral artery test, 93, 94
Neurologic injuries, 2, 17, 107, 114.
See also Cord syndromes;
entries beginning Neurologic
cervical spine, 107, 114
spinal cord injury, 2
thoracolumbar fracture–dislocation,
212–214
Neurologic sequelae, tuberculous
spondylitis, 42
Neurologic shock, 4
Neurologic status, 7–8, 12
complete cord syndrome, 12
flow sheet of changes in, 7–8
Newborn cervical spine, 131–132
Nonsteroidal anti-inflammatory drugs
(NSAIDs), 28, 31, 36, 277
low back pain, 277
Notches, 60
Notochord, malignant tumor from. See
Chordoma
NSAIDs. See Nonsteroidal anti-
inflammatory drugs
Nucha ligament, 80, 81
Nystagmus, 22

Obesity, 167, 241
lordosis and, increased, 241
Occipital headaches, 20, 30
Occipital nerve syndrome, greater, 80,
151
Occipital neuralgia, 125

Occipital neuritis, 151
Occipital pain, 141
Occupation, strenuous, 29
Odontoid fractures, 99, 107, 129–130,
132
pediatric, 132
Odontoid process, 61, 109
fractures, 109
Open-mouth view, 121
Oppenheim test, 184
Organ systems, 198, 208, 226
neurologic examination and, 198
Orotracheal intubation, 6, 7
Os odontoideum, 102
Osteoarthritis, 20, 29–32, 245
scoliosis and, 245
spine, 29–32
cervical spine, 29–30
clinical features, 29–30
complications, 30–31
diagnosis, 31
exercise and, 31
incidence, 29
lumbar spine, 30, 31
management and referral, 31–32
pathophysiology, 29
thoracic spine, 30
Osteoblastoma, 48–49, 103
Osteochondroma, 47, 48
Osteogenic sarcoma, 53, 54
Osteoid osteoma, 48
giant, 48
Osteomyelitis, 38–39, 40, 41, 178
chronic, 39
pyogenic, 38–39, 40, 41
age and, 38
incidence, 38
Osteoporosis, 34–36, 248, 269
age and, 34
clinical presentation, 34–35
definition, 34
diagnosis, 36
etiology, 34
exercise and, 36
immobilization, 34, 36
incidence, 34
pain, 34, 35
secondary to multiple myeloma, 51
sexual gender and, 34
treatment, 36
Osteoporotic wedge fractures, 167
Osteosarcoma, 51, 54
Oxacillin, 39

Pain. See also Back pain; Headaches;
Low back pain; entries beginning Pain
abdominal, 246
anal, 53

Pain (*cont.*)
  ankylosing spondylitis, 25, 28
  chest, 25
  deeper source, 179
  functional (nonorganic), 184, 198–
    200
    thoracolumbar, 184
  gluteal, 25
  hyperextension injury, 137
  hyperflexion sprain, cervical, 116
  intervertebral disc infection, 43
  ligaments, 84
  multiple myeloma, 51
  neck, 21, 29–30, 249
  occipital neuralgia, 125
  osteoporosis, 34, 35
  pleuritic component to, 239
  radiating, 140, 241, 248, 269
    to inguinal region, 248
    to occipital area, 141
    referred vs, 269
    to shoulders, 141
    to upper extremities, 140
  radiating vs. referred, 269
  radiosensitive myeloma, 51
  rectal, 53
  referred, 42, 269
    in lower extremities, 42
    radiating vs, 269
  tendons, 84
  thoracic spondylosis, 30
Pain sensation, decreased, 21
Pain syndrome, chronic, 120
Palpation, 76–80, 174–179
  atlas, 78
  bony structure, 76–79, 174–178
  carotid pulses, 79–80
  cervical spine, 76–80
  coccyx, 177–178
  cricoid ring, 78–79
  erector spinae muscles, 80
  facet joints, 78, 79, 254
  gluteal region, 179
  greater occipital nerve, 80, 81
  inion, 77
  ligamentum nuchae, 80, 81
  lymph nodes, 79
  mastoid processes, 77
  paraspinous muscles, 178–179, 180,
    248
  parotid gland, 80
  sacroiliac joints, 177
  scalene muscles, 80
  skull, 77
  soft tissue, 79–80, 178–179
  spine, 245
  spinous processes, 77, 78
  step-off, 174, 176
  sternocleidomastoid muscle, 79
  supraclavicular fossa, 80

  supraspinous ligament, 178, 179
  thoracolumbar spine, 174–179
  trapezius muscle, 80
Pancoast tumor, 80
Paralysis, 132, 244
  irreversible and permanent, 14
  paraplegia, 2, 42, 219, 228, 246
    congenital scoliosis, 246
  spastic, 249
  spinal cord injury and, 2
  upper extremities, 16
Paralytic ileus, 8
Paraplegia, 2, 42, 219, 228
  congenital scoliosis, 246
Pararenal space, 235
Paraspinous muscles, 26, 178–179,
    180, 239, 248
  palpation, 248
  spasm, 170, 239
Paraspinous soft tissues, 202
Paravertebral abscess, 42, 43
Paravertebral muscle spasm, 167, 169
Paresthesias, 21, 139, 199
  nonanatomic, 199
Parotid gland, palpation, 80
Pathology and symptoms, 169
Patient education, 142, 148, 243
  scalenus anticus syndrome, 148
Patient history, low back pain, 269
Patrick (FABERE) test, 194–196, 271–
    272, 274
Pectoralis muscles, 248
Pediatric patients. *See* Children
Pedicles, 60, 125, 133, 202, 206, 207,
    226, 228, 232
  distance between, 202, 206, 226,
    228
  fracture, 125, 132, 208, 232
Pelvic compression test, 194
Pelvic fractures, 226, 235
Pelvic ring, closed, 255
Pelvic rock test, 194, 271, 272
Pelvic rotation test, 200
Pelvic splay test, 191–193
Penetrating injuries, 17, 150, 207,
    235–236
  thoracolumbar spine, 235–236
Penicillamine, 28
Perched facets, 118
Percussion, 179–180
Pericarditis, 27, 39, 42
Phosphate in diet, high, 34
Physical examination, 76–93, 270–274
  Beevor's sign, 272, 274
  cervical spine, 76–93
    inspection, 76
    neurologic examination, 86–92
    palpation, 76–80
    range of motion, 84–85
  FABERE (Patrick) test, 194–196,

    271–272, 274
  Fajersztan test, 270
  Gaenslen's sign, 271, 273
  Hoover test, 271
  Kern test, 271
  Lasegue test, 270
  low back pain, 270–272
  Milgram test, 271
  pelvic rock test, 271, 272
  straight leg raising test, 30, 46, 54,
    189, 190, 199, 241, 256, 260–
    261, 262, 263, 266, 270
    acute disc herniation, 260–261,
      262, 263
    posterior facet syndrome, 254
    sitting, 199
    spinal stenosis, 256
    spondylosis, 266
  well-leg straight leg raising test, 270
Pia mater, 66
Pigmentation, 245
Pillar fracture, 121
Pinch test, superficial, 199–200
Plain film tomography, 103
Plain radiography, 96–103, 202–203
  cervical spine, 96–102
  thoracolumbar spine, 202–203
Plumb line, 166, 167
Pneumonia, 236
Pneumothorax, spontaneous, 239
Poliomyelitis, 152, 244
Popliteal pressure test, 189, 190
Posterior facet syndrome, 78, 254–255
  clinical features, 254
  radiographs, 254
  treatment, 254–255
Posture, 26, 76
  hunched over, 26
Pott's disease. *See* Tuberculous
    spondylitis
Powers ratio, 127
Pregnancy, 167, 241
Priapism, 12
Prostatitis, 38
Protein calorie malnutrition, 34
Proteinuria, 27
Pseudomonas, 265
Pseudo-subluxation, 102, 132
Psoas abscess, 39, 42
Psoriatic arthritis, 265
Pulmonary disease, chronic obstructive,
    198
Pulmonary embolism, 217
Pulmonary fibrosis, 27
Pulmonary hypertension, 246
Pulmonary *Mycobacterium tuberculo-
    sis*, 265
Pyogenic spondylitis, 38–39, 40, 41
  age and, 38
  clinical features, 38–39

complications, 39
diagnosis, 39
incidence, 38
management and referral, 39
pathophysiology, 38
risk factors for, 38
tuberculosis vs, 42
Pyogenic vertebral osteomyeolitis, 265

Quadriplegia, 2, 118, 123
  with normal cervical spine radiographs, 123

Radial fractures, 35
Radial nerve, neurologic examination, 89–90
Radial pulse, Adson maneuver, 93
Radiating pain, 255–263, 269
  low back with, 255–263
  posterior facet syndrome, 254–255
  referred pain vs, 269
Radiation therapy, 27, 49, 50, 51, 53, 56
  chordoma, 53
  spinal cord compression, 56
Radiography. *See also* X-rays
  acute disc herniation, 262–263
  aneurysmal bone cysts, 50
  ankylosing spondylitis, 27–28
  atlantoaxial disruption, 128
  atlanto-occipital disruption, 127
  atlas fractures, 123–124
  blow-out appearance, 50
  brachial plexus injuries, 150
  cervical disc disorders, 141
  cervical rib, 145–146
  cervical spine, 9, 96–103
    abnormal angulation, 98
    accuracy, 96
    alignment, 97–98, 100
    anteroposterior view, 100
    artifacts, 102
    axial traction, 96, 97
    bones, 99, 101
    cartilage, 99, 101
    computed tomography, 103
    congenital anomaly, 102
    cross-table lateral view, 96–100
    degenerative disease, 102
    disc, 141
    flexion–extension view, 101
    fracture–dislocation, 126
    hyperflexion, 108
    interpretation, 101
    lateral flexion, 127
    Mach effect, 102
    magnetic resonance imaging, 103
    myelography, 103
    normal anatomic variants, 102

oblique view, 100–101
open-mouth view, 100–101
pediatric, 130–131
physiologic subluxation, 102
pillar view, 101
pitfalls, 101–103
plain radiography, 96–102
prevertebral fat stripe, 100
scout film, 96
soft tissue space, 99–100
straight spine, 98
swimmer's view, 101
tomography, 102–103
Twining's view, 101
uncinate process, 102, 127
chondrosarcoma, 51
chordoma, 53
clay-shoveler fracture, 117
computed tomography, 103
computer assisted myelography (CAM), 103–104
cost, lumbar spine x-rays, 275
costoclavicular syndrome, 146
diagnosis, 246–248
disappearing vertebrae, 51
eosinophilic granuloma, 50
Ewing's sarcoma, 53
extension teardrop fracture of axis, 124
facet dislocation, 118, 120
facet subluxations, 240
fibrositis, 264
flexion–extension views, 109, 114, 126, 127, 129
flexion teardrop fracture, 119
giant cell tumor, 49
gonadal radiation exposure, 242, 275
greater occipital nerve syndrome, 151
hangman's fracture, 125, 126
hemangioma, 50
hyperabduction syndrome, 149
hyperextension injuries, 123, 124, 126, 137–138
  extension teardrop fracture, 124
  fracture–dislocation, 126
  sprain, 123
hyperflexion injuries, 116, 119, 140
  cervical, 116
  flexion teardrop fracture, 119
  sprain, 116
indications for emergency, 275
interpretation pitfalls, 101–102
intervertebral disc infection, 44
Jefferson burst fracture, 121–122
kyphosis, 49
laminar fracture, 125
low back pain, 275
lumbar spine, 242, 275
lumbosacral strains and sprains, 242

magnetic resonance imaging, 104
malignant lymphoma, 51
metastatic disease, 54, 57
multiple myeloma, 51
multiple trauma, 202
myelography, 103–104
myofascial sprain, 254
neoplasms of spine, 47, 268
neurologic injury and, 114
odontoid fracture, 129
open-mouth view, 121, 128
osteoblastoma, 49
osteochondroma, 47
osteoid osteoma, 48
osteoporosis, 36
osteosarcoma, 53
plain film tomography, 103
posterior facet syndrome, 254
pyogenic spondylitis, 39
rheumatoid cervical spondylitis, 24
sacroiliac sprain, 255
sacroiliitis, 265
scalenus anticus syndrome, 144, 147–148
scoliosis, 246
Scotty dog sign, 266, 267
simple wedge (compression) fractures of cervical spine, 117
soap bubble effect, 49
spinal cord compression, 57
spinal injury, 9–10
spinal stenosis, 256
spondylolisthesis of axis, 125
spondylolysis, 266, 267
spondylosis, 266–268
sunburst, 53
thoracic outlet syndromes, 145–146
thoracolumbar spine, 9, 202–210, 235–236, 239
  AP view, 202, 203
  axial load injuries, 226–228
    with rotation injuries, 229
  computed tomography, 207, 208, 209
  contusions, 239
  distraction injuries, 222–223
  flexion injuries, 216, 219–220, 221
    with rotation injuries, 219–220, 221
  fractures, 202, 203, 206
  fractures at other levels, 210
  lateral bending injuries, 233–234
    with axial load, 234
  lateral view, 203
  multiple trauma, 202
  myelography, 210
  normal, 204
  paraspinal hematoma, 206
  penetrating injuries, 235–236

Radiography (*cont.*)
thoracolumbar spine (*cont.*)
pitfalls, 210
plain radiography, 202–203
shearing injuries, 230–231, 232, 233
tomography, 210
tomography, 103, 210
torticollis, 153
tuberculous spondylitis, 42, 44
vertebral artery syndrome, 152
Radionuclide bone scan, 39, 265, 276
fibrositis, 265
low back pain, 275
pyogenic spondylitis, 39
Range of motion, 84–85, 169–174
cervical spine, 84–85
basic movements, 84
extension, 84, 85
flexion, 84, 85
lateral flexion, 85
rotation, 84, 85
thoracolumbar spine, 169–174
extension, 170
flexion, 170
lateral bending, 170, 172
symptoms and pathology, 169
Rectum, 53, 253
examination, low back pain, 253
rectal pain, 53
Referred pain, 254, 269
posterior facet syndrome, 254
radiating pain vs, 269
Reflex testing, 87, 88, 89, 183–184
ankle jerk, 183
C-5, 87
C-6, 88
C-7, 89
C-8, 89
knee jerk, 183
T-1, 89
thoracolumbar spine, 183–184
Reflexes, 12, 14, 141, 183–184, 188, 260. *See also* Reflex testing
abdominal, 184
anal wink, 184
Babinski sign, 184, 188
bulbocavernosus, 184, 184
Chaddock test, 184
complete cord syndrome, 12
cremasteric, 184, 188
cutaneous, 184
deep tendon, 183–184, 260
epigastric, 184
hypogastric, 184, 188
nerve root compression, 141
Oppenheim test, 184
pathologic, 184
Reiter's syndrome, 265
Relaxation exercises, 151

Renal failure, 38
Renal insufficiency, 27
Renal stones, 36
Respiration, 4, 120, 246
respiratory arrest, diving accident, 120
respiratory compromise, 246
respiratory insufficiency, 4
Respiratory tract infection, 152
Resuscitation, 4, 120
diving accident, 120
early efforts, 4
Retardation, 132
Reticulum cell sarcoma, 51
Retroperitoneum, 235
Retropharyngeal abscess, 39, 42
Retropharyngeal soft tissue swelling, 138
Rheumatoid arthritis, 20–24, 25, 109, 244, 265
spine, 20–24
ankylosing spondylitis, 24–29
atlantoaxial joint, 20–21, 22, 23
cervical spine, 20, 21
clinical features, 20–21
complications, 21–22
diagnosis, 22–23
incidence, 20
management and referral for, 23–24
pathophysiology, 20
radiographic changes, 24
subaxial cervical spine, 21, 23
thoracic spine, 21
trivial trauma and, 22
vascular compression, 21–22
vertical dislocations, 21
Rheumatoid spondylitis, 21, 22, 23–24
diagnosis, 22
management, 22, 23–24
radiographic changes, 24
Rib cage, scoliosis and, 245
Ribs, 156, 157, 159, 202, 245
Rifampin, 42
Right ventricular failure, 246
Rigid cervical collars, 4
Root compression syndromes, 262
Rotation injuries, 2, 84, 85
axial load with, 229
cervical spine, 107, 109, 110, 120
extension simultaneous with, 107, 110, 120–121
flexion simultaneous with, 107, 109, 120, 217, 218–221, 229
range of motion, 84, 85
thoracolumbar spine, 173, 174, 217, 218–221, 229
axial load with, 229
flexion with, 217, 218–221
Roundback, 248

Sacral pressure test, 194
Sacral spine, 60, 163, 164, 187, 212–214, 226
fractures, 226
innervation, 187
mixed injuries, 164
nerve roots, 163, 212–214
normal x-rays, 204, 205
Sacroiliac joint, 25, 26, 27, 184, 191–196, 254
ankylosing spondylitis, 25, 26, 27
palpation, 177
rheumatoid arthritis, 20, 21
sprain, 254
tests for, 184, 191–196
Sacroiliitis, 265
Sacrum, 60
Sandbags, 4, 5
Scalene muscle, 80, 123
palpation, 80
Scalenus anticus syndrome, 93, 144, 147–148
Scalp lacerations, 129, 130
Scapulae, 76, 245
asymmetry, 245
displacement, 76
Scapular approximation test, 198
Scheuermann's disease, 167
Schmorl's nodes, 36, 249
Sciatic nerve, 184, 189, 190
pain. *See* Sciatica
palpation, 179
root, 184, 189, 190
trunk, palpation, 179
Sciatica, 25, 256, 258, 261, 262, 266
acute disc herniation, 256, 258, 261, 262
spondylosis, 266
Scoliosis, 29, 48, 166–167, 168, 170, 172, 198, 236, 241, 242, 244–248
causes, 244
clinical features, 244–246
complications, 246
emergency management and referral, 246–248
humpback on skyline view, 170, 172, 245, 246
importance in emergency medicine, 244
incidence, 244
lumbar, 241
nonstructural, 166–167, 168, 179, 246, 247
paraspinous muscle spasm, 239
pathophysiology, 244
plumb line, 245
Seat belts, lap, 221, 222
Semiconscious patient, 4
Sensory deficits/loss, 7, 16, 141

acute disc herniation, 260
central cord syndrome, 16
nerve root compression, 141
Sensory examination, 8
Sensory innervation, thoracolumbar, 183
Sensory loss. *See* Sensory deficits/loss
Sensory testing, 86–92
axillary nerve, 92
C-1, 86
C-3, 87
C-4, 87
C-5, 87
C-6, 88
C-7, 88
C-8, 89
medial nerve, 92
musculocutaneous nerve, 92
radial nerve, 90
T-1, 89
ulnar nerve, 90
Sexual gender
chondrosarcoma, 51
giant cell tumor, 49
kyphosis, 248
lumbosacral strains and sprains, 240
malignant lymphoma, 51
multiple myeloma, 51
odontoid fractures, 129
osteochondroma, 47
osteoid osteoma, 48
osteoporosis and, 34
scoliosis, 244
Shaken infant syndrome, whiplash, 131–132
Shear fractures, 23
Shearing injuries, thoracolumbar spine, 230–231, 232, 233
Shock, 6–7, 235
hemorrhagic, 235
spinal, 6–7
Shoes, high-heeled, 241
Shoulder depression test, 93, 94
Shoulders, 76, 141, 150, 239, 245
asymmetry, 239, 245
dislocation, 150
pain radiating to, 141
symmetry, 76
Simple wedge fracture, 116–117
Sjögren's syndrome, 80
Skin, 38, 76
infections, 38
Skull, 77, 126
fracture, 126
palpation, 77
Slice fracture, 218, 219, 220, 229
Small intestines, 235
Sneezing, 216, 240, 241, 254, 257

acute disc herniation, 257
posterior facet syndrome, 254
Soap bubble effect, 49
Sodium fluoride, 36
Soft cervical collar, 4, 31, 116, 142, 152
hyperflexion sprain, 116
Soft disc, 140
Soft tissue injuries, 99, 100, 138, 178–179, 238–243
minor, 238–243
contusions, 238–239
lumbosacral, 240–243
thoracic strains and sprains, 239
palpation, 79–80, 178–179
radiography, 99–100
retropharyngeal, swelling, 138
Soft tissue space, radiography, 99, 100
Soto-Hall test, 196–197, 198
Space-occupying lesions, 257
Spasticity, 21
Spearguns, 235
Spina bifida, 178
Spinal abnormalities, asymptomatic, 242
Spinal accessory nerve, neuritis, 152, 153
Spinal cord. *See also* Spinal cord syndromes
age and, 2
anatomy, 12, 13
associated injuries, 6–7
blood flow changes, 6–7
causes/etiology, 2
cervical, 66–67, 71
circulation, 6–7
complications, 2
compression, 27, 39–42, 55–56, 118, 140
ankylosing spondylitis, 27
metastatic tumor, 54–57
osteoarthritis of spine, 29
contusion, 18
costs, 2
gastrointestinal considerations, 8
incidence, 2
knee hyperflexion test, 196, 197
lesions, incomplete, 114
mechanisms, 2–3
mortality, 2
motor examination, 9
nerve root damage vs, 214
normal cervical, 15
pathophysiology, 2–3
pelvic rock test, 194
radiographic evaluation, 9–10
respiratory complications, 6
sensory examination, 8
temperature regulation, 8
thoracolumbar, 162–163, 212

treatment, 10
vascular supply, 163
Spinal cord syndromes, 12–18, 114, 115, 248
anatomic considerations, 12
anterior cord syndrome, 14–15, 16, 114
Brown-Séquard syndrome, 17
cauda equina syndromes, 18
central cord syndrome, 15–17, 115
clinical features, 248
complete cord syndrome, 12–14, 17
contusio cervicalis posterior, 17
cord contusion, 18
nerve root injuries, 18
Spinal curvature. *See also* Kyphosis; Lordosis; Scoliosis
potential for progression, 248
Spinal fractures. *See* Fractures
Spinal infection, 244
Spinal injuries, 2–10, 17. *See also* Fractures
age at, 2
airway maintenance, 4
airway management, 6
associated injuries, 6–7
breathing, 6
causes/etiology, 2
circulation, 4, 6–7
complications, 2
compression injuries, 2
corticosteroids in treatment, 10
costs, 2
diuretics in treatment, 10
diving accident, patient in water, 4
emergency department management, 6–10
extension injuries, 2
extrication and movement of patient, 3, 4
flexion injuries, 2
gastrointestinal considerations, 8
genitourinary considerations, 8
helmet removal, 5
immobilization of patient, 4–5, 6
incidence, 2
indications for spinal precautions, 6
initial assessment, 3, 4
laboratory tests, 10
mechanisms, 2–3
mortality from, 2
motor examination, 9
neurologic status, flow sheet of changes in, 7–8
pathophysiology, 2–3
penetrating, 17
pre-hospital treatment, 3–5
primary assessment, 7–8
radiography, 9–10, 264
respiratory insufficiency in, 4

Spinal injuries (*cont.*)
  rotational injuries, 2
  scene of accident, 3
  semiconscious or unconscious
      patient, 4
  sensory examination, 8
  temperature regulation and, 8
  transport preparation, 5
  treatment, 10
  undressing patient, 7
Spinal irradiation, 27
Spinal malformation, 180
Spinal manipulation, 254, 276, 277
  low back pain, 276, 277
  posterior facet syndrome, 254
Spinal nerves, dermatome distribution,
    13
Spinal shock, 6–7
Spinal stenosis, 255–256
  clinical features, 255–256
  conditions associated with, 256
  radiographs, 256
  treatment, 256
Spinal tumors. *See* Neoplasms of spine
Spine. *See also* Cervical spine; Lumbar
    spine; Lumbosacral spine. Sacral
    spine; Thoracic spine; Thoraco-
    lumbar spine; entries beginning
    Spinal
  anatomy, 60, 61, 156, 214, 215
    lateral view, 156
    three-column concept, 215
    two-column concept, 214
  palpation, 245
  three-column concept, 162, 215
  two-column concept, 214
Spinous processes, 61, 77, 78, 116,
    174–177
  palpation, 77, 78, 174–177
  separation, 116
Spleen, 235
Spondylitis, rheumatoid, 21, 22
Spondylolisthesis, 109–112, 113, 170,
    174, 176, 265–266
  axis, 109–112, 113
  classification, 265
  clinical features, 265–266
  radiographs, 266
  treatment, 266
Spondylolysis, 265–266
  clinical features, 265–266
  four stages, 266, 267
  radiographs, 266
  treatment, 266
Spondylosis, 15, 29–30, 31, 78, 103,
    266–268
  cervical, 15, 29–30, 31, 140
  clinical features, 266
  degenerative, 241
  lumbar, 30, 31

  radiographs, 266–268
  thoracic, 30
  treatment, 268
Sports injuries, 2, 4, 16, 119–120,
    150
  diving, 4, 16, 119–120
Sprains, 100, 115–116, 136, 239,
    240–243, 255
  cervical, 136
  hyperflexion, 100, 116
  lumbar and lumbosacral, 240–243
    clinical features, 241
    complications, 242–243
    diagnosis, 240, 241–242
    emergency management and
        referral, 243
    mechanisms, 240
    predisposing circumstances, 241
    radiography, 242
  sacroiliac, 255
  thoracic, 239
Squat test, 181, 182
Stab wounds, 150, 235, 236
Stability, 14, 61–63, 107–114, 214
  cervical spine, 14, 61–63, 107–114
    neurologic damage, 107
    lower cervical spine, 112–114
    neurologic deficit, 14
    upper cervical spine, 108–112
  instability defined, 214
  thoracolumbar spine, 156–162, 215
    fracture–dislocation, 214
  two-column concept of spine, 61–63
Staphylococcus, 43, 45, 265
Steel's rule of thirds, 132
Step-off, 174, 176
Sternocleidomastoid muscle, 79, 123,
    152
Steroids, 10, 28, 31, 36, 56
  anabolic, 36
  intravenous high-dose, 56
Stiffness, 30
Stingers, 151
Straight leg raising test, 30, 46, 54,
    189, 190, 199, 241, 254, 256,
    260–261, 262, 263, 266, 270
  acute disc herniation, 260–261, 262,
    263
  posterior facet syndrome, 254
  sitting, 199
  spinal stenosis, 256
  spondylosis, 266
  well-leg, 270
Strains, 239, 240–243
  lumbar and lumbosacral, 240–243
    clinical features, 241
    complications, 242–243
    diagnosis, 240, 241–242
    emergency management and
        referral, 243

  mechanisms, 240
  predisposing circumstances, 241
  radiography, 242
  thoracic, 239
Streptomycin, 42
Stretching injuries, 150
Subarachnoid hemorrhage, intracranial,
    235
Subclavian artery, 144
Subluxations
  atlantoaxial, 20, 21, 22, 23, 24,
      132
    pediatric, 132
  cervical spine. *See* Cervical spine,
      fractures, dislocations, and
      subluxations
  facet, radiography, 240
  physiologic, 102
  respiratory tract infection in
      children, after, 152
  vertical, 23, 24
Sunburst, 53
Superficial pinch test, 199–200
Supraclavicular fossa, palpation, 80
Supraspinous ligament, palpation, 178,
    179
Swallowing, difficulty, 42
Swallowing test, 93
Symptoms and pathology, 169
Syndrome of sensory root of second
    cervical nerve, 151
Syringomyelia, 103

T-1 root stretch test, 197
Technitium bone scanning, 47
Temperature regulation, spinal injury, 8
Tendons, painful, 84
Tetanus prophylaxis, 236
Thiazides, 36
Thoracic injuries, intra-, 235
Thoracic kyphosis. *See* Kyphosis
Thoracic outlet syndromes, 80, 144–
    149
  cervical rib, 144, 145–146
  costoclavicular syndrome, 144, 146–
    147
  diagnostic tests, 144, 146
  factors associated with, 144
  hyperabduction syndrome, 144, 148–
    149
  mechanisms, 144
  scalenus anticus syndrome, 144,
    147–148
  symptoms, 144
Thoracic spine. *See also* Thoracolum-
    bar spine
  rheumatoid arthritis, 21
  strains and sprains, 239
Thoracic spondylosis, 30

Thoracolumbar spine
anatomy, 156–163
facet joints, 159, 161
functional anatomy, 156
ligaments, 156, 159, 161
mobility, 156–162
ribs, 156, 157, 159
spinal cord and nerve roots, 162–163
stability, 156–162
vascular supply, 163
vertebra, 156, 158, 160
lumbar, 160
typical, 156, 158
axial load injuries, 225–229, 234
lateral bending with, 234
pure axial load, 225–228
rotation with, 229
distraction (tension) injuries, 221–225
associated injuries, 222
clinical features, 222
complications, 223
emergency management and referral, 223–225
radiographs, 222–223
stability and mechanism, 221–222
extension injuries, 170, 230
flexion injuries, 107, 216–221
pure flexion, 216–217
rotation with, 217, 218–221
fracture–dislocations, 212–236
classification by mechanism of injury, 214–216
concepts, 212
diagnosis, delayed, 212
flexion, 216–221
mechanism of injury, classification by, 214–216
neurologic injury, 212–214
stability and, 214
fractures, minor, 234–235
kyphosis, 244, 248–249. See also Kyphosis
lateral bending, 233–234
with axial load, 234
ligaments, 215
penetrating injuries, 235–236
physical examination, 166–200
auscultation, 180
inspection, 166–167
neurologic examination, 180–200
palpation, 174–179
percussion, 179–180
range of motion, 169–174
skyline view of spine, 170, 172
T-12 to S-1 measurements, 170, 171
radiography, 9
scoliosis, 244–248. See also Scoliosis

shearing, 230–231, 232, 233
soft tissue injuries, minor, 238–243
contusions, 238–239
lumbosacral strains and sprains, 240–243
thoracic strains and sprains, 239
Thoracotomy, 244
Three-column spine concept, 162
Thromboembolism, 26, 147, 217, 243, 246
Thyrotoxicosis, 34
Thyrotropin releasing hormone for spinal injury, 10
Tinglers, 151
Tingling, 145, 146
Toe walk, 181, 182, 200
Tomography, 27, 103, 129. See also Computed tomography
computed tomography vs, 210
plain film, 103
thoracolumbar, 210
thoracolumbar axial load injuries, 228
Torticollis, 39, 54, 79, 152–153
clinical features, 152
congenital, 152
emergency management and referral, 153
radiography, 153
spasmodic, 152, 153
Tracheal tears, 137
Tracheotomy, 6
Traction, 118, 119, 275
axial, 118, 119
low back pain, 275
Transport of patient, 5
Transverse processes, 60, 61
Trapezius muscle, palpation, 8
Trendelenburg test, 197, 198
Triceps, 88, 89
Tricyclic antidepressants, fibrositis, 265
Trigger points, 31, 243, 254, 275
myofascial sprain, injection, 254
osteoarthritis of spine, 31
stretch and spray, 275
Tuberculosis, 27, 42, 178. See also Tuberculous spondylitis
pyogenic spondylitis vs, 42
spinal, 178
Tuberculous spondylitis (Pott's disease), 40–43, 167, 265
clinical features, 41–42
complications, 42
diagnosis, 42
incidence, 40
management and referral, 42–43
pathophysiology, 40–41
radiography, 44

Tuck-and-roll falls, 218, 219
Tumors, 17, 34, 80, 103, 150, 167, 179. See also Neoplasms of spine
computed tomography, 103
imaging modalities, 103
osteoporosis, 34
Pancoast, 80
spinal axis, 103
Twisting motion, 240

Ulnar nerve, neurologic examination, 90
Uncinate process, 102, 126–127
C-3, 102
fracture, 126–127
Unconscious patient, 4, 127
Undressing patient, 7
Upper extremities, 76, 139, 140
pain radiating to, 140
symmetry, 76
weakness in, 139
Urinary symptoms, 16, 21, 36, 38, 53, 262
acute disc herniation, 262
incontinence, 53
retention, 16, 21, 36
urinary tract infections, 38
Urinary tract infections, 38
Urinary tract instrumentation, 38
Uveitis, 27

Vacuum sign, 31
Valsalva maneuver, 93, 191, 239, 257
acute disc herniation, 257
Vascular claudication, 256
Vascular compression, rheumatoid arthritis of spine in, 21–22
Vascular supply, spinal cord, 163
Veins, cervical spine, 71, 75
Venous thrombosis, 147
Ventilation, assisted, 4, 5
Vertebrae, 36, 51, 60–61, 62, 112, 114, 156, 158, 241
anatomy, 60–61, 62
angular measurement between, 112, 114
cervical spine, 60–61, 62
codfish, 36
disappearing, 51
lumbar, extra, 241
thoracic, typical, 156, 158
Vertebral artery, 29, 30, 31, 32, 61, 71, 74, 93, 94, 142, 152
insufficiency, 93, 142, 152
osteoarthritis and, 29, 30, 31, 32
test, 93, 94
Vertebral artery test, 93, 94

Vertebral body, 35, 98–99, 101, 112, 170, 228
  compression injuries, 228
  computed tomography, 209
  degenerative fattening, 101
  distance between, 112
  fractures, 35, 98–99, 101, 170
    thoracic, 170
      radiography, 98–99, 101
  radiography, 98–99, 101
  thoracic, fractures, 170
Vertebral discs. See Intervertebral discs
Vertebral osteomyelitis, 265
Vertical compression, 121–122
Vertigo, 22, 116
Vision, 22, 27, 132, 149, 151
  blurred, 149, 151
  defects, 22, 132
  loss, 22, 27
Vital signs, 239
Vitamin D deficiency, 34

Vitamin D therapy, 36
Vomiting, 132, 246

Water, extrication in, 4
Weakness, 13, 21, 22
  upper extremities, 13
Wedge fractures, 116, 117, 167, 202, 203, 216, 220, 221, 234, 239
  anterior, thoracolumbar, 216
  burst fractures vs, 216
  lateral, 234
  ligamentous disruption with, 220, 221
  osteoporotic, 167
  thoracic, 239
Well-leg straight leg raising test, 270
Whiplash, 16
Whiplash shaken infant syndrome, 131–132
Wrist extension, 88

Wryneck. See Torticollis

X-rays. See also Plain radiography
  ankylosing spondylitis, 27
  lumbosacral, normal, 205
  neoplasms of spine, 47
  osteoarthritis, 31
  osteoporosis, 36
  pediatric cervical spine, 130–131
  pneumothorax presenting as thoracic strain, 239
  sacral, normal, 205
  sacroiliitis, 265
  spinal cord injury, indications for, 9
  spinal neoplasms, 268
  thoracic, normal, 204
  thoracolumbar flexion with rotation injuries, 221
  tuberculous spondylitis, 42
  vacuum sign, 31